Medicinal Plants - Harnessing the Healing Power of Plants

Edited by Viduranga Y. Waisundara

Published in London, United Kingdom

Medicinal Plants - Harnessing the Healing Power of Plants
http://dx.doi.org/10.5772/intechopen.1004662
Edited by Viduranga Y. Waisundara

Contributors
Abbad Abdelaziz, Abbad Imane, Abdellah Elyoussfi, Alfred Mutaramutswa, Amin Salhi, Ankita Wal, Ayoub Amssayef, Biplab Debnath, Cephas Mawere, Chahid Zannagui, Christine Midzi, Daniel Sule Bibinu, Donald T. Kapanga, Douglas O. Ochora, El Houssien Akichouh, Elliot Nyagumbo, Eneojo Ogu, Fabian Maunganidze, Fouad Mourabit, Gautier Roko, Godwins Ngorima, Hassan Amhamdi, Hassani Lahcen, Ifeoma Chidebe, Leroy Nhari, Lucy Mabaya, Mariana Babayeva, Martins Emeje, Marvellous Matsheza, Mbusiseni Mkwanazi, Mehtap Kilic, Michael Bhebhe, Michael Chimonyo, Mohd Masih Uzzaman Khan, Munira Abdullahi, M'hamed Ahari, Neha Verma, Nkanyiso Majola, Pranay Wal, Rahul Shivajirao Solunke, Rose Hayeshi, Sadaf Naeem, Sadia Suri Kashif, Saira Saeed Khan, Sithembile Z. Ndlela, Soufian El Barkany, Soulaimani Bouchra, Sumanta Bhattacharya, Thrineshen Moodley, Tracey Lynn Harney, Trust Nyirenda, William Pote, Yousra Shafiq, Zvi G. Loewy

First published in London, United Kingdom, 2024 by IntechOpen
IntechOpen is the global imprint of INTECHOPEN LIMITED, registered in England and Wales, registration number: 11086078, 167-169 Great Portland Street, London, W1W 5PF, United Kingdom

British Library Cataloguing-in-Publication Data
A catalogue record for this book is available from the British Library

Additional hard and PDF copies can be obtained from orders@intechopen.com

Medicinal Plants - Harnessing the Healing Power of Plants
Edited by Viduranga Y. Waisundara
p. cm.
Print ISBN 978-1-83769-640-6
Online ISBN 978-1-83769-639-0
eBook (PDF) ISBN 978-1-83769-641-3

For EU product safety concerns:
IN TECH d.o.o., Prolaz Marije Krucifikse Kozulić 3, 51000 Rijeka, Croatia,
info@intechopen.com or visit our website at intechopen.com.

Meet the editor

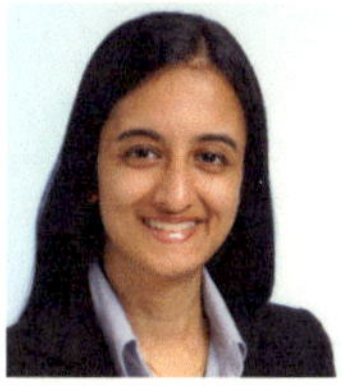

Dr. Viduranga Waisundara obtained her Ph.D. in Food Science and Technology from the Department of Chemistry, National University of Singapore, in 2010. She was a lecturer at Temasek Polytechnic, Singapore, from 2009 to 2013. Thereafter, she relocated to her motherland of Sri Lanka and spearheaded the Functional Food Product Development Project at the National Institute of Fundamental Studies during 2013–2016. She was a senior lecturer on a temporary basis at the Department of Food Technology, Faculty of Technology, Rajarata University of Sri Lanka. She is currently Deputy Principal of the Australian College of Business & Technology – Kandy Campus, Sri Lanka. She is also the current Global Harmonization Initiative (GHI) Ambassador to Sri Lanka.

Contents

Preface

Plants have long been humanity's primary source of medicine. From ancient civilizations to modern herbal practices, medicinal plants have played an essential role in healing and nurturing the human body. Whether growing in the wild, cultivated in gardens, or prepared in homes, plants possess remarkable properties that can alleviate ailments, restore balance, and promote overall well-being. In many parts of the world, the knowledge of their healing power has been passed down through generations, forming a bridge between traditional wisdom and modern health care.

The use of medicinal plants is not only a testament to nature's ingenuity but also a recognition of the vital relationship between humans and the natural world. This book, *Medicinal Plants – Harnessing the Healing Power of Plants*, is a celebration of this relationship and an in-depth exploration of how plants have been used for health and healing across cultures and time. This book provides readers with a comprehensive understanding of the medicinal properties of plants, blending historical knowledge with contemporary scientific research.

With an increasing number of people turning to natural remedies to complement conventional treatments, medicinal plants are enjoying a resurgence in popularity. This book is written for those who wish to reconnect with nature and discover how the plants around them can support health, prevent illness, and restore balance to the body. It is a guide not only for a scientific audience but also for herbalists, health enthusiasts, and individuals interested in natural healing methods.

Each chapter of this book is dedicated to exploring different medicinal plants, their unique properties, and their applications in everyday health practices. From well-known herbs to more exotic plants with specialized uses, the chapters delve into how these plants can be harnessed for various health benefits, including boosting the immune system, treating common ailments, and improving mental clarity.

The growing body of scientific research supporting the use of medicinal plants lends further credibility to their benefits. By integrating modern science with centuries of herbal wisdom, how plant compounds interact with the human body to facilitate healing can be better understood. This blend of old and new knowledge empowers readers to make informed decisions about incorporating plant-based remedies into their lives.

At its core, *Medicinal Plants – Harnessing the Healing Power of Plants* seeks to honor the legacy of traditional plant medicine while advocating for its place in the future of health care. In an age where synthetic pharmaceuticals dominate, it is vital to remember that the earth provides an abundant pharmacy, rich with healing potential.

The use of medicinal plants is not about rejecting modern medicine but complementing it. By reconnecting with the natural world and understanding the medicinal properties of plants, we can enrich our lives and foster a more holistic approach to health.

I would like to take this opportunity to extend my appreciation to the authors who have contributed so many wonderful chapters. Also, I express my gratitude to the publisher, IntechOpen, with whom I have worked on many book projects. Finally, I wish to thank Publishing Process Manager Mr. Josip Knapic, for his invaluable support in putting the material together.

It is my hope that this book will inspire readers to embrace the healing power of plants, encouraging a deeper connection to nature and greater wellbeing in their daily lives. Whether you are new to herbal medicine or an experienced practitioner, the wisdom contained within these pages will guide you on a journey toward natural health and healing.

Dr. Viduranga Y. Waisundara
Deputy Principal,
Australian College of Business and Technology,
Kandy Campus,
Kandy, Sri Lanka

Section 1

Bioactive Compounds in Medicinal Plants

Chapter 1

Cannabis Compounds: Potential Therapy for Neurological Disease

Mariana Babayeva and Zvi G. Loewy

Abstract

Identification and development of pharmaceuticals for neurological disorders is associated with several unique challenges. The primary weakness of candidate neurological compounds is the poor penetration efficacy across the blood-brain barrier (BBB). The BBB is the bottleneck in nervous system drug development and is the paramount factor that limits success in neurotherapeutics. Findings suggest cannabinoids might overcome the limiting effects of the BBB and play a key role in improving neurological dysfunctions. This supports the therapeutic potential of cannabidiol for the treatment of ischemic and inflammatory diseases of the central nervous system (CNS). The potential application of cannabinoids for Parkinson's disease, Autism, and childhood Epilepsy is explored in this chapter.

Keywords: neurological disorders, Parkinson disease, autism, epilepsy, cannabis, CBD, THC

1. Introduction: ethnobotanical aspects of *Cannabis sativa*

Geographically, Central Asia and South-East Asia are believed to be the regions of origin for *Cannabis sativa.* Various forms of *C. sativa* were identified in medieval Europe, however, *Cannabis* was unknown in the Americas until the arrival and settlement of the European colonists. In the 18th century Carl Linnaeus, a Swedish botanist introduced the name *Cannabis sativa*. The primary use of the plant historically was in textile manufacturing. Of note, the psychotropic application of the plant was in fact discovered by accident. In the 19th century, medical applications for treating pain and inflammation were introduced. More recently, there has been extensive interest in the medical use of cannabis for pain, gastrointestinal disorders, anti-microbial, multiple sclerosis (MS), nausea and vomiting, anorexia, sleep disorders, anxiety, Tourette syndrome, and several neurological diseases—epilepsy, Parkinson's, autism, and Alzheimer's.

Over 500 compounds have been identified in *Cannabis sativa* of which approximately 100 have been characterized as phytocannabinoids. The phytocannabinoid composition of *C. sativa* is influenced by environmental conditions including humidity, temperature, ultraviolet radiation, soil nutrients, and parasites. Phytocannabinoids include the neutral cannabinoids (absence of carboxyl group) and the cannabinoid acids (presence of carboxyl group). The phytocannabinoids are segmented into 10 subclasses as shown in **Figure 1**. Trans-Δ-9-tetrahydrocannabinol

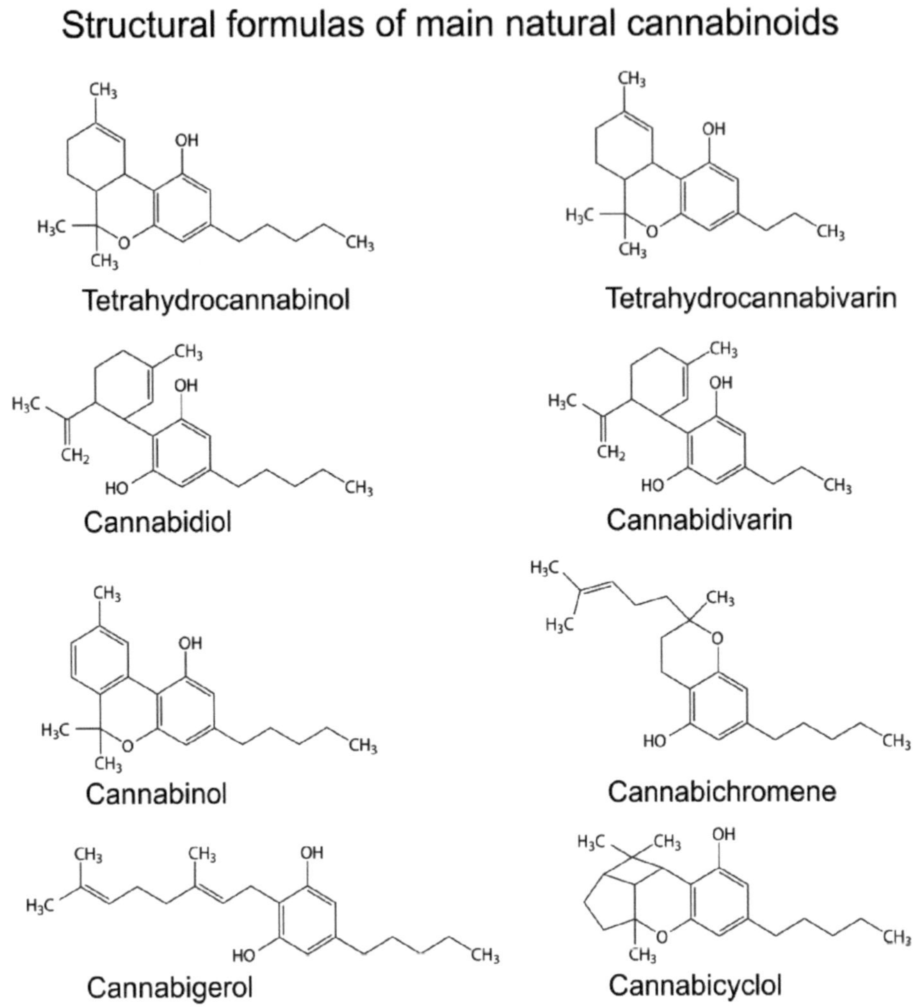

Figure 1.
Chemical structures of primary natural cannabinoids.

is the primary *C. sativa* associated with psychoactive effects including anxiety, paranoia, perceptual alterations, and cognitive deficiency. Cannabidiol (CBD) is the most abundant phytocannabinoid in *Cannabis* species cultivated for textile use.

2. Cannabinoids

Neurological disorders are a group of illnesses influencing the central and peripheral nervous systems. Depending on the part of the nervous system, a person may experience difficulties with movement, sensations, breathing, speech, learning, memory, mood, and more. Triggers of neurological conditions are genetic disorders, congenital abnormalities, infections, and brain injuries.

Recently, cannabis and its substances (cannabinoids) began using as therapeutic agents in some disease states [1]. CBD and delta-9-tetrahydrocannabinol (THC) are the most researched compounds found in cannabis plants. The effects of CBD and

THC on the body are different. THC is psychoactive and affects mood, perception, and other mental processes. THC also has neuroprotective, analgesic, antiemetic, and antiglaucoma impacts [2, 3]. CBD is a nonpsychoactive ingredient and exhibits anti-inflammatory, antioxidant, anticonvulsant, and neuroprotective effects as well as decreases the THC psychoactivity [4, 5]. Epidiolex, a pharmaceutical grade-CBD, is used to treat seizures of Dravet syndrome, Lennox–Gastaut syndrome and tuberous sclerosis complex. Sativex containing CBD (50%) and THC (50%) is employed to treat multiple sclerosis [1]. THC-containing medications, dronabinol, and nabilone are utilized for chemotherapy-induced nausea and vomiting as well as for anorexia in AIDS patients [6]. Another cannabinoid, cannabidivarin (CBDV) also manifests the medicinal effects of cannabis. CBDV is similar to CBD structurally and functionally. CBDV is a nonpsychotropic phytocannabinoid with anti-inflammatory and anticonvulsant activities [7]. Recently, the FDA and EMA granted an orphan designation to CBDV for both fragile X and Rett syndromes.

The cannabinoids interact with is the endocannabinoid system (ECS). The ECS controls some biological operations and incorporates the endocannabinoids, the cannabinoid receptors, and the endocannabinoid enzymes. Endocannabinoids, ECBs assist in regulation of memory, pleasure, concentration, thinking, movement and coordination, sensory and time perception, and pain [8]. Endocannabinoids are produced by cultured neurons, microglia, and astrocytes [9]. The key ECBs are arachidonoyl ethanolamide (anandamide, AEA) and 2-arachidonoyl glycerol (2-AG) [9]. The ECBs activate the G-protein coupled (GPR55), the cannabinoid 1 (CB1) and 2 (CB2) receptors [10]. AEA has agonistic action on TRPV1 as well [11]. CB1 is mostly localized in the central and peripheral nerve cells, specifically in glutamatergic and gamma-aminobutyric neurons and is responsible for the neurotransmitter release [12, 13]. The CB2 receptors were primarily detected in the immune system: T and B cells and macrophages [8]. CB2 was also found in the brain microglial cells and in peripheral nerves [8]. Both CB1 and CB2 were also discovered in cardiovascular, reproductive, and gastrointestinal systems. Levels of endocannabinoids, AEA and 2-AG are controlled by enzymes. N-acylphosphatidylethanolamine phospholipase D (NAPE-PLD) and diacylglycerol lipase (DAGL) modulate synthesis of the endocannabinoids, while fatty acid amide hydrolase (FAAH) and monoacylglycerol lipase (MAGL) are responsible for their degradation [1].

Cannabinoids interact with ECS in the body. THC relates to CB1, CB2, and GPR55 receptors as a partial agonist [4]. THC administration creates an overexcitation of the endocannabinoid system that results in altered perceptions, pleasure, and mood [8]. CBD exhibits just minor attraction to CB1 and CB2 and functions as an indirect antagonist of cannabinoid agonists and inverse CB2 agonist [4]. CBD was connected to indirect modulation of the CB1 and CB2 via FAAH inhibition, which results in increased levels of agonist AEA [14]. CBD might also interact with GPR55, TRPV, TRPA, and TRPM [15]. CBD functions as an agonist of TRPVs and as an antagonist of GPR55 [16–18].

3. Parkinson's disease

Research results suggest the key role of the endocannabinoid system in Parkinson's disease (PD). Endocannabinoids contribute a major role in regulating transmission at synapses between cortical and striatal neurons, in influencing basal ganglia activity, and in controlling the induction of a particular form of synaptic plasticity and motor functions [19]. PD patients have an evolving deficiency of dopaminergic nerve cells leading to decreased striatal dopamine concentrations, which in turn produces variations of the balance related to basal ganglia paths and endocannabinoid signaling [8]. The endocannabinoid signaling manifests two-phase alterations in the evolution of this disease [20]. Premature phases are correlated with CB1 desensitization and downregulation as well as with aggravation of excitotoxicity, oxidative stress, and glial activation [21]. More progressive phases with deeper nigral deterioration have up regulatory reactions of CB1 ligands [21]. PD laboratory animals had enhanced CB1 density and concentrations of endogenic ligands, both of which led to increased basal ganglia CB1 binding [8]. Further signs of a major position of ECS in PD entail inhibition of the neurotransmitters by cannabinoids and deviations in the endocannabinoid's transmission [8, 22]. These findings may define CB1 as a therapeutic target in easing PD signs.

An additional receptor controlling movement and interacting with ECS is TRPV1, which was found in sensory neurons and basal ganglia circuitry of dopaminergic neurons [23]. AEA is one of the key activators of TRPV1 [24, 25]. Several investigations reported that motor behavior could be controlled by the activation of TRPV1 [26, 27], suggesting that this receptor might play a role in the control of motor function.

3.1 Endocannabinoid system in Parkinson's disease

The correlation of the ECS with motor functions was well confirmed. Studies have shown that not only endocannabinoids but also synthetic and plant-derived cannabinoids regulate the ECS and exert a powerful motor effect [8, 24]. Activation of CB1 receptors in neurons of the basal ganglia mediated a hypokinetic effect [28–31]. In animal PD model cannabinoid HU-210 reduced glutamatergic activity and decreased pharmacologically induced spins by interaction with CB1 [32, 33]. THC and synthetic cannabinoids WIN 55,212–2 and CP 55,940 elevated dopamine levels and diminished contralateral rotations in PD rats [8]. THC generated increased tyrosine activity in parkin-null animals and emitted motor inhibition, catalcpsy, antinociception, and ring immobility in other animal models [8]. Additional animal studies reported that THC decreased the motor disfunction triggered by 6- hydroxydopamine and intensified the hypokinetic impact of reserpine [34, 35]. However, THC has not influenced motor function in PD primates [36]. Conversely, the synthetic agonist levonantradol decreased general and locomotor activity and increased bradykinesia in a primate model of Parkinson's disease [36]. WIN 55,212-2 demonstrated a dose-dependent reduction of the spontaneous motor activity and catalepsy in mutant Syrian hamsters and markedly reduced the anti-kinetic effects produced by quinpirole in reserpine animals [37]. WIN 55,212-2 has lowered levodopa-made dyskinesias, weakened axial, limb, and orolingual abnormal activities in 6-OHDA animals [38, 39]. Endocannabinoid agonist oleoylethanolamide, OAE developed lessening of involuntary rotary motions and reduction of molecular associates of induced dyskinesia [40]. Nabilone, a synthetic cannabinoid agonist, co-administered with levodopa significantly lowered total dyskinesia and extended the duration of antiparkinsonian action of levodopa in PD marmosets [41]. Endocannabinoid agonist AEA increased the extracellular dopamine levels in the nucleus accumbens shell of rats and induced hypokinesia [42]. Additionally, AEA constrained ambulation and stereotypical activities and blocked the influence of VR1 agonist livanil on motor functions [42]. Treatment with AEA reduced motor activity with the maximal inhibition by approximately 85% in mice and extended the inactivity time, lowered the ambulation and the frequency of spontaneous non-ambulatory activities in rats [8]. AEA also generated similar to THC decrease in impulsive motor activity in PD animals [8, 42].

Activities of AEA and 2-AG can be affected by inhibition of the FAAH enzyme. Studies have confirmed that FAAH inhibition remarkably increases AEA tissue level but reduces 2- AG level [43, 44]. Animal studies have shown that the FAAH enzyme inhibitor URB597 intensified and prolonged a dopamine increase produced by AEA [45]. Moreover, URB597 raised AEA blood concentrations, dropped the hyperactivity and prevented induced motor deficiency [46, 47]. Some other FAAH blockers (JNJ1661010 and TCF2) have anticataleptic ability as well [47]. In general, the findings indicate endogenous or exogenous cannabinoid agonists activate the dopaminergic system and play an important role in the regulation of motor behavior.

The CB1 receptor antagonists can also influence movement syndromes of Parkinson's disease. In a study with PD rats and marmosets rimonabant (SR141716A), a selective antagonist of the CB1 receptor was functioning as a potential anti-hypokinetic agent [48, 49]. This compound blocked the THC impact on dopamine release and improved the locomotive movement in animals pre-exposed to THC [50]. SR141716A drastically reduced levodopa-induced dyskinesia, overturned the impact of the agonist WIN 55,212-2 and recovered the locomotive motions in PD animals [49, 51]. Administration of SR141716A dropped AEA and 2AG concentrations in the brain, promoted the locomotive power of quinpirole, and rebuilt movements in laboratory models [8, 49]. Moreover, SR141716A and additional CB1 receptor antagonist AM251 generated antiparkinsonian effects in rats with severe nigral degeneration [8, 52] (Fernandez-Espejo, 2005). A second CB1 antagonist, CE-178253, generated a 30% increase in motor behavior responses to L-DOPA in MPTP-treated rhesus monkeys [53]. THCV enabled modifications in glutamatergic transmission and reduced the motor obstruction [34]. Taken together, the discoveries advocate CB1 antagonists could be successful in controlling PD symptoms.

The activation of CB2 receptors may also contribute to the potential of cannabinoids in PD treatment [54]. CBD has also demonstrated significant effects in preclinical models of neurodegenerative disorders in combination with other cannabinoids [34, 55]. CBD and THCV, which is a CB2 partial agonist, reduced the loss of tyrosine hydroxylase-positive neurons in the substantia nigra of PD rats [34]. The two compounds acted by means of neuroprotective and antioxidant mechanisms [34, 54], suggesting that CB2 receptor agonists may have a promising pharmacological profile for delaying disease progression. Therefore, CB1 antagonists may produce antiparkinsonian results, whereas CB agonists might be beneficial as a therapy of motor problems in PD.

3.2 Cannabinoids as a potential therapy for Parkinson's disease

Cannabis and related compounds have generated a major research interest as a potential therapy in neurodegenerative and movement disorders. Cannabinoids have demonstrated healing properties in the management of Tourette, Huntington's, and Parkinson's disorders [8]. In a study with 339 PD patients, smoked cannabis created substantial upgrading of typical signs in almost half of the affected people. The patients noticed alleviation in resting tremor, rigidity, bradykinesia, and dyskinesias [56]. The same study connected high urine levels of 11-HO-THC (THC active metabolite) with decline of PD indications [56]. In other PD patients who smoked cannabis developed substantial positive transformation in tremor, rigidity, and bradykinesia [57, 58]. The dose and frequency of the cannabis administrations were key factors in relieving PD symptoms. A single smoked cannabis process resulted in tree-hours signs removal [58]. The investigations also demonstrated meaningful improvements in sleep and pain, which are common nonmotor PD signs [57, 58]. In contrast, PD patients and patients with levodopa-induced dyskinesia displayed no improvement after administration of oral cannabis extract [59].

Some reports described the impacts of CBD on Parkinson's disease indicators. CBD reduced Unified Parkinson Disease Rating Scale (UPDRS) results and notably lowered signs of psychosis in PD individuals with psychotic disorder [60]. CBD ameliorated tremor and hypokinesia in patients with Parkinson's disease [61]. However, in a second study CBD administration resulted in no improvement in measures of motor and general PD symptoms [62, 63]. Interestingly, in PD population CBD produced substantially different Parkinson Disease Questionnaire results compared to placebo treatment [62, 63].

More investigations were performed to examine cannabinoid nabilone. Nabilone has markedly alleviated abnormal involuntary movements in individuals with deep levodopa-induced dyskinesia [64, 65]. Nabilone was also effective against bradykinesia [64]. Other cannabinoid-associated substances CE178253, OEA, and HU-210 were also effective in treatment of levodopa-induced dyskinesia and bradykinesia [8, 66]. But the American Academy of Neurology (AAN) review deemed marijuana "probably ineffective" for treating L-DOPA-induced dyskinesia [67].

The impact of cannabis on dystonia was investigated as well. Cannabis generated significant alleviation of dystonia and pain lessening in dystonic patients with severe pain. The patients were able to withdraw opioids [68]. Cannabis eased idiopathic and generalized dystonia in patients with Wilson's disorder [69]. CBD improved dystonia by 20–50% in dystonic patients and CBD withdrawal resulted in severe generalized dystonia in PD patients [8, 61]. Another cannabinoid, THC generated a reduction of abnormal movement patterns in patients with dystonia and athetosis [70].

The potential benefits of medical cannabis and cannabinoids for the treatment of another neurodegenerative disorder, Huntington's disease (HD) has also been evaluated. A study reported that nabilone compared to placebo showed a treatment difference for total motor score, chorea, Unified Huntington's Disease Rating Scale (UHDRS) cognition and behavior, and for the neuropsychiatric inventory in HD patients [71]. AAN recommended nabilone for moderate lessening of chorea in HD patients [72]. Research reports regarding CBD value in treatment of HD are lacking consistency. An investigation stated that CBD lowered chorea in 20–40% of patients with HD [73]. Conversely, more recent research did not verify this discovery [74]. CBD did not produce any meaningful results on chorea difficulty in HD individuals [74]. It was reported cannabis and THC may lessen tics and behavior conditions in patients with Tourette's syndrome (TS) [75–77]. These patients informed consumption of cannabis/THC improved or in some cases completely revised motor and vocal tics as well as premonitory urges and obsessive-compulsive signs [76, 77].

Collectively, no powerful verification was obtained to suggest cannabis as a therapy for Parkinson's disease. Though, prospective values were discovered in easing tremor, anxiety, pain, and sleep disorder [78]. Given the relative lack of investigations, there is a recognized necessity for additional well-designed studies.

4. Autism

Autism spectrum disorders (ASD) are neurodevelopment disorders characterized by difficulty in social communication and atypical patterns of activities and behaviors.

The frequency of ASD is almost 4.5 times greater in boys than in girls [79]. The exact trigger of autism is unidentified. Up to 20% of ASD cases were linked to genetic alterations [80]. Other factors include immune dysfunction, inflammation, and embryonic exposure to anticonvulsant drugs [1]. Though the frequency of autism is growing, no medicine has been developed for the therapy of the ASD core symptoms [79].

Autism has been associated with disfunction of the endocannabinoid system [81, 82]. The ECS disorder was linked to the pathology of neurological disorders and to the behavioral deficits and neuroinflammation detected in autism [83, 84]. Pathophysiological processes generating the autistic neurobehavioral disfunction involve irregular synaptic plasticity and immune and metabolic disorders that are controlled by ECS [85]. The ECS plays a significant role in the development of the central nervous system (CNS) [17, 86]. In the CNS, CB1 receptors were found in the cerebellum, hippocampus, and the basal ganglia, which are zones of dysfunction in ASD [87, 88]. Autism was also correlated with dysregulation of the immune system [89, 90]. Localization of CB2 receptors in the immune cells, microglia and astrocytes has been associated with ASD-allied neuroinflammation [87, 91–93]. Raised autoimmune activity and increased levels of inflammatory cytokines and chemokines were correlated with microglial activation in ASD patients and were results of the pro-inflammatory status of the immune system [1, 18]. Alteration in monocyte and macrophage reactions, abnormal T helper cytokine and immunoglobulin levels, and decreased level of lymphocytes were detected in ASD children [1, 94]. Besides, elevated level of pro-inflammatory cytokines was linked to regressive forms of autism and typical behavior deficits [18].

4.1 Changes in the endocannabinoid system in autism

Research confirmed involvement of the ECS in ASD [1]. The endocannabinoid system impacts neuromodulation, emotional responses, behavioral reactivity, and social interaction [1, 95]. Disorder of the ECS might damage social play and reciprocity [95]. Dropped CB1 expressions were discovered in the brains of ASD individuals [18]. Motivation of the CB1 directly by agonist WIN55212-2 or indirectly by 2-AG inhibitor has increased the spatial memory in laboratory animals [96]. Polymorphism in CNR1 gene, encoding the CB1 receptor was related to modulation of striatal responses and gaze duration to social reward [97, 98], suggesting that altered affinity to the CB1 receptors could produce deficits in social rewards detected in autism. Animal studies have shown social play increases AEA concentrations in some brain regions [82]. Elevated AEA levels created the CB1 activation and improved social play [99], advising social play behavior deficit might be produced by low AEA levels in critical brain zones. Conversely, it was reported that excitement of CB1 receptors inhibited the typical excitation of complex social actions by affecting cognitive functions [99, 100]. Furthermore, a downregulation of alternative receptors involved in social play behaviors, GPR55 and PPAR, was displayed in animal model of autism [95]. The behavioral alterations could be facilitated by activation of PPARγs by endogenous agonists, OEA or PEA, as stimulation of hippocampal PPARγ improves cognitive performance [101]. PEA's intestinal anti-inflammatory property is important since a portion of autistic inflammatory disorder is produced by gastrointestinal immune system [1]. The anti-inflammatory impact of PEA is utilized by stimulation CB2, GPR55, and PPARγ receptors [102].

Alteration of the ECS influences ASD-associated social and cognitive impairments in animal genetic models. CB1 density in the hippocampus of mice with autism-like phenotype (BTBR mice) was increased by 15–20%. Interaction of CB1 agonist CP55940 to Gi/o-coupled receptors in the BTBR models was also higher, demonstrating increased sensitivity [103, 104]. In the same animals enhanced AEA activity at CB1 targets improved social deficiency and decreased locomotive function [105]. The therapy of BTBR mice with the FAAH inhibitor, URB597, and THC improved the social behavior deficit [105, 106]. The BTBR models have also upregulated mRNA CB2 levels and elevated CB2 expression in their brain [106, 107]. A clinical investigation displayed upregulation of CB2 gene expression in peripheral blood mononuclear cells in ASD patients [108], which might be a compensatory mechanism of the autism-associated inflammation [1]. The augmentation of CB2 could be negative response to decrease the proinflammatory reactions since AEA suppresses the release of proinflammatory cytokines through CB2-mediated mechanism. In the FXS autistic animal model, URB597 enhanced AEA activity, improved memory, and anxiety-like behavior, and inverted the social impairment [109]. In Shank3B−/− mice ZL184 (MAGL inhibitor) produced an increase of 2-AG levels and improved social interaction deficits [110]. Alteration in neuroligin-3, 4 gene, NLGN 3,4 was correlated with intelligent debility, seizures, and ASD behavior [111]. Findings in genetic animal models with a neuroligin-3 substitution and a neuroligin-3 deletion showed neuroligin-3 is essential for EC signaling [112]. A study has reported WIN55212-2 might decrease aggressive behavior of neuroligin-3 R451C mouse model of autism via modification of CB1 receptor [113]. Another animal model, VPA model has alterations in ECS and corresponding ASD-like anomalies [95, 114]. Decreased expressions of mRNA PPARα and GPR55 in hippocampus and cortex, reduced amounts of FAAH and unusual AEA activity facilitate autistic behaviors in VPA animals [95, 114]. In the VPA rats the FAAH inhibitor PF3845 increased AEA signaling and impaired the difference in social behavior [95]. Another FAAH inhibitor, URB597 improved social conditions, repetitive and emotional behaviors in VPA animals [18]. Raised 2-AG levels have corrected behavior weaknesses in VPA rats [115]. The reduced endocannabinoid and enzymes levels and upregulation of CB receptors lead to lowered endocannabinoid signaling and link alterations in the ECS with ASD. Based on this finding, the ECS can be recommended as a novel target for ASD therapy.

4.2 Cannabinoids as a potential therapy of ASD

Cannabis and cannabinoids have been shown to be efficient as a therapy for some neurological disorders including ASD. In animal ASD models, CBD inversed the behavioral disorders by increasing AEA plasma concentrations and strengthening AEA signaling [116, 117]. In C57BL/6 J mice, CBD diminished marble-burying behavior that is similar to repetitive and compulsive behaviors in ASD [18]. Moreover, CBD weakened autism-like social behavior and cognitive disorders in animal models of Dravet syndrome and schizophrenia [118–120].

Phytocannabinoid CBDV can also produce anti-autistic effects. A clinical study showed CBDV corrected atypical striatal circuitry toward neurotypical function in ASD patients [121]. In genetic Mecp2 animal model, CBDV improved AEA and OEA levels and decreased DAGL and CB1 and CB2 receptor expressions [1, 122, 123]. The compromised general health, behavioral disorders, memory deficits, sociability, and brain weight were repaired [122, 123]. CBDV also restored neurotrophic factor level and ribosomal protein phosphorylation, which are damaged in autism [123].

In VPA animals, cannabidivarin produced hippocampal microglia activation, rebuilt endocannabinoid signaling and reduced neuroinflammation [124]. Outcomes of the CBDV administration were repaired social deficiencies, memory shortages, repetitive behaviors and hyperlocomotion [124]. THC also has a therapeutic impact on autism. THC administration improved locomotor behavior and depressogenic aspect in animals with an autism-like phenotype [106]. Other studies have confirmed the association between behavioral disorders and alteration of the ECS as well as the ability of some cannabinoids to treat autistic symptoms, providing more support for the cannabinoids as an ASD therapy [1].

Cannabis usage as an ASD therapy gained a rising attraction in public media. Anecdotal cases demonstrated autistic children failing conventional treatment have responded to cannabis therapy. Parents of the children noticed significant symptoms lessening. An ASD boy spoke his first words after taking cannabis oil and then obtained substantial talking ability [1]. In a 10-year-old boy with ASD the FDA-approved drugs created life-threatening toxicities. He was started on cannabis and in 6 years the child was sociable and successful [1]. Other autistic children have also shown remarkable improvement in communications after treatment with cannabis [1].

There are lacking clinical data on the effect of cannabis on ASD. Numerous studies demonstrated cannabis is safe and successful in decreasing disruptive behaviors and improving social communication. In a single-case-study, dronabinol (THC) has reduced hyperactivity, irritability, stereotyped behaviors, and improved speech in a boy with autism [125]. Another study has reported that dronabinol alleviated self-injurious behavior of mentally retarded adolescents [126].

Optimistic outcomes in ASD patients treated with cannabinoids and raising anecdotal commentaries of cannabis positive effects directed to more scientific assessment. A clinical trial was initiated to assess the safety and efficacy of cannabinoids (CBD:THC, 20:1) in 150 ASD children [127]. This cannabinoid treatment caused a reduction of disrupting behavior. Another effect was a reduction in body weight in obese patients. This is important since antipsychotics accompany significant weight gain. No substantial adverse events were shown [127]. Although this study displayed cannabis might correct ASD disrupting behaviors, efficiency data were lacking. An additional investigation was suggested.

A recent clinical trial assessed the effect of cannabis extract intense in CBD in 60 children with autism. Significant improvements were found for social interaction, anxiety, psychomotor agitation, and concentration. Only three children in the treatment group had mild adverse effects [128]. In another investigation, cannabis oil containing CBD and THC (20:1) was administered to 188 autistic patients. Significant improvements were noticed in 30.1%, moderate in 53.7%, minor in 6.4% and no adjustment in 8.6% of the patients [129]. Same cannabinoids concentrations were used in a study with 53 ASD patients [130]. Self-injury, rage attacks, hyperactivity, and sleep troubles were bettered in most of these patients [130]. In 110 children and teenagers with autism CBD-rich cannabis generated a significant improvement in social communication [131]. ASD patients treated with CBD/THC mixture (75:1) showed improvement of core ASD symptoms. Adverse outcomes were mild and infrequent [132].

Overall, cannabinoids were found to be successful in relieving ASD symptoms. The cannabinoid therapy was associated with low incidents of adverse events and reductions in concomitant medications. However, it is essential to conduct more large-scale and long-term clinical trials to support these conclusions.

5. Epilepsy

Epilepsy is neurological illness that causes seizures or unusual sensations and behaviors. One third of the patients diagnosed with epilepsy are children. Epilepsy can affect children of all races and ethnic backgrounds and might have different reasons, although most of the cases have idiopathic origin [133]. Genetic alterations and brain damage as well as some illnesses may trigger epilepsy [133]. Treatment of pediatric epilepsy is challenging and includes pharmacologic, non-pharmacologic, and surgical options [134]. Unfortunately, childhood epilepsies are generally coupled with therapy-resistant seizures. Such severe seizures might produce long-term defects in perception, behaviors, and some other activities [135]. Resistance to epilepsy regimens has created real challenge in treatment of Dravet, Lennox-Gastaut, Doose, and West syndromes [136].

Dravet syndrome (DS) is a severe and pharmaco-resistant type of epilepsy. Certain anti-epileptic drugs (AED) can even aggravate seizures and should be avoided in patients with Dravet syndrome. Infants being treated for status epilepticus with phenobarbital developed cerebral atrophy with dramatic neurological worsening [137].

Lennox-Gastaut syndrome (LGS) is a severe, chronic, epileptic encephalopathy, primarily with childhood onset [138]. LGS syndrome begins in childhood, worsens during latency, and persists frequently into adulthood. The syndrome is refractory to anti-epileptic medications. Most patients develop moderate intellectual disability within a few years of onset of the syndrome [139].

Doose syndrome (DS) or Myoclonic-Astatic Epilepsy (MAE) is an uncommon childhood epilepsy with frequent myoclonic and myoclonic-atonic seizures. Children with MAE may also have other types of seizures. MAE outcomes depend on seizures severity and may vary from normal or severe developmental and learning delays [140].

West syndrome (WS) is a rare epileptic disorder happening in infants and characterized by infantile spasms, hypsarrhythmia, and developmental regression [141]. Neurodevelopment is normal in only 10–15% of affected patients [142]. Pharmacologic agents used to treat WS are not always effective.

Pediatric epilepsies are generally linked to treatment-resistant seizures. Management of these disorders needs more efficient treatment to prevent development-related neurological conditions.

5.1 Cannabinoid's effect on epilepsy molecular targets and syndromes

Medical cannabis has created a significant research interest as a potential therapy option in epilepsy treatment. Studies investigated the effects of cannabinoids on molecular targets in animal models of seizure and epilepsy. The results of these studies are summarized in **Table 1** [143].

The data demonstrated mixed efficacy in various acute seizure animal models [143]. CBD exerts its antiepileptic effects through several different mechanisms. Main molecular target responsible for the antiepileptic effect of CBD is still unclear. Some authors reported the role of the cannabinoid CB1 receptor in modulating seizure activity [144]. Other investigations indicated that cannabinoids produce anticonvulsant effects via non-CB1/CB2 mechanisms [145]. At low micromolar concentrations, CBD worked as a blocker of ENT and TRPM8 channels. Conversely, CBD enhanced the activity of 5-HT1a receptor, a3 and a1 glycine receptors, and TRPA1 channel [12, 146]. At higher micromolar concentrations, CBD activated the nuclear TRPV1 and TRPV2 channels and inhibited cellular uptake and degradation of AE [12, 147].

Cannabinoid	Molecular target(s)
D9-Tetrahydrocannabinol (THC)	CB_1R, CB_2R, TRPV1, TRPV2
D9-Tetrahydrocannabivarin (THCV)	CB1, CB2, TRPV1, TRPV3, TRPV4
Cannabidiol (CBD)	GPR55, TRPV1, TRPV2, TRPV3, TRPA1, FAAH, TRPM8
Cannabidivarin (CBDV)	TRPV4, DAGLa
Cannabinol (CBN)	CB_1R, TRPV4, TRPA1

Table 1.
Cannabinoid's molecular targets studied in animal models of seizure.

Additionally, CBD has a good affinity toward GPR55, which is involved in the modulation of synaptic transmission. CBD agonist action may weaken the synaptic transmission and produce antiepileptic effects [118]. Cannabinoids THCV and CBDV also produce anticonvulsant effects, most probably not via CB1 or CB2 pathways [34]. Similar to CBD, THCV and CBDV have an affinity to TRPV1, 2, TRPA1, and TRPM8, but processes of the relations are not identified. Cannabinoids have been demonstrated to be beneficial in experimental models of several neurologic disorders, including seizure and epilepsy (**Table 2**).

CBD has been shown to have anticonvulsant effect in different animal seizure prototypes [148, 149]. In pilocarpine animals, CBD radically lowered fraction of rodents with very intense seizures. In the penicillin animals, CBD substantially reduced the intensity of seizures, corresponding mortality, and number of rodents with critical tonic-clonic seizures. Besides, CBD decreased seizure intensity and number of death cases in generalized seizure model [149, 150]. CBD caused concentration-related and region-dependent attenuation of chemically induced epileptiform activity in hippocampal brain slices [150]. Other cannabinoids, THCV and CBDV were also effective in lessening seizures and generated anticonvulsant effects in animal models of epilepsy [34].

Unfortunately, seizures remain refractory to pharmacological treatments in a substantial portion of pediatric patients. After unsuccessful antiepileptic treatment, parents initiated epilepsy therapy with cannabis containing products. More than 84% of the parents noted a reduction in the frequency of seizures and 11% reported that their children became seizure-free [151]. The parents highlighted some of the additional beneficial outcomes such as better sleep patterns, increased alertness, and an overall positive change in mood [151].

Several randomized, double-blind, placebo-controlled studies evaluated the activity of a new anti-epileptic formulation of purified CBD. Studies have shown that CBD was beneficial in decreasing seizure frequency in children with treatment-resistant epilepsy [152, 153]. In open label study in patients with drug-resistant seizures, CBD given as add-on therapy reduced seizure frequency [153]. CBD also greatly diminished convulsive-seizure rate in DS patients [153]. CBD was very well tolerated and did not produce psychotic symptoms even at high doses. As a result, the first CBD drug (Epidiolex) was authorized in 2018 as a therapy for LGS-, DS-, and tuberous sclerosis complex (TCS) -associated seizures [154]. This approval ensured the safety and effectiveness of CBD in seizure disorders.

THC also helps in reducing epileptic seizures. In animal seizure models THC, AEA, and WIN55212-2 exhibited potent anticonvulsant effects via CB1 activation [155, 156]. A clinical study reported that THC (Dronabinol, Marinol) reduced spasticity,

Cannabinoid	Model	Efficacy
D9-Tetrahydrocannabinol (THC)	Generalized seizure	Y
	Temporal lobe epilepsy	Y
Synthetic CB1R agonists (e.g., WIN55-212)	Generalized seizure	Y
	Partial seizure with secondary generalization	Y
	Temporal lobe epilepsy	Y
	Absence epilepsy	Mixed effect
Synthetic CB1R antagonists (e.g., SR141716A)	Generalized seizure	N[a]
	Absence epilepsy	N
	Partial seizures with secondary generalization	N[a]
	Epileptogenesis	Y
D9-Tetrahydrocannabivarin (THCV)	Generalized seizure	Y
Cannabidiol (CBD)	Generalized seizure	Y
	Temporal lobe convulsions/status epilepticus	Y
	Partial seizures with secondary generalization	Y
Cannabidivarin (CBDV)	Generalized seizure	Y
	Temporal lobe convulsions/status epilepticus	Y
	Partial seizures with secondary generalization	Y
Cannabinol (CBN)	Generalized seizure	Y

[a]*Indicates a proconvulsant effect.*

Table 2.
Cannabinoid efficacy in animal models of seizure and epilepsy [143].

improved dystonia, increased interest in the surrounding, and produced anticonvulsive action [70]. However, the results of THC experiments are inconsistent. Some studies informed THC did not exhibit any value as a seizure therapy. Other investigations demonstrated that THC even potentiates convulsions and provokes the epileptiform activity [157]. Recent study reported that administration of THC-like substances calmed seizures but leaded to post-seizure oxygen deprivation in the brain [158].

6. Additional effects of cannabinoids in neurological disorders

6.1 Neuroprotection

Cannabinoids have demonstrated neuroprotective, immunomodulatory, anxiolytic, and antidepressant benefits. Cannabis and related compounds exhibit the neuroprotection mostly because of their ant-inflammatory, the anti-oxidative, and the anti-excitotoxicity properties. Both THC and CBD provide neuroprotection against the *in vivo* and *in vitro* toxicity of 6-hydroxydopamine (6-OHDA) [159]. In a study, CBD regained 6-OHDA-made dopamine drop and reduced oxidative stress [8]. CBD also lessened a rise in NADPH-oxidase levels and reduced indicators of oxidation, inflammation, as well as cell mortality [160]. The mechanism by which CBD reduces NADPH oxidase expression and inhibits oxidative injury suggests a straightforward association involving CB1 and mitochondrial brain activity [161]. Cannabinoid's phenolic ring plays an important role in an anti-oxidative action *versus* glutamate-persuaded neurotoxicity [162]. Moreover, CBD greatly diminished oxidative destruction produced by hydroperoxide and was more defensive to glutamate-associated neurotoxicity than alpha-tocopherol [163]. These findings support the hypothesis that the treatment with cannabinoids having antioxidant effects may modulate mitochondrial reactive oxygen production.

Several studies showed that cannabinoids have anti-inflammatory properties and may attenuate neuroinflammation and produce beneficial effects in acute inflammation and chronic neuropathic states [143]. Inflammation has been shown to be a crucial pathological factor responsible for the death of dopaminergic neurons [164, 165]. Individuals with neurodisorders have elevated expression of active microglia suggesting deep involvement of the glial chambers in neuroinflammation [166]. Cannabinoids overcome stimulation of microglia and cytokine production and as a result, reduce the inflammation [167, 168]. Cannabinoids also activate the CB2 receptor, which mediates the anti-inflammatory effect and preserve cells from excessive apoptosis [34, 169]. Moreover, a recent study reported that CBD stimulates neurogenesis [170]. In contrast, THC produces its anti-inflammation impact by CB1 stimulation [171, 172]. Cannabis/cannabinoids also produce anti-inflammatory influence via reduction of blood vessels constriction and repair blood stream to the affected zones [173]. Based on the information, it is possible to conclude cannabinoids are hypothetically valuable as neuroinflammation therapy.

Moreover, cannabis might deter brain injury via protection against neural damage. Cannabinoid's protective processes involve CB2 stimulation and regulation of neuronal homeostasis [174]. Activation of CB1 receptors is another mechanism of neuroprotection. Cannabinoids activating the CB1 receptor are anti-excitotoxic due to suppression of glutamatergic activity with a subsequent decrease in nitric oxide creation [175, 176]. The mixture of THC and CBD exhibited neuroprotection impact interacting with CB1 and CB2 [177]. Additionally, THC lowered tyrosine hydroxylase-positive neurons death and demonstrated neuroprotection result via PPARγ stimulation [34, 178]. Cannabis/cannabinoids have potential to suspend/block ongoing brain dopaminergic deterioration and have neuroprotective value in management of neurodegeneration.

6.2 Analgesic effect of cannabinoids

Pain is a significant and often underestimated symptom of neurological disorders. Medications to treat pain include *analgesics*, opioids, and, in some cases, antiseizures. Unfortunately, the drugs do not have comprehensive effectiveness and can produce substantial adverse effects. Cannabis has pain-dismissing value. It was reported that CB receptors in CNS have ability to modify pain sensitivity [179]. In medical investigations Sativex and smoked cannabis greatly decreased pain feeling in neuropathic patients [180–182]. In another study, cannabis substantially demoted pain in patients with distal symmetrical polyneuropathic disorder [183]. Additional studies reinforced that cannabis-based medicine significantly decreases chronic pain intensity in patients with neurological disorders [8]. These findings are supporting the efficacy of cannabis in relieving pain in various disease states including neurological disorders.

6.3 Antidepressant effect of cannabinoids

Depression and mood disorders are the common symptoms of neurological disorders. Therapy of co-occurring depression and mood conditions is complex and standard pharmacotherapy may be ineffective. It was reported that mood and emotional activities are under control of the endocannabinoid system and deficit or obstruction of the EC signaling system may produce depressing signs [184]. For instance, rimonabant, CB1 antagonist promoted anxiety and depression [8]. Moreover, CB1 gene mutations were linked to depression in PD patients [185]. In genetic animals, THC has stimulated CB1, intensified serotonergic action, and generated antidepressant effect [186]. Other investigations showed AEA hydrolysis blockage produces antidepressive impact due to enhanced serotogenic and norepinephric neuronic action [187].

Cannabinoids have possibility to lower depression and mood conditions indicators. CBD shows antidepressive and antipsychotic impacts in depression, and some other mental conditions [1]. THC in mixture with CBD also produces neuroleptic effect [188]. But consumption of cannabis herb produced controversial outcomes on depression and mood disorders [189]. Some studies reported anxiety and increased symptoms of depression. Conversely, many cannabis users describe an improvement in mood [190]. Understanding long-term consequences of cannabis use is important in managing neurological conditions, especially in pediatric patients. The advances of cannabis should be evaluated *versus* the dangers/harmful outcomes.

6.4 Antianxiety effect of cannabinoids

Many patients with neurological disorders have anxiety. The current anxiety treatment is cognitive-behavioral therapy together with antianxiety medicines. Administration of these drugs lead to dependence and tolerance with increasingly larger doses needed and produces many overdose-related fatalities. Cannabinoids impact on anxiety is complicated since cannabinoids antagonistically influence brain functions [1]. THC psychotropic stimulation is transient and could create retention and intellectual destruction [191]. THC was also linked to psychosis and severe anxiety [192]. Oppositely, CBD generates anxiolytic impact and blocks THC anxiogenic/psychotogenic influence [193]. CBD increases AEA concentrations via inhibition of FAAH [1]. Elevated AEA concentrations are associated with lowered depression and nervousness. Additionally, CBD anti-anxiogenic impact might be due to modulation of serotonin, adenosine, TRPV1, GABAA and PPAR receptors [1]. CBD exhibited effectiveness as anxiolytic agent in genetic animals [194, 195]. Animal studies advocate CBD has value as a prospective medicine for various anxiety disorders and as an inhibitor of lifelong anxiogenic outcomes [196, 197]. Medical research proves results of animal studies. CBD radically weakened anxiety, intellectual and speaking failings and improved remembrances in patients with common anxiety syndromes [1]. Brain examinations demonstrated alteration of blood circulation in limbic brain regions after CBD administration. This finding was associated with CBD anti-anxiety effect [198]. In another study, CBD as add-on treatment reduced anxiety in 79.2% patients. However, 15.3% of the patients faced intensified anxiety [199]. Some additional investigations have also informed that CBD produces anxiolytic effect in various populations [1]. Nonetheless, extra studies are needed to confirm the value of CBD as a therapy for anxiety.

6.5 Effect of cannabinoids on sleep disorders

Various sleep problems are the very frequent syndromes in neurological disorders [200]. Pharmacologic treatment of sleep conditions involves drugs most of which are hypnotic. These medications are a source of severe adverse effects. Cannabis has demonstrated slight calming validity in animals and humans [201]. A medical study revealed that cannabis administration bettered sleep quality and decreased sleep length in 79% individuals [202]. Nabiximols improved subjective sleep factors in 2000 patients with pain [203]. THC and CBD affect sleep differently. In an early clinical research, THC generated sleepy result [1]. Conversely, in a later study THC did not create an impact on nighttime sleep and enhanced daytime sleep [204]. Another trial reported that THC reduced nocturnal sleep length due to developed tolerance to its sedative impact [205]. CBD opposes THC action via activation of the brain awaken-related areas and increasing dopamine concentrations [1]. CBD augmented sleeplessness throughout light-on time, improved lights-off sleep, and inhibited sleep rebound after sleep absence [1]. In study with 72 individuals CBD improved sleep results in 66.7% of the patients [199]. CBD appears to optimize sleep and improve associated sleep problems and may have a beneficial value in some sleep conditions.

7. Summary

Cannabis and related compounds have recently been studied as promising therapeutic agents in treatment of neurological disorders. Research studies have provided evidence for the potential effectiveness of medical marijuana and its components in the treatment of these disorders. Cannabis may offer a viable alternative or addition to the current treatment of neurological diseases. However, cannabis and related compounds may create not only the medicinal consequences but also generate threatening conditions. Constant cannabis consumption was correlated with several mental difficulties. Additional worries are relative absence of standardizations and regulations, inaccurate dosage, and potential adverse results. More investigations are required to obtain additional information on medicinal value and safety of cannabinoids.

Author details

Mariana Babayeva[1] and Zvi G. Loewy[1,2*]

1 Department of Biomedical and Pharmaceutical Sciences, Touro College of Pharmacy, New York, NY, United States

2 New York Medical College, Valhalla, NY, United States

*Address all correspondence to: zvi.loewy@touro.edu

References

[1] Babayeva M, Assefa H, Basu P, Loewy Z. Autism and associated disorders: Cannabis as a potential therapy. Frontiers in Bioscience. 2022;**14**:1. DOI: 10.31083/j.fbe1401001

[2] Fishbein M, Gov S, Assaf F, Gafni M, Keren O, Sarne Y. Long-term behavioral and biochemical effects of an ultra-low dose of Δ9-tetrahydrocannabinol (THC): Neuroprotection and ERK signaling. Experimental Brain Research. 2012;**221**(4):437-448. DOI: 10.1007/s00221-012-3186-5

[3] Nahas G, Harvey DJ, Sutin K, Turndorf H, Cancro R. A molecular basis of the therapeutic and psychoactive properties of cannabis (delta9-tetrahydrocannabinol). Progress in Neuro-Psychopharmacology & Biological Psychiatry. 2002;**26**(4):721-730. DOI: 10.1016/s0278-5846(01)00245-7

[4] Babayeva M, Loewy ZG. Cannabis pharmacogenomics: A path to personalized medicine. Current Issues in Molecular Biology. 2023;**45**(4):3479-3514. DOI: 10.3390/cimb45040228

[5] Furgiuele A, Cosentino M, Ferrari M, Marino F. Immunomodulatory potential of cannabidiol in multiple sclerosis: A systematic review. Journal of Neuroimmune Pharmacology. 2021;**16**(2):251-269. DOI: 10.1007/s11481-021-09982-7

[6] Badowski ME. A review of oral cannabinoids and medical marijuana for the treatment of chemotherapy-induced nausea and vomiting: A focus on pharmacokinetic variability and pharmacodynamics. Cancer Chemotherapy and Pharmacology. 2017;**80**:441-449. DOI: 10.1007/s00280-017-3387-5

[7] National Library of Medicine Cannabidivarin. C19H26O2-PubChem (nih.gov). Available from: https://pubchem.ncbi.nlm.nih.gov/compound/Cannabidivarin [Accessed: January 28, 2024]

[8] Babayeva M, Assefa H, Basu P, Chumki S, Loewy Z. Marijuana compounds: A nonconventional approach to Parkinson's disease therapy. Parkinson's Disease. 2016;**2016**:1279042. DOI: 10.1155/2016/1279042

[9] Ivanov I, Borchert P, Hinz B. A simple method for simultaneous determination of N-arachidonoylethanolamine, N-oleoylethanolamine, N-palmitoylethanolamine and 2-arachidonoylglycerol in human cells. Analytical and Bioanalytical Chemistry. 2015;**407**(6):1781-1787. DOI: 10.1007/s00216-014-8384-5

[10] Hiley CR. Endocannabinoids and the heart. Journal of Cardiovascular Pharmacology. 2009;**53**(4):267-276. DOI: 10.1097/FJC.0b013e318192671d

[11] Pertwee RG, Howlett AC, Abood ME, Alexander SP, Di Marzo V, Elphick MR, et al. International union of basic and clinical pharmacology. LXXIX. Cannabinoid receptors and their ligands: Beyond CB1 and CB2. Pharmacological Reviews. 2010;**62**(4):588-631. DOI: 10.1124/pr.110.003004

[12] Pertwee RG. The diverse CB 1 and CB 2 receptor pharmacology of three plant cannabinoids: Δ 9-tetrahydrocannabinol, cannabidiol and Δ 9-tetrahydrocannabivarin. British Journal of Pharmacology. 2008;**153**(2):199-215. DOI: 10.1038/sj.bjp.0707442

[13] Xu J-Y, Chen C. Endocannabinoids in synaptic plasticity and neuroprotection.

The Neuroscientist. 2015;**21**(2):152-168. DOI: 10.1177/1073858414524632

[14] Lim K, See YM, Lee J. A systematic review of the effectiveness of medical cannabis for psychiatric, movement and neurodegenerative disorders. Clinical Psychopharmacology and Neuroscience. 2017;**15**:301-312. DOI: 10.9758/cpn.2017.15.4.301

[15] Zou S, Kumar U. Cannabinoid receptors and the endocannabinoid system: Signaling and function in the central nervous system. International Journal of Molecular Sciences. 2018;**19**:833. DOI: 10.3390/ijms19030833

[16] Gray RA, Whalley BJ. The proposed mechanisms of action of CBD in epilepsy. Epileptic Disorders. 2020;**22**(S1):10-15. DOI: 10.1684/epd.2020.1135

[17] Cheung KA, Mitchell MD, Heussler HS. Cannabidiol and neurodevelopmental disorders in children. Frontiers in Psychiatry. 2021;**12**:643442. DOI: 10.3389/fpsyt.2021.643442

[18] Nezgovorova V, Ferretti CJ, Taylor BP, Shanahan E, Uzunova G, Hong K, et al. Potential of cannabinoids as treatments for autism spectrum disorders. Journal of Psychiatric Research. 2021;**137**:194-201. DOI: 10.1016/j.jpsychires.2021.02.048

[19] Heifets BD, Castillo PE. Endocannabinoid signaling and long-term synaptic plasticity. Annual Review of Physiology. 2009;**71**:283-306. DOI: 10.1146/annurev.physiol.010908.163149

[20] More SV, Choi D-K. Promising cannabinoid-based therapies for Parkinson's disease: Motor symptoms to neuroprotection. Molecular Neurodegeneration. 2015;**10**(1, article 17). DOI: 10.1186/s13024-015-0012-0

[21] García-Arencibia M, García C, Fernández-Ruiz J. Cannabinoids and Parkinson's disease. CNS & Neurological Disorders Drug Targets. 2009;**8**(6):432-439. DOI: 10.2174/187152709789824642

[22] Pérez-Rial S, García-Gutiérrez MS, Molina JA, Pérez-Nievas BG, Ledent C, Leiva C, et al. Increased vulnerability to 6-hydroxydopamine lesion and reduced development of dyskinesias in mice lacking CB1 cannabinoid receptors. Neurobiology of Aging. 2011;**32**(4):631-645. DOI: 10.1016/j.neurobiolaging.2009.03.017

[23] Batista LA, Gobira PH, Viana TG, Aguiar DC, Moreira FA. Inhibition of endocannabinoid neuronal uptake and hydrolysis as strategies for developing anxiolytic drugs. Behavioural Pharmacology. 2014;**25**(5-6):425-433. DOI: 10.1097/FBP.0000000000000073

[24] de Lago E, de Miguel R, Lastres-Becker I, Ramos JA, Fernández-Ruiz J. Involvement of vanilloid-like receptors in the effects of anandamide on motor behavior and nigrostriatal dopaminergic activity: In vivo and in vitro evidence. Brain Research. 2004;**1007**(1-2):152-159. DOI: 10.1016/j.brainres.2004.02.016

[25] Dos Anjos-Garcia T, Ullah F, Falconi-Sobrinho LL, Coimbra NC. CB_1 cannabinoid receptor-mediated anandamide signalling reduces the defensive behaviour evoked through $GABA_A$ receptor blockade in the dorsomedial division of the ventromedial hypothalamus. Neuropharmacology. 2017;**113**(Pt. A):156-166. DOI: 10.1016/j.neuropharm.2016.04.003

[26] Di Marzo V, Berrendero F, Bisogno T, González S, Cavaliere P, Romero J, et al. Enhancement of anandamide formation in the limbic forebrain and reduction

of endocannabinoid contents in the striatum of delta9-tetrahydrocannabinol-tolerant rats. Journal of Neurochemistry. 2000;**74**(4):1627-1635. DOI: 10.1046/j.1471-4159.2000.0741627.x

[27] Di Marzo V, Hill MP, Bisogno T, Crossman AR, Brotchie JM. Enhanced levels of endogenous cannabinoids in the globus pallidus are associated with a reduction in movement in an animal model of Parkinson's disease. The FASEB Journal. 2000;**14**(10):1432-1438. DOI: 10.1096/fj.14.10.1432

[28] Herkenham M, Lynn AB, Little MD, Johnson MR, Melvin LS, de Costa BR, et al. Cannabinoid receptor localization in brain. Proceedings of the National Academy of Sciences of the United States of America. 1990;**87**(5):1932-1936. DOI: 10.1073/pnas.87.5.1932

[29] Herkenham M, Lynn AB, Johnson MR, Melvin LS, de Costa BR, Rice KC. Characterization and localization of cannabinoid receptors in rat brain: A quantitative in vitro autoradiographic study. The Journal of Neuroscience. 1991;**11**(2):563-583. DOI: 10.1523/JNEUROSCI.11-02-00563.1991

[30] Hohmann AG, Herkenham M. Localization of cannabinoid CB1 receptor mRNA in neuronal subpopulations of rat striatum: A double-label in situ hybridization study. Synapse. 2000;**37**(1):71-80. DOI: 10.1002/(sici)1098-2396(200007)37:1<71:aid-syn8>3.0.co;2-k

[31] Romero J, Lastres-Becker I, de Miguel R, Berrendero F, Ramos JA, Fernández-Ruiz J. The endogenous cannabinoid system and the basal ganglia. Biochemical, pharmacological, and therapeutic aspects. Pharmacology & Therapeutics. 2002;**95**(2):137-152. DOI: 10.1016/s0163-7258(02)00253-x

[32] Gubellini P, Picconi B, Bari M, Battista N, Calabresi P, Centonze D, et al. Experimental parkinsonism alters endocannabinoid degradation: Implications for striatal glutamatergic transmission. The Journal of Neuroscience. 2002;**22**(16):6900-6907. DOI: 10.1523/JNEUROSCI.22-16-06900.2002

[33] Gilgun-Sherki Y, Melamed E, Mechoulam R, Offen D. The CB1 cannabinoid receptor agonist, HU-210, reduces levodopa-induced rotations in 6-hydroxydopamine-lesioned rats. Pharmacology & Toxicology. 2003;**93**(2):66-70. DOI: 10.1034/j.1600-0773.2003.930202.x

[34] García C, Palomo-Garo C, García-Arencibia M, Ramos J, Pertwee R, Fernández-Ruiz J. Symptom-relieving and neuroprotective effects of the phytocannabinoid Δ^9-THCV in animal models of Parkinson's disease. British Journal of Pharmacology. 2011;**163**(7):1495-1506. DOI: 10.1111/j.1476-5381.2011.01278.x

[35] Moss DE, McMaster SB, Rogers J. Tetrahydrocannabinol potentiates reserpine-induced hypokinesia. Pharmacology, Biochemistry and Behavior. 1981;**15**(5):779-783. DOI: 10.1016/0091-3057(81)90022-8

[36] Meschler JP, Howlett AC, Madras BK. Cannabinoid receptor agonist and antagonist effects on motor function in normal and 1-methyl-4-phenyl-1,2,5,6-tetrahydropyridine (MPTP)-treated non-human primates. Psychopharmacology. 2001;**156**(1):79-85. DOI: 10.1007/s002130100728

[37] Maneuf YP, Crossman AR, Brotchie JM. The cannabinoid receptor agonist WIN 55,212-2 reduces D_2, but not D_1, dopamine receptor-mediated alleviation of akinesia in the reserpine-treated rat model of Parkinson's

disease. Experimental Neurology. 1997;**148**(1):265-270. DOI: 10.1006/exnr.1997.6645

[38] Morgese MG, Cassano T, Gaetani S, Macheda T, Laconca L, Dipasquale P, et al. Neurochemical changes in the striatum of dyskinetic rats after administration of the cannabinoid agonist WIN55,212-2. Neurochemistry International. 2009;**54**(1):56-64. DOI: 10.1016/j.neuint.2008.10.007

[39] Segovia G, Mora F, Crossman AR, Brotchie JM. Effects of CB1 cannabinoid receptor modulating compounds on the hyperkinesia induced by high-dose levodopa in the reserpine-treated rat model of Parkinson's disease. Movement Disorders. 2003;**18**(2):138-149. DOI: 10.1002/mds.10312

[40] González-Aparicio R, Moratalla R. Oleoylethanolamide reduces L-DOPA-induced dyskinesia via TRPV1 receptor in a mouse model of Parkinson's disease. Neurobiology of Disease. 2014;**62**:416-425. DOI: 10.1016/j.nbd.2013.10.008

[41] Fox SH, Henry B, Hill M, Crossman A, Brotchie J. Stimulation of cannabinoid receptors reduces levodopa-induced dyskinesia in the MPTP-lesioned nonhuman primate model of Parkinson's disease. Movement Disorders. 2002;**17**(6):1180-1187. DOI: 10.1002/mds.10289

[42] Di Marzo V, Lastres-Becker I, Bisogno T, De Petrocellis L, Milone A, Davis JB, et al. Hypolocomotor effects in rats of capsaicin and two long chain capsaicin homologues. European Journal of Pharmacology. 2001;**420**(2-3):123-131. DOI: 10.1016/s0014-2999(01)01012-3

[43] Maccarrone M. Fatty acid amide hydrolase: A potential target for next generation therapeutics. Current Pharmaceutical Design. 2006;**12**(6):759-772. DOI: 10.2174/138161206775474279

[44] Di Marzo V, Maccarrone M. FAAH and anandamide: Is 2-AG really the odd one out? Trends in Pharmacological Sciences. 2008;**29**(5):229-233. DOI: 10.1016/j.tips.2008.03.001

[45] Solinas M, Justinova Z, Goldberg SR, Tanda G. Anandamide administration alone and after inhibition of fatty acid amide hydrolase (FAAH) increases dopamine levels in the nucleus accumbens shell in rats. Journal of Neurochemistry. 2006;**98**(2):408-419. DOI: 10.1111/j.1471-4159.2006.03880.x

[46] Johnston TH, Huot P, Fox SH, Wakefield JD, Sykes KA, Bartolini WP, et al. Fatty acid amide hydrolase (FAAH) inhibition reduces L-3,4-dihydroxyphenylalanine-induced hyperactivity in the 1-methyl-4-phenyl-1,2,3,6-tetrahydropyridine-lesioned non-human primate model of Parkinson's disease. The Journal of Pharmacology and Experimental Therapeutics. 2011;**336**(2):423-430. DOI: 10.1124/jpet.110.169532

[47] Celorrio M, Fernández-Suárez D, Rojo-Bustamante E, Echeverry-Alzate V, Ramírez MJ, Hillard CJ, et al. Fatty acid amide hydrolase inhibition for the symptomatic relief of Parkinson's disease. Brain, Behavior, and Immunity. 2016;**57**:94-105. DOI: 10.1016/j.bbi.2016.06.010

[48] García-Arencibia M, Ferraro L, Tanganelli S, Fernández-Ruiz J. Enhanced striatal glutamate release after the administration of rimonabant to 6-hydroxydopamine-lesioned rats. Neuroscience Letters. 2008;**438**(1):10-13. DOI: 10.1016/j.neulet.2008.04.041

[49] van der Stelt M, Fox SH, Hill M, Crossman AR, Petrosino S, Di Marzo V,

et al. A role for endocannabinoids in the generation of parkinsonism and levodopa-induced dyskinesia in MPTP-lesioned non-human primate models of Parkinson's disease. The FASEB Journal. 2005;**19**(9):1140-1142. DOI: 10.1096/fj.04-3010fje

[50] Huang P, Liu-Chen LY, Unterwald EM, Cowan A. Hyperlocomotion and paw tremors are two highly quantifiable signs of SR141716-precipitated withdrawal from delta9-tetrahydrocannabinol in C57BL/6 mice. Neuroscience Letters. 2009;**465**(1):66-70. DOI: 10.1016/j.neulet.2009.08.073

[51] Ferrer B, Asbrock N, Kathuria S, Piomelli D, Giuffrida A. Effects of levodopa on endocannabinoid levels in rat basal ganglia: Implications for the treatment of levodopa-induced dyskinesias. The European Journal of Neuroscience. 2003;**18**(6):1607-1614. DOI: 10.1046/j.1460-9568.2003.02896.x

[52] Fernández-Espejo E, Caraballo I, Fonseca FR, Banoua FE, Ferrer B, Flores JA, et al. Cannabinoid CB1 antagonists possess antiparkinsonian efficacy only in rats with very severe nigral lesion in experimental parkinsonism. Neurobiology of Disease. 2005;**18**(3):591-601. DOI: 10.1016/j.nbd.2004.10.015

[53] Cao X, Liang L, Hadcock JR, Iredale PA, Griffith DA, Menniti FS, et al. Blockade of cannabinoid type 1 receptors augments the antiparkinsonian action of levodopa without affecting dyskinesias in 1-methyl-4-phenyl-1,2,3,6-tetrahydropyridine-treated rhesus monkeys. The Journal of Pharmacology and Experimental Therapeutics. 2007;**323**(1):318-326. DOI: 10.1124/jpet.107.125666

[54] García-Arencibia M, González S, de Lago E, Ramos JA, Mechoulam R, Fernández-Ruiz J. Evaluation of the neuroprotective effect of cannabinoids in a rat model of Parkinson's disease: Importance of antioxidant and cannabinoid receptor-independent properties. Brain Research. 2007;**1134**(1):162-170. DOI: 10.1016/j.brainres.2006.11.063

[55] Fernández-Ruiz J, Moreno-Martet M, Rodríguez-Cueto C, Palomo-Garo C, Gómez-Cañas M, Valdeolivas S, et al. Prospects for cannabinoid therapies in basal ganglia disorders. British Journal of Pharmacology. 2011;**163**(7):1365-1378. DOI: 10.1111/j.1476-5381.2011.01365.x

[56] Venderová K, Růzicka E, Vorísek V, Visnovský P. Survey on cannabis use in Parkinson's disease: Subjective improvement of motor symptoms. Movement Disorders. 2004;**19**(9):1102-1106. DOI: 10.1002/mds.20111

[57] Lotan I, Treves TA, Roditi Y, Djaldetti R. Cannabis (medical marijuana) treatment for motor and non-motor symptoms of Parkinson disease: An open-label observational study. Clinical Neuropharmacology. 2014;**37**(2):41-44. DOI: 10.1097/WNF.0000000000000016

[58] Lotan I, Treves T, Roditi Y, Djaldetti R. Medical marijuana (cannabis) treatment for motor and non-motor symptoms in Parkinson's disease. An open-label observational study. Movement Disorders. 2013;**28**(1):448

[59] Carroll CB, Bain PG, Teare L, Liu X, Joint C, Wroath C, et al. Cannabis for dyskinesia in Parkinson disease: A randomized double-blind crossover study. Neurology. 2004;**63**(7):1245-1250. DOI: 10.1212/01.wnl.0000140288.48796.8e

[60] Zuardi AW, Crippa JA, Hallak JE, Pinto JP, Chagas MH, Rodrigues GG,

et al. Cannabidiol for the treatment of psychosis in Parkinson's disease. Journal of Psychopharmacology. 2009;**23**(8):979-983. DOI: 10.1177/0269881108096519

[61] Consroe P, Sandyk R, Snider SR. Open label evaluation of cannabidiol in dystonic movement disorders. International Journal of Neuroscience. 1986;**30**(4):277-282. DOI: 10.3109/00207458608985678

[62] Chagas MH, Eckeli AL, Zuardi AW, Pena-Pereira MA, Sobreira-Neto MA, Sobreira ET, et al. Cannabidiol can improve complex sleep-related behaviours associated with rapid eye movement sleep behaviour disorder in Parkinson's disease patients: A case series. Journal of Clinical Pharmacy and Therapeutics. 2014;**39**(5):564-566. DOI: 10.1111/jcpt.12179

[63] Chagas MH, Zuardi AW, Tumas V, Pena-Pereira MA, Sobreira ET, Bergamaschi MM, et al. Effects of cannabidiol in the treatment of patients with Parkinson's disease: An exploratory double-blind trial. Journal of Psychopharmacology. 2014;**28**(11):1088-1098. DOI: 10.1177/0269881114550355

[64] Sieradzan KA, Fox SH, Hill M, Dick JP, Crossman AR, Brotchie JM. Cannabinoids reduce levodopa-induced dyskinesia in Parkinson's disease: A pilot study. Neurology. 2001;**57**(11):2108-2111. DOI: 10.1212/wnl.57.11.2108

[65] Sieradzan KA, Fox SH, Dick J, Brotchie JM. The effects of the cannabinoid receptor agonist nabilone on L-DOPA induced dyskinesia in patients with idiopathic Parkinson's disease. Movement disorders. 1998;**13**(Supplement 2):29

[66] Consroe P. Brain cannabinoid systems as targets for the therapy of neurological disorders. Neurobiology of Disease. 1998;**5**(6):534-551. DOI: 10.1006/nbdi.1998.0220

[67] Koppel BS, Brust JC, Fife T, Bronstein J, Youssof S, Gronseth G, et al. Systematic review: Efficacy and safety of medical marijuana in selected neurologic disorders: Report of the guideline development Subcommittee of the American Academy of Neurology. Neurology. 2014;**82**(17):1556-1563. DOI: 10.1212/WNL.0000000000000363

[68] Chatterjee A, Almahrezi A, Ware M, Fitzcharles MA. A dramatic response to inhaled cannabis in a woman with central thalamic pain and dystonia. Journal of Pain and Symptom Management. 2002;**24**(1):4-6. DOI: 10.1016/s0885-3924(02)00426-8

[69] Uribe Roca MC, Micheli F, Viotti R. Cannabis sativa and dystonia secondary to Wilson's disease. Movement Disorders. 2005;**20**(1):113-115. DOI: 10.1002/mds.20268

[70] Lorenz R. On the application of cannabis in paediatrics and epileptology. Neuroendocrinology Letters. 2004;**25**(1-2):40-44

[71] Curtis A, Mitchell I, Patel S, Ives N, Rickards H. A pilot study using nabilone for symptomatic treatment in Huntington's disease. Movement Disorders. 2009;**24**(15):2254-2259. DOI: 10.1002/mds.22809

[72] Armstrong MJ, Miyasaki JM, American Academy of Neurology. Evidence-based guideline: Pharmacologic treatment of chorea in Huntington disease: Report of the guideline development subcommittee of the American Academy of Neurology. Neurology. 2012;**79**(6):597-603. DOI: 10.1212/WNL.0b013e318263c443

[73] Sandyk R, Consroe P, Stern L, Snider SR, Bliklen D, Chesher G, et al. Marijuana: An international research report. In: National Campaign against Drug Monograph Series n° 7. Australia: Australian Government Publication Service; 1988

[74] Consroe P, Laguna J, Allender J, Snider S, Stern L, Sandyk R, et al. Controlled clinical trial of cannabidiol in Huntington's disease. Pharmacology, Biochemistry, and Behavior. 1991;**40**(3):701-708. DOI: 10.1016/0091-3057(91)90386-g

[75] Kogan NM, Mechoulam R. Cannabinoids in health and disease. Dialogues in Clinical Neuroscience. 2007;**9**(4):413-430. DOI: 10.31887/DCNS.2007.9.4/nkogan

[76] Hasan A, Rothenberger A, Münchau A, Wobrock T, Falkai P, Roessner V. Oral delta 9-tetrahydrocannabinol improved refractory Gilles de la Tourette syndrome in an adolescent by increasing intracortical inhibition: A case report. Journal of Clinical Psychopharmacology. 2010;**30**(2):190-192. DOI: 10.1097/JCP.0b013e3181d236ec

[77] Brunnauer A, Segmiller FM, Volkamer T, Laux G, Müller N, Dehning S. Cannabinoids improve driving ability in a Tourette's patient. Psychiatry Research. 2011;**190**(2-3):382. DOI: 10.1016/j.psychres.2011.05.033

[78] Urbi B, Corbett J, Hughes I, Owusu MA, Thorning S, Broadley SA, et al. Effects of cannabis in Parkinson's disease: A systematic review and meta-analysis. Journal of Parkinson's Disease. 2022;**12**(2):495-508. DOI: 10.3233/JPD-212923

[79] Volkmar FR, editor. ASD (Autism Spectrum Disorder). In: Encyclopedia of Autism Spectrum Disorders. Cham: Springer; 2021. DOI: 10.1007/978-3-319-91280-6_300130 [Accessed: January 12, 2024]

[80] Ghosh A, Michalon A, Lindemann L, Fontoura P, Santarelli L. Drug discovery for autism spectrum disorder: Challenges and opportunities. Nature Reviews. Drug Discovery. 2013;**12**(10):777-790. DOI: 10.1038/nrd4102

[81] Lutz B. Endocannabinoid signals in the control of emotion. Current Opinion in Pharmacology. 2009;**9**(1):46-52. DOI: 10.1016/j.coph.2008.12.001

[82] Marco EM, Scattoni ML, Rapino C, Ceci C, Chaves N, Macrì S, et al. Emotional, endocrine and brain anandamide response to social challenge in infant male rats. Psychoneuroendocrinology. 2013;**38**(10):2152-2162. DOI: 10.1016/j.psyneuen.2013.04.004

[83] Zamberletti E, Gabaglio M, Parolaro D. The endocannabinoid system and autism spectrum disorders: Insights from animal models. International Journal of Molecular Sciences. 2017;**18**(9):1916. DOI: 10.3390/ijms18091916

[84] Pietropaolo S, Bellocchio L, Bouzón-Arnáiz I, Yee BK. The role of the endocannabinoid system in autism spectrum disorders: Evidence from mouse studies. Progress in Molecular Biology and Translational Science. 2020;**173**:183-208. DOI: 10.1016/bs.pmbts.2020.04.016

[85] Careaga M, Water J, Ashwood P. Immune dysfunction in autism: A pathway to treatment. Neurotherapeutics. 2010;**7**:283-292. DOI: 10.1016/j.nurt.2010.05.003

[86] Anavi-Goffer S, Mulder J. The polarised life of the endocannabinoid system in CNS development.

Chembiochem. 2009;**10**(10):1591-1598. DOI: 10.1002/cbic.200800827

[87] Drysdale AJ, Platt B. Cannabinoids: Mechanisms and therapeutic applications in the CNS. Current Medicinal Chemistry. 2003;**10**(24):2719-2732. DOI: 10.2174/0929867033456387

[88] Courchesne E, Pierce K, Schumann CM, Redcay E, Buckwalter JA, Kennedy DP, et al. Mapping early brain development in autism. Neuron. 2007;**56**(2):399-413. DOI: 10.1016/j.neuron.2007.10.016

[89] Onore C, Careaga M, Ashwood P. The role of immune dysfunction in the pathophysiology of autism. Brain, Behavior, and Immunity. 2012;**26**(3):383-392. DOI: 10.1016/j.bbi.2011.08.007

[90] TonhajzerovaI,OndrejkaI,MestanikM, MikolkaP, HrtanekI, Mestanikova A, et al. Inflammatory activity in autism spectrum disorder. Advances in Experimental Medicine and Biology. 2015;**861**:93-98. DOI: 10.1007/5584_2015_145

[91] Lunn CA, Reich EP, Bober L. Targeting the CB2 receptor for immune modulation. Expert Opinion on Therapeutic Targets. 2006;**10**(5):653-663. DOI: 10.1517/14728222.10.5.653

[92] Cencioni MT, Chiurchiù V, Catanzaro G, Borsellino G, Bernardi G, Battistini L, et al. Anandamide suppresses proliferation and cytokine release from primary human T-lymphocytes mainly via CB2 receptors. PLoS One. 2010;**5**(1):e8688. DOI: 10.1371/journal.pone.0008688

[93] Xu N, Li X, Zhong Y. Inflammatory cytokines: Potential biomarkers of immunologic dysfunction in autism spectrum disorders. Mediators of Inflammation. 2015;**2015**:531518. DOI: 10.1155/2015/531518

[94] Li X, Chauhan A, Sheikh AM, Patil S, Chauhan V, Li XM, et al. Elevated immune response in the brain of autistic patients. Journal of Neuroimmunology. 2009;**207**(1-2):111-116. DOI: 10.1016/j.jneuroim.2008.12.002

[95] Kerr DM, Downey L, Conboy M, Finn DP, Roche M. Alterations in the endocannabinoid system in the rat valproic acid model of autism. Behavioural Brain Research. 2013;**249**: 124-132. DOI: 10.1016/j.bbr.2013.04.043

[96] Morena M, De Castro V, Gray JM, Palmery M, Trezza V, Roozendaal B, et al. Training-associated emotional arousal shapes endocannabinoid modulation of spatial memory retrieval in rats. Journal of Neuroscience. 2015;**35**:13962-13974. DOI: 10.1523/JNEUROSCI.1983-15.2015

[97] Chakrabarti B, Baron-Cohen S. Variation in the human cannabinoid receptor CNR1 gene modulates gaze duration for happy faces. Molecular Autism. 2011;**2**:10. DOI: 10.1186/2040-2392-2-10

[98] Chakrabarti B, Kent L, Suckling J, Bullmore E, Baron-Cohen S. Variations in the human cannabinoid receptor (CNR1) gene modulate striatal responses to happy faces. European Journal of Neuroscience. 2006;**23**:1944-1948. DOI: 10.1111/j.1460-9568.2006.04697.x

[99] Trezza V, Vanderschuren LJ. Bidirectional cannabinoid modulation of social behavior in adolescent rats. Psychopharmacology. 2008;**197**(2):217-227. DOI: 10.1007/s00213-007-1025-3

[100] Trezza V, Damsteegt R, Manduca A, Petrosino S, Van Kerkhof LW, Pasterkamp RJ, et al. Endocannabinoids in amygdala and nucleus accumbens mediate social play reward in adolescent rats. The Journal of

Neuroscience. 2012;**32**(43):14899-14908. DOI: 10.1523/JNEUROSCI.0114-12.2012

[101] Denner LA, Rodriguez-Rivera J, Haidacher SJ, Jahrling JB, Carmical JR, Hernandez CM, et al. Cognitive enhancement with rosiglitazone links the hippocampal PPARγ and ERK MAPK signaling pathways. The Journal of Neuroscience. 2012;**32**(47):16725-1635a. DOI: 10.1523/JNEUROSCI.2153-12.2012

[102] Gao F, Zhang LH, Su TF, Li L, Zhou R, Peng M, et al. Signaling mechanism of cannabinoid receptor-2 activation-induced β-endorphin release. Molecular Neurobiology. 2016;**53**(6):3616-3625. DOI: 10.1007/s12035-015-9291-2

[103] Howlett AC, Abood ME. CB_1 and CB_2 receptor pharmacology. Advances in Pharmacology. 2017;**80**:169-206. DOI: 10.1016/bs.apha.2017.03.007

[104] Gould GG, Burke TF, Osorio MD, Smolik CM, Zhang WQ, Onaivi ES, et al. Enhanced novelty-induced corticosterone spike and upregulated serotonin 5-HT1A and cannabinoid CB1 receptors in adolescent BTBR mice. Psychoneuroendocrinology. 2014;**39**:158-169. DOI: 10.1016/j.psyneuen.2013.09.003

[105] Wei D, Dinh D, Lee D, Li D, Anguren A, Moreno-Sanz G, et al. Enhancement of anandamide-mediated endocannabinoid signaling corrects autism-related social impairment. Cannabis and Cannabinoid Research. 2016;**1**(1):81-89. DOI: 10.1089/can.2015.0008

[106] Onaivi ES, Benno R, Halpern T, Mehanovic M, Schanz N, Sanders C, et al. Consequences of cannabinoid and monoaminergic system disruption in a mouse model of autism spectrum disorders. Current Neuropharmacology. 2011;**9**(1):209-214. DOI: 10.2174/157015911795017047

[107] Liu QR, Pan CH, Hishimoto A, Li CY, Xi ZX, LlorenteBerzal A, et al. Species differences in cannabinoid receptor 2 (CNR2gene): Identification of novel human and rodent CB2 isoforms, differential tissue expression and regulation by cannabinoid receptor ligands. Genes, Brain and Behavior. 2009;**8**:519-530. DOI: 10.1111/j.1601-183X.2009.00498.x

[108] Siniscalco D, Sapone A, Giordano C, Cirillo A, de Magistris L, Rossi F, et al. Cannabinoid receptor type 2, but not type 1, is up-regulated in peripheral blood mononuclear cells of children affected by autistic disorders. Journal of Autism and Developmental Disorders. 2013;**43**:2686-2695. DOI: 10.1007/s10803-013-1824-9

[109] Carbone E, Manduca A, Cacchione C, Vicari S, Trezza V. Healing autism spectrum disorder with cannabinoids: A neuroinflammatory story. Neuroscience & Biobehavioral Reviews. 2021;**121**:128-143. DOI: 10.1016/j.neubiorev.2020.12.009

[110] Folkes OM, Báldi R, Kondev V, Marcus DJ, Hartley ND, Turner BD, et al. An endocannabinoid-regulated basolateral amygdala–nucleus accumbens circuit modulates sociability. Journal of Clinical Investigation. 2020;**130**:1728-1742. DOI: 10.1172/JCI131752

[111] Jamain S, Quach H, Betancur C, Råstam M, Colineaux C, Gillberg IC, et al. Mutations of the X-linked genes encoding neuroligins NLGN3 and NLGN4 are associated with autism. Nature Genetics. 2003;**34**(1):27-29. DOI: 10.1038/ng1136

[112] Földy C, Malenka RC, Südhof TC. Autism-associated neuroligin-3 mutations commonly disrupt tonic endocannabinoid signaling. Neuron. 2013;**78**:498-509. DOI: 10.1016/j.neuron.2013.02.036

[113] Hosie S, Malone DT, Liu S, Glass M, Adlard PA, Hannan AJ, et al. Altered amygdala excitation and CB1 receptor modulation of aggressive behavior in the Neuroligin-3^{R451C} mouse model of autism. Frontiers in Cellular Neuroscience. 2018;**12**:234. DOI: 10.3389/fncel.2018.00234

[114] Servadio M, Melancia F, Manduca A, di Masi A, Schiavi S, Cartocci V, et al. Targeting anandamide metabolism rescues core and associated autistic-like symptoms in rats prenatally exposed to valproic acid. Translational Psychiatry. 2016;**6**:e902-e902. DOI: 10.1038/tp.2016.182

[115] Zou M, Liu Y, Xie S, Wang L, Li D, Li L, et al. Alterations of the endocannabinoid system and its therapeutic potential in autism spectrum disorder. Open Biology. 2021;**11**(2):200306. DOI: 10.1098/rsob.200306

[116] Schultz S, Gould GG, Antonucci N, Brigida AL, Siniscalco D. Endocannabinoid system dysregulation from acetaminophen use may lead to autism spectrum disorder: Could cannabinoid treatment be efficacious? Molecules. 2021;**26**:7. DOI: 10.3390/molecules26071845

[117] Loss CM, Teodoro L, Rodrigues GD, Moreira LR, Peres FF, Zuardi AW, et al. Is cannabidiol during neurodevelopment a promising therapy for schizophrenia and autism spectrum disorders? Frontiers in Pharmacology. 2021;**11**:635763. DOI: 10.3389/fphar.2020.635763

[118] Kaplan J, Stella N, Catterall WA, Westenbroek RE. Cannabidiol attenuates seizures and social deficits in a mouse model of Dravet syndrome. Proceedings of the National Academy of Sciences. 2017;**114**:11229-11234. DOI: 10.1073/pnas.1711351114

[119] Osborne AL, Solowij N, Weston-Green K. A systematic review of the effect of cannabidiol on cognitive function: Relevance to schizophrenia. Neuroscience and Biobehavioral Reviews. 2017;**72**:310-324. DOI: 10.1016/j.neubiorev.2016.11.012

[120] Patra PH, Serafeimidou-Pouliou E, Bazelot M, Whalley BJ, Williams CM, McNeish AJ. Cannabidiol improves survival and behavioural co-morbidities of Dravet syndrome in mice. British Journal of Pharmacology. 2020;**177**(12):2779-2792. DOI: 10.1111/bph.15003

[121] Pretzsch CM, Floris DL, Voinescu B, Elsahib M, Mendez MA, Wichers R, et al. Modulation of striatal functional connectivity differences in adults with and without autism spectrum disorder in a single-dose randomized trial of cannabidivarin. Molecular Autism. 2021;**12**(1):49. DOI: 10.1186/s13229-021-00454-6

[122] Vigli D, Cosentino L, Raggi C, Laviola G, Woolley-Roberts M, De Filippis B. Chronic treatment with the phytocannabinoid cannabidivarin (CBDV) rescues behavioural alterations and brain atrophy in a mouse model of Rett syndrome. Neuropharmacology. 2018;**140**:121-129. DOI: 10.1016/j.neuropharm.2018.07.029

[123] Zamberletti E, Gabaglio M, Piscitelli F, Brodie JS, Woolley-Roberts M, Barbiero I, et al. Cannabidivarin completely rescues cognitive deficits and delays neurological and motor defects in male *Mecp2* mutant mice. Journal of Psychopharmacology. 2019;**33**(7):894-907. DOI: 10.1177/0269881119844184

[124] Zamberletti E, Gabaglio M, Woolley-Roberts M, Bingham S, Rubino T, Parolaro D. Cannabidivarin treatment ameliorates autism-like

behaviors and restores hippocampal endocannabinoid system and glia alterations induced by prenatal valproic acid exposure in rats. Frontiers in Cellular Neuroscience. 2019;**13**:367. DOI: 10.3389/fncel.2019.00367

[125] Kurz R, Blaas K. Use of dronabinol (delta-9-THC) in autism: A prospective single-case-study with an early infantile autistic child. Cannabinoids. 2010;**5**:4-6. Corpus ID: 4844281

[126] Kruger T, Christophersen E. An open label study of the use of Dronabinol (Marinol) in the management of treatment resistant self-injurious behavior in 10 retarded adolescent patients. Journal of Developmental & Behavioral Pediatrics. 2006;**27**:433. DOI:10.1097/00004703-200610000-00029

[127] Aran A, Harel M, Cassuto H, Polyansky L, Schnapp A, Wattad N, et al. Cannabinoid treatment for autism: A proof-of-concept randomized trial. Molecular Autism. 2021;**12**(1):6. DOI: 10.1186/s13229-021-00420-2

[128] Junior S, EAD, Medeiros WMB, Santos JPMD, Sousa JMM, Costa FBD, Pontes KM, et al. Evaluation of the efficacy and safety of cannabidiol-rich cannabis extract in children with autism spectrum disorder: Randomized, double-blind and controlled placebo clinical trial. Trends in Psychiatry and Psychotherapy. 2022;**44**. DOI: 10.47626/2237-6089-2021-0396

[129] Bar-Lev Schleider L, Mechoulam R, Saban N, Meiri G, Novack V. Real life experience of medical cannabis treatment in autism: Analysis of safety and efficacy. Scientific Reports. 2019;**9**:200. DOI: 10.1038/s41598-018-37570-y

[130] Barchel D, Stolar O, De-Haan T, Ziv-Baran T, Saban N, Fuchs DO, et al. Oral cannabidiol use in children with autism spectrum disorder to treat related symptoms and co-morbidities. Frontiers in Pharmacology. 2019;**9**:1521. DOI: 10.3389/fphar.2018.01521

[131] Hacohen M, Stolar OE, Berkovitch M, Elkana O, Kohn E, Hazan A, et al. Children and adolescents with ASD treated with CBD-rich cannabis exhibit significant improvements particularly in social symptoms: An open label study. Translational Psychiatry. 2022;**12**(1):375. DOI: 10.1038/s41398-022-02104-8

[132] Fleury-Teixeira P, Caixeta FV, Ramires da Silva LC, Brasil-Neto JP, Malcher-Lopes R. Effects of CBD-enriched *Cannabis sativa* extract on autism Spectrum disorder symptoms: An observational study of 18 participants undergoing compassionate use. Frontiers in Neurology. 2019;**10**:1145. DOI: 10.3389/fneur.2019.01145

[133] Epilepsy. Nemours Kids Health. Available from: Epilepsy (for Parents) - Nemours KidsHealth [Accessed: November. 27, 2023]

[134] Wheless JW. Managing severe epilepsy syndromes of early childhood. Journal of Child Neurology. 2009;**24**(8 Suppl.):24S-32S. quiz 33S-6S. DOI: 10.1177/0883073809338153

[135] Bromfield EB, Cavazos JE, Sirven JI, editors. An Introduction to Epilepsy. West Hartford (CT): American Epilepsy Society; 2006. PMID: 20821849

[136] Ceulemans B, Boel M, Leyssens K, Van Rossem C, Neels P, Jorens PG, et al. Successful use of fenfluramine as an add-on treatment for Dravet syndrome. Epilepsia. 2012;**53**(7):1131-1139. DOI: 10.1111/j.1528-1167.2012.03495.x

[137] Chiron C. Current therapeutic procedures in Dravet syndrome. Developmental Medicine and Child

Neurology. 2011;**53**(Suppl. 2):16-18. DOI: 10.1111/j.1469-8749.2011.03967.x

[138] Widdess-Walsh P, Dlugos D, Fahlstrom R, Joshi S, Shellhaas R, Boro A, et al. Lennox-Gastaut syndrome of unknown cause: Phenotypic characteristics of patients in the epilepsy phenome/genome project. Epilepsia. 2013;**54**(11):1898-1904. DOI: 10.1111/epi.12395

[139] Crumrine PK. Management of seizures in Lennox-Gastaut syndrome. Paediatric Drugs. 2011;**13**(2):107-118. DOI: 10.2165/11536940-000000000-00000

[140] Inoue T, Ihara Y, Tomonoh Y, Nakamura N, Ninomiya S, Fujita T, et al. Early onset and focal spike discharges as indicators of poor prognosis for myoclonic-astatic epilepsy. Brain & Development. 2014;**36**(7):613-619. DOI: 10.1016/j.braindev.2013.08.009

[141] Asadi-Pooya AA, Sharifzade M. West syndrome in South Iran: Electro-clinical manifestations. Iranian Journal of Child Neurology. 2013;7:40-44

[142] Cvitanović-Sojat L, Gjergja R, Sabol Z, Hajnzić TF, Sojat T. Lijecenje Westovog sindroma [treatment of west syndrome]. Acta Medica Croatica. 2005;**59**(1):19-29. Croatian

[143] Babayeva M, Fuzailov M, Rozenfeld P, Basu P. Marijuana compounds: A non-conventional therapeutic approach to epilepsy in children. Journal of Addiction and Neuropharmacology. 2014;**1**:002

[144] Wallace MJ, Martin BR, DeLorenzo RJ. Evidence for a physiological role of endocannabinoids in the modulation of seizure threshold and severity. European Journal of Pharmacology. 2002;**452**(3):295-301. DOI: 10.1016/s0014-2999(02)02331-2

[145] Devinsky O, Cilio MR, Cross H, Fernandez-Ruiz J, French J, Hill C, et al. Cannabidiol: Pharmacology and potential therapeutic role in epilepsy and other neuropsychiatric disorders. Epilepsia. 2014;**55**(6):791-802. DOI: 10.1111/epi.12631

[146] Ryan D, Drysdale AJ, Lafourcade C, Pertwee RG, Platt B. Cannabidiol targets mitochondria to regulate intracellular Ca2+ levels. The Journal of Neuroscience. 2009;**29**(7):2053-2063. DOI: 10.1523/JNEUROSCI.4212-08.2009

[147] Leweke FM, Piomelli D, Pahlisch F, Muhl D, Gerth CW, Hoyer C, et al. Cannabidiol enhances anandamide signaling and alleviates psychotic symptoms of schizophrenia. Translational Psychiatry. 2012;**2**(3):e94. DOI: 10.1038/tp.2012.15

[148] Karler R, Cely W, Turkanis SA. Anticonvulsant properties of delta 9-tetrahydrocannabinol and other cannabinoids. Life Sciences. 1974;**15**(5):931-947. DOI: 10.1016/0024-3205(74)90009-5

[149] Jones NA, Glyn SE, Akiyama S, Hill TD, Hill AJ, Weston SE, et al. Cannabidiol exerts anti-convulsant effects in animal models of temporal lobe and partial seizures. Seizure. 2012;**21**(5):344-352. DOI: 10.1016/j.seizure.2012.03.001

[150] Jones NA, Hill AJ, Smith I, Bevan SA, Williams CM, Whalley BJ, et al. Cannabidiol displays antiepileptiform and antiseizure properties in vitro and in vivo. The Journal of Pharmacology and Experimental Therapeutics. 2010;**332**(2):569-577. DOI: 10.1124/jpet.109.159145

[151] Porter BE, Jacobson C. Report of a parent survey of cannabidiol-enriched cannabis use in pediatric

treatment-resistant epilepsy. Epilepsy & Behavior. 2013;**29**(3):574-577. DOI: 10.1016/j.yebeh.2013.08.037

[152] Huntsman RJ, Tang-Wai R, Shackelford AE. Cannabis for Pediatric epilepsy. Journal of Clinical Neurophysiology. 2020;**37**(1):2-8. DOI: 10.1097/WNP.0000000000000641

[153] Madan Cohen J, Checketts D, Dunayevich E, Gunning B, Hyslop A, Madhavan D, et al. Time to onset of cannabidiol treatment effects in Dravet syndrome: Analysis from two randomized controlled trials. Epilepsia. 2021;**62**(9):2218-2227. DOI: 10.1111/epi.16974

[154] Silvinato A, Floriano I, Bernardo WM. Use of cannabidiol in the treatment of epilepsy: Lennox-Gastaut syndrome, Dravet syndrome, and tuberous sclerosis complex. Revista da Associação Médica Brasileira (1992). 2022;**68**(10):1345-1357. DOI: 10.1590/1806-9282.2022D689

[155] Ibeas Bih C, Chen T, Nunn AV, Bazelot M, Dallas M, Whalley BJ. Molecular targets of cannabidiol in neurological disorders. Neurotherapeutics. 2015;**12**(4):699-730. DOI: 10.1007/s13311-015-0377-3

[156] Rosenberg EC, Tsien RW, Whalley BJ, Devinsky O. Cannabinoids and epilepsy. Neurotherapeutics. 2015;**12**(4):747-768. DOI: 10.1007/s13311-015-0375-5

[157] Epilepsy Foundation. Treatment options. Available from: https://epilepsycoloradowyoming.org/what-is-epilepsy/treatment-options [Accessed: May 01, 2024]

[158] Stanford Medicine. News Center. Available from: https://med.stanford.edu/news/all-news/2021/07/marijuana-like-brain-substance-calms-seizures-but-increases-afte.html [Accessed: January 18, 2024]

[159] Lastres-Becker I, Molina-Holgado F, Ramos JA, Mechoulam R, Fernández-Ruiz J. Cannabinoids provide neuroprotection against 6-hydroxydopamine toxicity in vivo and in vitro: Relevance to Parkinson's disease. Neurobiology of Disease. 2005;**19**(1-2):96-107. DOI: 10.1016/j.nbd.2004.11.009

[160] Pan H, Mukhopadhyay P, Rajesh M, Patel V, Mukhopadhyay B, Gao B, et al. Cannabidiol attenuates cisplatin-induced nephrotoxicity by decreasing oxidative/nitrosative stress, inflammation, and cell death. The Journal of Pharmacology and Experimental Therapeutics. 2009;**328**(3):708-714. DOI: 10.1124/jpet.108.147181

[161] Hebert-Chatelain E, Reguero L, Puente N, Lutz B, Chaouloff F, Rossignol R, et al. Cannabinoid control of brain bioenergetics: Exploring the subcellular localization of the CB1 receptor. Molecular Metabolism. 2014;**3**(4):495-504. DOI: 10.1016/j.molmet.2014.03.007

[162] Yamaori S, Ebisawa J, Okushima Y, Yamamoto I, Watanabe K. Potent inhibition of human cytochrome P450 3A isoforms by cannabidiol: Role of phenolic hydroxyl groups in the resorcinol moiety. Life Sciences. 2011;**88**(15-16):730-736. DOI: 10.1016/j.lfs.2011.02.017

[163] Hampson AJ, Grimaldi M, Axelrod J, Wink D. Cannabidiol and (−)Delta9-tetrahydrocannabinol are neuroprotective antioxidants. Proceedings of the National Academy of Sciences of the United States of America. 1998;**95**(14):8268-8273. DOI: 10.1073/pnas.95.14.8268

[164] Amor S, Peferoen LA, Vogel DY, Breur M, van der Valk P, Baker D, et al.

Inflammation in neurodegenerative diseases–An update. Immunology. 2014;**142**(2):151-166. DOI: 10.1111/imm.12233

[165] Clark LF, Kodadek T. The immune system and neuroinflammation as potential sources of blood-based biomarkers for Alzheimer's disease, Parkinson's disease, and huntington's disease. ACS Chemical Neuroscience. 2016;**7**(5):520-527. DOI: 10.1021/acschemneuro.6b00042

[166] McGeer PL, McGeer EG. Glial reactions in Parkinson's disease. Movement Disorders. 2008;**23**(4):474-483. DOI: 10.1002/mds.21751

[167] Sayd A, Antón M, Alén F, Caso JR, Pavón J, Leza JC, et al. Systemic administration of oleoylethanolamide protects from neuroinflammation and anhedonia induced by LPS in rats. The International Journal of Neuropsychopharmacology. 2014;**18**(6):pyu111. DOI: 10.1093/ijnp/pyu111

[168] More SV, Kumar H, Kim IS, Song S-Y, Choi D-K. Cellular and molecular mediators of neuroinflammation in the pathogenesis of Parkinson's disease. Mediators of Inflammation. 2013;**2013**:12. DOI: 10.1155/2013/952375.952375

[169] Singh R, Kisku A, Kungumaraj H, Nagaraj V, Pal A, Kumar S, et al. Autism spectrum disorders: A recent update on targeting inflammatory pathways with natural anti-inflammatory agents. Biomedicine. 2023;**11**(1):115. DOI: 10.3390/biomedicines11010115

[170] Valeri A, Mazzon E. Cannabinoids and neurogenesis: The promised solution for neurodegeneration? Molecules. 2021;**26**(20):6313. DOI: 10.3390/molecules26206313

[171] Assaf F, Fishbein M, Gafni M, Keren O, Sarne Y. Pre- and post-conditioning treatment with an ultra-low dose of Δ9-tetrahydrocannabinol (THC) protects against pentylenetetrazole (PTZ)-induced cognitive damage. Behavioural Brain Research. 2011;**220**(1):194-201. DOI: 10.1016/j.bbr.2011.02.005

[172] Fishbein-Kaminietsky M, Gafni M, Sarne Y. Ultralow doses of cannabinoid drugs protect the mouse brain from inflammation-induced cognitive damage. Journal of Neuroscience Research. 2014;**92**(12):1669-1677. DOI: 10.1002/jnr.23452

[173] Sagredo O, García-Arencibia M, de Lago E, Finetti S, Decio A, Fernández-Ruiz J. Cannabinoids and neuroprotection in basal ganglia disorders. Molecular Neurobiology. 2007;**36**(1):82-91. DOI: 10.1007/s12035-007-0004-3

[174] Price DA, Martinez AA, Seillier A, Koek W, Acosta Y, Fernandez E, et al. WIN55,212-2, a cannabinoid receptor agonist, protects against nigrostriatal cell loss in the 1-methyl-4-phenyl-1,2,3,6-tetrahydropyridine mouse model of Parkinson's disease. The European Journal of Neuroscience. 2009;**29**(11):2177-2186. DOI: 10.1111/j.1460-9568.2009.06764.x

[175] Martínez-Orgado J, Fernández-López D, Lizasoain I, Romero J. The seek of neuroprotection: Introducing cannabinoids. Recent Patents on CNS Drug Discovery. 2007;**2**(2):131-139. DOI: 10.2174/157488907780832724

[176] Romero J, Martínez-Orgado J. Cannabinoids and neurodegenerative diseases. CNS and Neurological Disorders – Drug Targets. 2009; **8**(6): 440-450. DOI: 10.2174/187152709789824589

[177] Valdeolivas S, Satta V, Pertwee RG, Fernández-Ruiz J, Sagredo O. Sativex-like combination of phytocannabinoids is neuroprotective in malonate-lesioned rats, an inflammatory model of Huntington's disease: Role of CB1 and CB2 receptors. ACS Chemical Neuroscience. 2012;**3**(5):400-406. DOI: 10.1021/cn200114w

[178] Zeissler M, Hanemann C, Zajicek J, Carroll C. FAAH inhibition is protective in a cell culture model of Parkinson's disease. Journal of Neurology, Neurosurgery & Psychiatry. 2012;**83**(Supplement 2):A15. DOI: 10.1136/jnnp-2012-304200a.56

[179] Greenbaum L, Tegeder I, Barhum Y, Melamed E, Roditi Y, Djaldetti R. Contribution of genetic variants to pain susceptibility in Parkinson disease. European Journal of Pain. 2012;**16**(9):1243-1250. DOI: 10.1002/j.1532-2149.2012.00134.x

[180] Ellis RJ, Toperoff W, Vaida F, van den Brande G, Gonzales J, Gouaux B, et al. Smoked medicinal cannabis for neuropathic pain in HIV: A randomized, crossover clinical trial. Neuropsychopharmacology. 2009;**34**(3):672-680. DOI: 10.1038/npp.2008.120

[181] Nurmikko TJ, Serpell MG, Hoggart B, Toomey PJ, Morlion BJ, Haines D. Sativex successfully treats neuropathic pain characterised by allodynia: A randomised, double-blind, placebo-controlled clinical trial. Pain. 2007;**133**(1-3):210-220. DOI: 10.1016/j.pain.2007.08.028

[182] Wilsey B, Marcotte T, Tsodikov A, Millman J, Bentley H, Gouaux B, et al. A randomized, placebo-controlled, crossover trial of cannabis cigarettes in neuropathic pain. The Journal of Pain. 2008;**9**(6):506-521. DOI: 10.1016/j.jpain.2007.12.010

[183] Abrams DI, Jay CA, Shade SB, Vizoso H, Reda H, Press S, et al. Cannabis in painful HIV-associated sensory neuropathy: A randomized placebo-controlled trial. Neurology. 2007;**68**(7):515-521. DOI: 10.1212/01.wnl.0000253187.66183.9c

[184] Gorzalka BB, Hill MN. Putative role of endocannabinoid signaling in the etiology of depression and actions of antidepressants. Progress in Neuro-Psychopharmacology and Biological Psychiatry. 2011;**35**(7):1575-1585. DOI: 10.1016/j.pnpbp.2010.11.021

[185] Barrero FJ, Ampuero I, Morales B, et al. Depression in Parkinson's disease is related to a genetic polymorphism of the cannabinoid receptor gene (CNR1). The Pharmacogenomics Journal. 2005;**5**(2):135-141. DOI: 10.1038/sj.tpj.6500301

[186] Bambico FR, Hattan PR, Garant JP, Gobbi G. Effect of delta-9-tetrahydrocannabinol on behavioral despair and on pre- and postsynaptic serotonergic transmission. Progress in Neuro-Psychopharmacology & Biological Psychiatry. 2012;**38**(1):88-96. DOI: 10.1016/j.pnpbp.2012.02.006

[187] Gobbi G, Bambico FR, Mangieri R, Bortolato M, Campolongo P, Solinas M, et al. Antidepressant-like activity and modulation of brain monoaminergic transmission by blockade of anandamide hydrolysis. Proceedings of the National Academy of Sciences of the United States of America. 2005;**102**(51):18620-18625. DOI: 10.1073/pnas.0509591102

[188] Cuttler C, Spradlin A, McLaughlin RJ. A naturalistic examination of the perceived effects of cannabis on negative affect. Journal of Affective Disorders. 2018;**235**:198-205. DOI: 10.1016/j.jad.2018.04.054

[189] van Laar M, van Dorsselaer S, Monshouwer K, de Graaf R. Does cannabis use predict the first incidence of mood and anxiety disorders in the adult population? Addiction. 2007;**102**(8):1251-1260. DOI: 10.1111/j.1360-0443.2007.01875.x

[190] Womack SR, Shaw DS, Weaver CM, Forbes EE. Bidirectional associations between cannabis use and depressive symptoms from adolescence through early adulthood among At-risk young men. Journal of Studies on Alcohol and Drugs. 2016;**77**(2):287-297. DOI: 10.15288/jsad.2016.77.287

[191] Harvard Health Publishing. Medical Marijuana. 2018. Available from: https://www.health.harvard.edu/mind-and-mood/medical-marijuana-and-the-mind [Accessed: January 23, 2024]

[192] Bhattacharyya S. Induction of psychosis byΔ9- tetrahydrocannabinol reflects modulation of prefrontal and striatal function during attentional salience processing. Archives of General Psychiatry. 2012;**69**:27. DOI: 10.1001/archgenpsychiatry.2011.161

[193] Bhattacharyya S, Morrison PD, Fusar-Poli P, Martin-Santos R, Borgwardt S, Winton-Brown T, et al. Opposite effects of delta9-tetrahydrocannabinol and cannabidiol on human brain function and psychopathology. Neuropsychopharmacology. 2010;**35**:764-774. DOI: 10.1038/npp.2009.184

[194] Lemos JI, Resstel LB, Guimarães FS. Involvement of the prelimbic prefrontal cortex on cannabidiol-induced attenuation of contextual conditioned fear in rats. Behavioural Brain Research. 2010;**207**:105-111. DOI: 10.1016/j.bbr.2009.09.045

[195] de Mello Schier AR, de Oliveira Ribeiro NP, Coutinho DS, Machado S, Arias-Carrión O, Crippa JA, et al. Antidepressant-like and anxiolytic-like effects of cannabidiol: A chemical compound of Cannabis sativa. CNS & Neurological Disorders Drug Targets. 2014;**13**(6):953-960. DOI: 10.2174/1871527313666140612114838

[196] Blessing EM, Steenkamp MM, Manzanares J, Marmar CR. Cannabidiol as a potential treatment for anxiety disorders. Neurotherapeutics. 2015;**12**:825-836. DOI: 10.1007/s13311-015-0387-1

[197] Papagianni EP, Stevenson CW. Cannabinoid regulation of fear and anxiety: An update. Current Psychiatry Reports. 2019;**21**(6):38. DOI: 10.1007/s11920-019-1026-z

[198] Crippa JA, Derenusson GN, Ferrari TB, Wichert-Ana L, Duran FL, Martin-Santos R, et al. Neural basis of anxiolytic effects of cannabidiol (CBD) in generalized social anxiety disorder: A preliminary report. Journal of Psychopharmacology. 2011;**25**(1):121-130. DOI: 10.1177/0269881110379283

[199] Shannon S, Lewis N, Lee H, Hughes S. Cannabidiol in anxiety and sleep: A large case series. The Permanente Journal. 2019;**23**:18-04. DOI: 10.7812/TPP/18-041

[200] Trotti LM, Bliwise DL. Treatment of the sleep disorders associated with Parkinson's disease. Neurotherapeutics. 2014;**11**(1):68-77. DOI: 10.1007/s13311-013-0236-z

[201] Pickens J. Sedative activity of cannabis in relation to its delta trans THC and cannabidiol content. British Journal of Pharmacology. 1981;**72**:649-656. DOI: 10.1111/j.1476-5381.1981.tb09145.x

[202] Tringale R, Jensen C. Cannabis and Insomnia. O'Shaughnessy's. Autumn; 5E9EC245-448E-17B2-16 C7CA-21C6BDC6852D.pdf (webydo.com). 2011. [Accessed: January 14, 2024]

[203] Russo EB, Guy GW, Robson PJ. Cannabis, pain, and sleep: Lessons from therapeutic clinical trials of Sativex, a cannabis-based medicine. Chemistry & Biodiversity. 2007;**4**(8):1729-1743. DOI: 10.1002/cbdv.200790150

[204] Nicholson AN, Turner C, Stone BM, Robson PJ. Effect of delta 9 THC and cannabidiol on nocturnal sleep and early-morning behavior in young adults. Journal of Clinical Psychopharmacology. 2004;**24**:305-313. DOI: 10.1097/01.jcp.0000125688.05091.8f

[205] Gorelick DA, Goodwin RS, Schwilke E, Schroeder JR, Schwope DM, Kelly DL, et al. Around-the-clock oral THC effects on sleep in male chronic daily cannabis smokers. The American Journal on Addictions. 2013;**22**(5):510-514. DOI: 10.1111/j.1521-0391.2013.12003.x

Chapter 2

Resveratrol and Curcumin: Extending the Frontier of Phytomedicine

Tracey Lynn Harney

Abstract

The health of the oral cavity is a starting point for overall health, and systemic inflammation can arise when the oral health is compromised, leading to an increased risk of developing cardiovascular, metabolic, autoimmune, and neurodegenerative disease or cancer. Fortunately, nature has provided us with bioactive molecules like polyphenols, such as curcumin and resveratrol, which have demonstrated a capacity for immunomodulation, regeneration, and repair. One of the challenges for the biomedical scientific community that has delayed the actualization of the full potential of phytochemicals like curcumin and resveratrol as potent therapeutic agents is the fact that they display low oral bioavailability, instability, and rapid clearance, making them unsuitable as medicines by modern pharmacological standards. Thankfully, the application of nanotechnological design has provided a viable solution to the poor pharmacological profile of curcumin and resveratrol, making their clinical translation a feasible emergence in the near future.

Keywords: polyphenols, resveratrol, curcumin, phamacognosy, nanotechnology, periodontitis, inflammation

1. Introduction

Inflammation is a natural immunological response that protects us from invasion in the short term, but if unresolved and persistent for the long term, it can become destructive to tissues. In general, diseases that are governed by inflammation contribute to decreased quality of life and premature aging and have become an area of focus in research to determine the best approach for their prevention, treatment, and management [1]. The development of chronic systemic inflammatory conditions is multifaceted including factors such as immune resilience, genetics, age, lifestyle, and socioeconomics. For example, chronic periodontitis, a complex inflammatory condition originating in the oral cavity, has been associated with an array of conditions spanning the physiological systems, including, but not limited to, cardiovascular, neurological, pulmonary, metabolic, autoimmune disease, adverse pregnancy outcomes, and cancer [2–4]. Fortunately, the reported crosstalk between a spectrum of inflammatory conditions has led researchers to some common biochemical targets that hold potential for the mitigation of chronic systemic inflammation and/or the stimulation of the restoration of tissue [5–7]. Interestingly, certain phytochemicals, called polyphenols, have been found to modulate these significant biochemical targets involved in the promotion of chronic deregulated inflammation [7]. Consequently, polyphenolic phytochemicals such as curcumin and resveratrol have been reported to be prospective therapeutics for the adjunct treatment of periodontitis [7–10]. Unfortunately, one of the obstacles presented by many polyphenolic phytonutrients is their inadequate clinical translation, often due to low bioavailability, rapid metabolism, and/or low stability, which has earned them a reputation for having a poor pharmacological profile [11, 12]. This is further evidenced by the many studies being conducted to enhance the bioavailability and stability of curcumin and resveratrol, thus optimizing their therapeutic potential and improving their translatability into clinical practice [13–15]. An example of a cutting-edge enhancement tool is the integration of nanotechnology, which has been shown to increase the drug profile of a multitude of therapeutics used in pharmacognosy [13, 15]. Moreover, both curcumin and resveratrol are available internationally as supplements, but the purity varies from product to product, and dosing for specific ailments can be complicated, because like many bioactive phytochemicals, curcumin and resveratrol display a biphasic dose-response drug profile [16, 17]. This chapter surveys the therapeutic application of phytochemical polyphenols curcumin and resveratrol, using chronic periodontitis as a framework for their potential therapeutic application, and some common systemic inflammatory-mediated conditions with which it is associated.

2. Periodontitis: a framework for exploring inflammatory disease

Chronic periodontitis is a globally prevalent inflammatory condition that involves an unresolved persistent pathogenic biofilm, chronic inflammation, and gradual destruction of the tissues supporting the tooth [18, 19]. The clinical diagnostic parameters for periodontitis include probing pocket depth (PPD), relative attachment level (RAL), plaque index (PI), and bleeding on probing (BoP). The severity of the condition is determined by the practitioner via the interpretation of the extent of gingival detachment, periodontal ligament destruction, and alveolar bone loss parameters. Risk factors, such as age, genetics, smoking, and extraoral inflammatory conditions, are also taken into consideration [20]. Here, the gingival crevice transmutes into a pathogenic periodontal pocket. If left untreated, periodontitis can lead to edentulism and an increased risk of developing systemic inflammatory disease [18, 19]. **Figure 1** shows a summary of the conditions linked to periodontitis.

2.1 Pathogenesis of periodontitis

The pathogenesis of periodontitis is complex and involves an unfavorable shift in the normal oral microbiota resulting in the gradual development and maturation of a dysbiotic pathogenic biofilm that is disproportionately populated with opportunistic pathogens referred to as a red complex of bacteria (e.g., *Tannerella forsythia, Treponema dentolitica, and Porphyromonas gingivalis*) [18–20].

Over time, periodontal pockets form in regions where the gingiva has become detached from the tooth due to chronic inflammatory damage. Periodontal pockets provide an optimal anaerobic environment for the destructive red complex bacteria to thrive. This is one mechanism through which the cycle of immune dysregulation and tissue destruction observed in periodontitis is perpetuated [18–20].

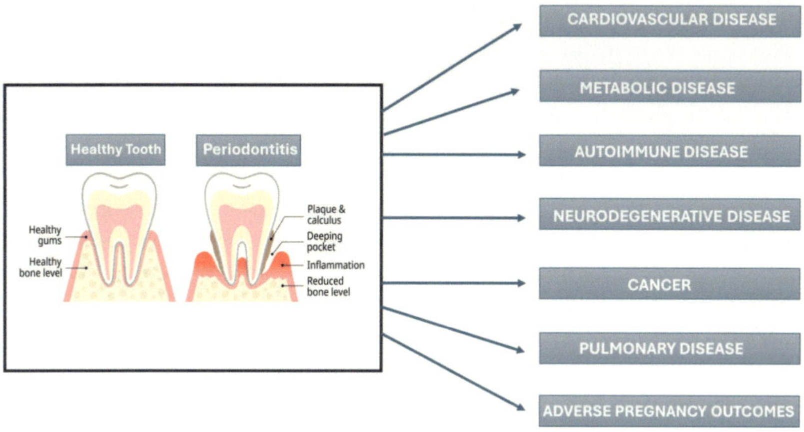

Figure 1.
Diseases that are associated with periodontitis.

Periodontal pockets may also act as reservoirs from which pathogenic bacterial cells and their virulence factors can be disseminated throughout the body. For example, periodontal pathogenic bacteria have been found in the systemic circulation of periodontitis patients following chewing or brushing [21, 22]. This frequent transient bacteremia is a key factor linking the local oral inflammatory process with systemic inflammation. It is also important to note that Gram-negative cell walls have an outer membrane, with lipopolysaccharide (LPS), also known as endotoxin, which presents as a pathogen-associated molecular pattern (PAMP), triggering pattern recognition receptors (PRRs) such as Toll-Like Receptor (e.g., TLR4) pathways which produce pro-inflammatory factors when the bacteria are killed or disrupted. For example, when LPS binds to TLR4, it activates signaling pathways (e.g., Mitogen-activated protein kinase (MAPK) and nuclear factor kappa-light-chain-enhancer of B cells (NF-kB)) which result in the release of pro-inflammatory cytokines such as interleukin-1β (IL-1β), IL-6, and tumor necrosis factor-α (TNF-α). Additionally, the innate and adaptive host immune responses lose homeostasis and become distorted due to the negative influence of the dysbiotic pathogenic microbiota and their virulence factors on the host's immune system. Such immune dysregulation results in the deleterious evolution of innate immune cells (e.g., polymorphonuclear cells (neutrophils) and macrophages) as well as the deregulated activation of formed elements that govern adaptive immunity (e.g., B and T lymphocytes), resulting in the secretion of more pro-inflammatory cytokines such as interferon-ϒ (IFN-ϒ), IL-1, IL-6, TNF-α, and IL-17. Furthermore, the perpetuity of inflammation observed in chronic periodontitis is supported by IL-17 and the destructive proteolytic enzymes, matrix metalloproteases (e.g., MMP-9) remain active, resulting in further tissue damage. Moreover, once tissue destruction occurs, even further inflammation is perpetuated from the activation of TLRs via the release of damage-associated molecular patterns (DAMPs) from injured tissues [18, 19, 23].

2.2 Comorbidities of periodontitis

Common comorbidities of chronic periodontitis include, but are not limited to, autoimmune disease, pulmonary disease, neurodegenerative disease, metabolic disease, adverse pregnancy outcomes, and cancer [24]. The highly intricate relationship between periodontitis and systemic inflammation is evident by the fact that patients with type 2 diabetes mellitus (DMII) have altered microbiomes and a noted susceptibility to developing periodontitis [25]. Moreover, since patients with chronic periodontitis have a higher chance of presenting with insulin resistance, the relationship between the risk of DMII and periodontitis is likely bidirectional [26].

It is also worth noting that many studies have reported the presence of red complex bacteria and/or their DNA in the distal tissues of patients with periodontitis. For example, red complex bacterial cells, which have been found inside local cells of the oral cavity, have also been discovered within the atherosclerotic plaques of coronary artery disease patients, cancerous tumors, and the amyloid beta plaques of Alzheimer's patients [27–30]. Moreover, since Gram-negative bacteria, such as those identified as members of the red complex of periodontitis, constitutively release outer membrane vesicles (OMVs), (virulence factor-loaded membrane-bound nanoparticles, approximately 50–250 nm in size), they can easily enter any local or distal cell where they alter cellular processes with potency. Therefore, dramatic alterations in the immune response of distal tissues and organs can take place without the red complex bacteria themselves being present [27].

Hence, the interplay between local and systemic immune dysregulation may be partly due to the dissemination of bacteria and their damaging products throughout the body, in addition to the long-term release of locally produced pro-inflammatory molecules into the systemic circulation from the locally inflamed area within the oral cavity [2, 5]. Interestingly, a causal relationship between periodontitis and the diseases that it has been linked to has not yet been confirmed. This is partly due to the inconsistency in the reporting of the degree to which periodontitis contributes as a risk factor for a given condition [2, 5, 31]. Nonetheless, because both periodontitis and systemic inflammatory diseases are governed by deregulated molecular pathways, it is feasible to consider that therapeutic agents that are found to ameliorate any of these conditions via the modulation of key biomolecular targets may act as promising therapeutics for their resolution [2, 7].

2.3 Treatment of periodontitis

Conventional treatment of periodontitis involves the removal of the pathogenic biofilm and diseased tissue through scaling and root planing (SRP), antibiotics, comprehensive care, and, in some cases, adjunct therapy to reduce the probability of recurrence [32, 33]. A novel approach to SRP includes periodontal endoscopy, where the bacterial colonies are gently removed with the assistance of a tiny camera called a periscope that inserts into the subgingival periodontal region for gentle removal of all infected colonies and material. PE-assisted SRP, which requires specialized skills through intensive training, has been reported to have effective outcomes [34–37].

In addition to SRP (with or without the assistance of PE), adjunct therapies such as host modulation, which aims to suppress the destruction of connective tissue hence supporting regeneration of both soft and bony tissues, have been used as an adjunct therapy with success [33, 37]. For example, the host-modulating drug, Perisostat®, which consists of a sub-antibiotic dose of doxycycline (SDD), has demonstrated improved outcomes, partly due to its ability to inhibit destructive proteolytic enzymes such as MMP-9, encouraging restoration of the periodontium and gingival reattachment. Since the molecular mechanism of MMP-9 inhibition (MMP-9 inhibition active site) is elucidated, novel host modulators are being investigated, based on their molecular structure [33, 37, 38]. Hence, three generations of host-modulating molecules have been explored since their dawn in the late twentieth century. Interestingly, since it was the polyphenolic region of the doxycycline that was interacting with the MMP-9 inhibitory active site, the third generation of host-modulating molecules being currently investigated includes polyphenolic phytochemicals, curcumin, and resveratrol [33].

3. Pharmacological action of curcumin

Curcumin, (1E,6E)-1,7-bis (4-hydroxy-3-methoxyphenyl)-1,6-heptadiene-3,5-dione, is a bioactive polyphenolic compound sourced from the rhizome of the plant *Curcuma longa*, also known as turmeric. Curcumin is what gives turmeric its deep orange color. **Figure 2** shows the molecular structure of curcumin and a photograph of the rhizome of turmeric.

Curcumin has been found to demonstrate a breadth of beneficial effects including but not limited to antimicrobial, antioxidant, antitumorigenic, antiviral, antidiabetic, anti-inflammatory, antilipidemic, cardioprotective, hepatoprotective, neuroprotective, and vulnerary action [39, 40]. The mechanism of the anti-inflammatory action of curcumin has been reported to involve the inhibition of pro-inflammatory pathway mediators such as NF-kB and the attenuation of inflammatory enzymes like cyclooxygenase-2 (COX-2), lipoxygenase (LOX), and inducible nitric oxide synthase (iNOS). The pleiotropic effects of curcumin have made it a molecule of interest for the treatment and prevention of many conditions [39, 40].

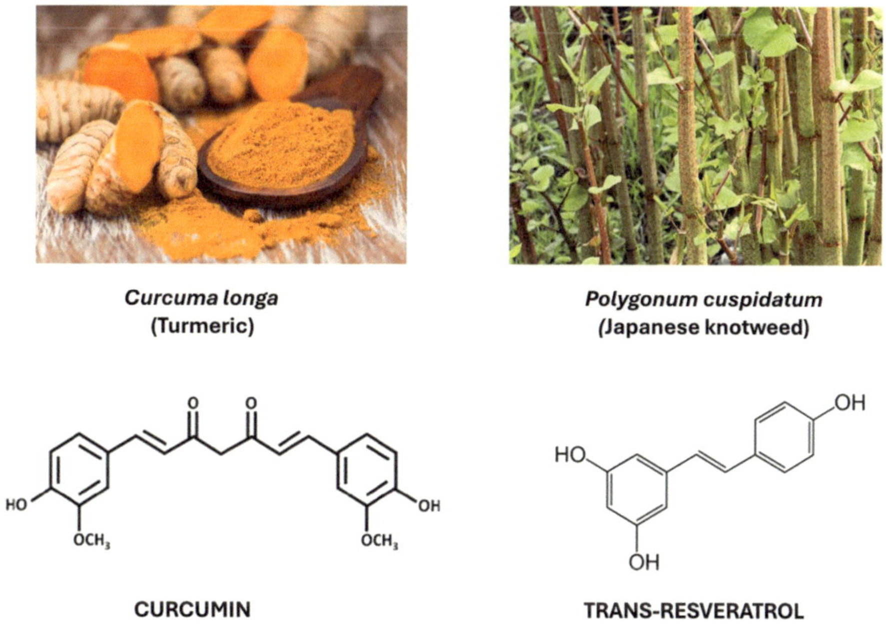

Figure 2.
Molecular structure and plant sources for curcumin and trans-resveratrol.

3.1 Curcumin and periodontitis

Assessed for its efficacy in pre-clinical ligature-induced periodontitis animal model studies, *in vitro* assays, and, to a lesser extent, clinical trials, curcumin has been found to inhibit destructive collagenase enzyme MMP-9, reduce alveolar bone loss whilst supporting osteogenesis, decrease pro-inflammatory cytokine production, and resolve red complex bacterial infection and biofilm formation [33, 41, 42]. For example, a 2022 histological study, comparing tetracycline to curcumin as adjunct treatments to SRP, concluded that the decreased inflammation and bone loss resulting from curcumin was comparable to that of tetracycline [43]. Details of the mechanisms of action regarding the mitigation of periodontitis by curcumin are highly complex and still being established but have been reported to be partly due to its suppression of pro-inflammatory pathways governed by molecular targets such as MAPK, NF-kB, and Janus kinase/signal transducers and activators of transcription (JAK/STAT) pathways [8]. Interestingly, curcumin has also been reported to manage the pathogenic dysbiotic biofilm displayed in periodontitis by way of its antimicrobial action. An *in vitro* study found that curcumin inhibited the cytotoxic effects of *P. gingivalis* (OMZ314 strain, which is highly invasive) by preventing the adhesion and entry of OMVs into human gingival epithelial cells. Because OMVs are highly complex stealth virulence factors that can easily disseminate and enter cells throughout the body, they are major contributors to the pathogenesis of periodontitis, and this study provides evidence for the preventative application of curcumin [44]. There have also been studies reporting curcumin as a safe and efficacious adjunct to SLP and has been found to be as effective as chlorohexidine (i.e., an antiseptic) in improving clinical parameters (e.g., BI, CAL, and PPD) [45].

3.2 Curcumin and cardiovascular disease

An increased risk of heart disease such as myocardial infarction, stroke, and atherosclerosis has been associated with poor oral health for decades and curcumin has demonstrated cardioprotective action by way of the attenuation of molecular pathways that govern oxidative stress, apoptosis, and inflammation. The effect of curcumin has been reported to include, but not be limited to, preventing the development of foam cells (formed as a part of the disease process of atherosclerosis), supporting the remodeling of the ventricular chambers of the heart, and reducing scar tissue formation via the inhibition of myocardial hypertrophy and fibrosis [46, 47]. Oxidative stress is often observed in cardiovascular disease because it induces inflammation and destruction of myocardial cells. Additionally, abnormally elevated free fatty acid in the systemic circulation, which is often the result of obesity and/or a high-fat diet, induces inflammatory pathways governed by the transcription factor, NF-kB, which results in the increased expression of pro-inflammatory cytokines, IL-1β, TNF-α, and IL-6. Animal studies have also shown that curcumin has been found to suppress high-fat diet-induced cardiac inflammation via the inhibition of NF-kB. Further to this, the anti-atherosclerotic action of curcumin has been reported to be due to its activation of the enzyme 5′ adenosine monophosphate-activated protein kinase (AMPK), which leads to the activation of NAD-dependent deacetylase sirtuin-1 (SIRT1) and subsequently, liver X receptor alpha (LXR-α), ultimately resulting in the efflux of cholesterol and a reduction in the accumulation of lipids in foam cells [46, 47]. Further protection of the myocardium is denoted from AMPK activation via optimized metabolism, the stimulation of mitochondrial biogenesis, and the suppression of myocardial apoptosis. Even though specific targets are yet to be fully elucidated, the potential mechanism for the cardioprotective action of curcumin has been reported to be the result of its regulation of various signaling pathways (e.g., AMPK, Nrf2, JAK/STAT, NF-κB, phosphatidyl inositol 3-kinase (PI3k)/protein kinase B (Akt), MAPK, Notch, mammalian target of rapamycin (mTOR), peroxisome proliferator-activated receptor (PPARs), and arachidonic acid) [48, 49].

3.3 Curcumin and cancer

Anticancer action of curcumin, which has been observed from *in vitro* and *in vivo* animal studies, is related to its ability to affect signaling pathways resulting in diminished cancer cell proliferation, migration, and invasion, as well as induction of cancer cell autophagy (natural cell self-recycling) and apoptosis (i.e., programmed cell death) [50, 51]. Further to this, malignant tumors often grow their own blood supply via a process called angiogenesis. Curcumin has been found to inhibit this process, thus slowing tumor formation. The majority of randomized clinical trials investigating curcumin as a cancer therapy have set up curcumin as an adjunct to conventional therapy, where it has been reported to improve survival and/or improve quality of life for various cancers. Interestingly, the results of a 2019 randomized clinical trial on prostate cancer patients suggested that curcumin (1440 mg/day orally) significantly suppressed PSA progression during the curcumin treatment period ($p = 0.0259$) [51].

Epigenetics, which contributes to the regulation of gene expression, is the study of changes in genetic expression which are brought about in the absence of any change in the gene sequence. Epigenetic mechanisms include methylation of DNA, histone modification (e.g., acetylation/deacetylation), and micro-RNA (miRNA) expression. DNA methylation suppresses the expression of a given gene due to the hydrophobic effect of the methyl groups. Further to this, cancer cells can express irregular hypo- and/or hypermethylation of DNA. For example, abnormal hypermethylation may turn off anticancer genes (e.g., tumor suppressor genes) whilst abnormal hypomethylation may turn on cancer-supporting genes (e.g., oncogenes) [52]. Acting as a modulator, curcumin has been found to restructure irregular DNA methylation patterns via demethylation. Since carcinogenesis has been linked to the irregular activity of enzymes histone acetyltransferases (HATs) and histone deacetylases (HDACs), which govern histone acetylation and deacetylation, respectively, molecules that inhibit HDACs have been a target for new cancer drug discovery. Interestingly, it has been suggested that curcumin restores balance in the activity of HDACs/HATs and it has been found to attenuate HATs/HDACs in a tissue-specific manner. Curcumin has also been found to boost p53 acetylation via its inhibition of HDAC1, resulting in tumor suppression and apoptosis. The expression of miRNA, which exerts epigenetic control of gene expression, is also modulated by curcumin according to the tissue and the nature of the imbalance. Over recent decades, there have been some successful anticancer drugs designed based on epigenetic principles and there is a body of research emerging noting that phytonutrients work at this level [52, 53].

3.4 Curcumin and metabolic disease

The antilipidemic effect of curcumin has been examined via studies of its effect on non-alcoholic fatty liver disease (NAFLD). A randomized placebo-controlled clinical trial was conducted on 50 patients diagnosed with NAFLD where they compared the effect of lifestyle modification vs. curcumin supplementation only. The results showed that curcumin supplementation significantly decreased hepatic fibrosis ($p > 0.001$) and NF-kB ($p > 0.05$) [54]. Further to this, a 2022 systemic review and meta-analysis of over 20 years of controlled trials were conducted, which concluded that curcumin significantly improved NAFLD severity ($P = 0.02$), demonstrated liver steatosis improvement ($p = 0.004$), and improved liver function as evidenced by the significant reduction in AST and ALT ($p < 0.001$). Furthermore, the BMI and total serum cholesterol were also significantly reduced ($p = 0.004$ and $p = 0.04$, respectively) with curcumin supplementation [55].

In addition to its antilipidemic effect, curcumin has been found to have an antidiabetic effect. This is evidenced by studies commenced with DMII patients, who commonly present with insulin resistance and poor glucose management which was found to be improved by curcumin supplementation [56, 57]. For example, a 2021 systemic review exploring the effect of various curcumin supplementation formulations on DMII concluded that curcumin should be considered as a therapeutic for DMII because it was found to significantly suppress oxidative stress, the inflammatory process whilst significantly reducing BMI, blood glucose concentration (fasting), and glycated hemoglobin (Hb-A1c) [56]. Moreover, a systemic review and meta-analysis of randomized controlled trials reported similar findings for the amelioration of DMII parameters via curcumin supplementation. In this study, the homeostasis model assessment insulin-resistance (HOMA-IR), Hb-A1c, triglycerides (TG), and total cholesterol (TC) values were gathered, and the findings indicated that HOMA-IR values were significantly lower than those of the control in Middle Eastern and Asian subgroups ($p < 0.00001$ and $p = 0.02$, respectively). Additionally, Hb-A1c was significantly reduced ($p < 0.0001$) as were the TC and TG ($p = 0.006$ and $p = 0.01$, respectively, in the Asian subgroup) values [57].

3.5 Curcumin and neurodegenerative disorders

Further to this, curcumin has been assessed as a therapeutic for neurodegenerative conditions, which have a complex array of contributing factors such as oxidative stress, neuroinflammation, and damage to neurons as key features of their pathogenesis [58]. Additionally, curcumin has been reported to aid in the prevention and slowing of the progression of neurodegenerative diseases by way of the modulation of significant biochemical pathways that reduce oxidative stress and neuroinflammation [58–60]. For example, curcumin has been reported to reduce the progression of Alzheimer's disease (AD) by inhibiting the formation of amyloid beta peptide (Aβ) (murine model), which forms plaques. It has been proposed that curcumin interferes with the pathogenesis of AD via the downregulation of BACE1, which executes the aberrant cleavage of amyloid precursor peptide (APP), which forms insoluble and therefore aggregation-sensitive Aβ monomers that contribute to the formation of plaques [59]. Interestingly, curcumin supplementation applied to murine models of Parkinson's disease (induction via rotenone treatment) demonstrated improvement via the reduction in Lewy bodies. It is also worth noting that curcumin is being considered as a potential mitigator of multiple sclerosis, a neuroinflammatory demyelinating autoimmune disease affecting young people. *In vitro* studies pre-treating human astrocytes (U375-MG cell line) with LPS found that curcumin significantly reduced the release of pro-inflammatory cytokine IL-6 and inhibited the activity of destructive proteolytic enzyme MMP-9, which has been found to be involved in the breakdown of the blood-brain barrier [61].

3.6 Curcumin and autoimmune disease

The current conventional pharmacological interventions for the mitigation of autoimmune conditions, such as rheumatoid arthritis (RA), include a lot of deleterious side effects. Fortunately, with the intention of finding less-toxic approaches, curcumin has been explored as a treatment with reports of improvement. For example, a systematic meta-analysis from 2023 examining the effects of oral curcumin supplementation on RA reported that curcumin supplementation significantly reduced erythrocyte sedimentation rate (ESR), C-reactive protein (CRP), disease activity scale (DAS), rheumatoid factor (RF), visual analogue scale (VAS), tender joint counts (TJC), and swollen joint counts (SJC) in RA patients [62].

Moreover, curcumin has shown some promise as a treatment for the autoimmune disease, systemic lupus erythematosus (SLE). Although there are little data available regarding clinical trials, pre-clinical animal model studies have demonstrated promise. For example, a 2020 study employing an established induced SLE model in mice (i.e., NZBWF1 mice) examined the attenuation of autoimmunity and renal damage via the administration of an oral gavage (500 mg/Kg/day in corn oil) of curcumin over 14 days. The early treatment group started at 26 weeks old, and the later treatment group commenced at 32 weeks of age. The results demonstrated that SLE-curcumin-treated mice preserved lean body mass compared to the control group (NZBWF1 mice + corn oil only) at a temporal juncture where cachexia would have typically occurred (i.e., 32–34 weeks old). Additionally, the spleen mass, which was used as an index for immune activity, was significantly lower ($p > 0.0001$) in the early treatment group of SLE-curcumin-treated mice (i.e., commenced at 26 weeks old). Further to this, the SLE mice treated at 32 weeks old demonstrated a significant reduction in renal damage ($p = 0.05$) [63].

3.7 Curcumin and pulmonary disease

Chronic obstructive pulmonary disease (COPD), such as emphysema, or chronic bronchitis is a condition of chronic inflammation and tissue damage deleteriously affecting lung function. Interestingly, a 2022 systemic review on the effects of curcumin on COPD concluded that although there was a shortage of randomized clinical trials available, according to the nine included articles examined, curcumin could exert anti-inflammatory actions within the pulmonary tissues and was reported to impede the thickening of alveolar tissue and prevent complications leading to local ischemia from lack of blood supply to tissues [64].

3.8 Curcumin and adverse pregnancy outcomes

Additionally, adverse pregnancy outcomes like preterm births, gestational diabetes, and low birth weight have been linked to poor oral health due to the dissemination of pathogenic bacteria and/or their destructive virulence factors through the maternal bloodstream to the placental tissues. Curcumin has been reported to prevent and improve the incidence of negative pregnancy outcomes [65–67]. A review in *Antioxidants* which examined a collection of *in vitro* (mostly animal) and *in vivo* (animal) studies assessing the viability of curcumin as a supplement to reduce adverse pregnancy outcomes was conducted in 2021. The study reported that curcumin supplementation beneficially modulated key biochemical aspects of the pathogenesis of common adverse pregnancy outcomes such as gestational diabetes, preterm births, preeclampsia, teratogenicity, and slow fetal growth restriction [67].

4. Pharmacological action of trans-resveratrol

Trans-resveratrol, trans-3,5,4′-trihydroxystilbene, is the bioactive isomer of the polyphenolic bioactive molecule found in many plants which is popularly known to be sourced from red grape skins, but its richest source is from the rhizome of the Japanese knotweed (*Polygonum cuspidatum*) [68, 69]. Additionally, it is the trans-isomer that has been found to possess bioactivity and therefore trans-resveratrol has been the focus of resveratrol studies. Trans-resveratrol has been extensively studied for its cardioprotective, neuroprotective, hepatoprotective, antitumorigenic, anti-oxidant, anti-inflammatory, immunomodulatory, and beneficial metabolic effects. Trans-resveratrol has been found to modulate deregulated inflammation via the attenuation of the arachidonic acid (AA), NF-kB, MAPK, and activator protein-1 (AP-1) signaling pathways. It has been suggested that the mechanism through which trans-resveratrol exerts its anti-inflammatory action via the AA pathway is by inhibiting cyclooxygenase enzymes, COX-1 and COX-2. Further to this, the mechanism of action of trans-resveratrol as an antioxidant is executed via the direct scavenging of free radicals and the inhibition of the production of free radicals. For example, in vitro studies have shown that trans-resveratrol scavenges superoxide, hydroxyl free radical, hydrogen peroxide, and peroxynitrite. Additionally, trans-resveratrol exerts antioxidant action by way of upregulating antioxidant enzymes such as superoxide dismutase (SOD), glutathione peroxidase, and the antioxidant glutathione [68–70]. **Figure 2** shows the molecular structure of trans-resveratrol and a photograph of *Polygonum cuspidatum* (Japanese knotweed).

4.1 Trans-resveratrol and periodontitis

Trans-resveratrol has been investigated as a viable treatment for periodontitis due to its ability to attenuate deregulated inflammation, reduce free radical damage, and support the regeneration of tissues [71–75]. For example, there are several pre-clinical reports using the ligature-induced periodontitis animal model that demonstrated the decrease in the expression of pro-inflammatory cytokines such as IL-1β, TNF-α, IL-6, IL-8, interferon-gamma (IFN-ϒ), and IL-17, with the concomitant increase in anti-inflammatory cytokines such as IL-4 in the periodontal tissue [71–73]. Further to this, it was also reported through immunobinding assays, the reduction in destructive proteases such as MMP-9, MMP-2, the decrease in both oxidative and nitrosive stress markers (e.g., dityrosine and NOx, respectively) in the local tissues [74]. Moreover, RT-PCR demonstrated an increase in the expression of antioxidants (e.g., SOD, SIRT1, and Nrf2) in the periodontal tissues, elucidating some of the mechanisms of the antioxidant action of trans-resveratrol [72, 74]. Furthermore, the observed decrease in NF-kB expression, which is accompanied by an increase in the expression of AMPK, has given rise to further information about the mechanism of anti-inflammatory action [72]. Animal model studies also consistently found that trans-resveratrol significantly reduced alveolar bone loss, as indicated by morphometric analysis and Micro-CT [73, 74]. Interestingly, a 2023 *in vitro* study employing human gingival-derived mesenchymal stem cells (hGMSCs) from periodontitis patients, which incubated the cells for 12 hours in medium with or without trans-resveratrol, and qRT-PCR showed that the experimental group had a significantly lower expression of the NF-kB gene. Additionally, trans-resveratrol was found to increase the proliferation of the hGMSCs, showing its restorative action [75].

4.2 Trans-resveratrol and cardiovascular disease

The pathophysiological process of cardiovascular diseases such as myocardial infarction, hypertension [76, 77], atherosclerosis [77], and congestive heart failure [78] involves oxidative stress as well as cardiac remodeling [76]. The cardioprotective mechanism of trans-resveratrol involves the activation of signaling pathways that support the metabolism and repair of cardiomyocytes, optimizing endothelial function and inhibiting cardiac remodeling [77]. Furthermore, it has been suggested that the anti-atherosclerotic action of trans-resveratrol may be executed via its downregulation of PI3K/Akt/mTOR signaling pathways, which prevents the overproduction of endothelial cells, a key feature of the pathogenesis of atherosclerosis [79]. Moreover, trans-resveratrol may attenuate cardiac fibrosis (seen in post-MI patients) by way of the inhibition of TGF-β/Smad pathways and alleviate oxidative stress via the activation of Nrf2 signaling pathway which inhibits the pro-oxidant enzyme NADPH oxidase whilst activating antioxidant enzymes [80, 81].

4.3 Trans-resveratrol and cancer

There have been thousands of pre-clinical studies reporting on the anticancer effects of trans-resveratrol and the body of evidence has demonstrated that its mechanism of antitumorigenic action is pleotropic. That is, trans-resveratrol has been found to be a useful cancer therapeutic for many cancers (e.g., breast, colon, prostate, and multiple myeloma) due to its action on many modes of carcinogenesis including, metastasis, invasion, migration, and angiogenesis [82–85]. Moreover, when combined with other therapeutics, trans-resveratrol demonstrates chemosensitization of resistant tumor cells as well as the protection of healthy cells from the cytotoxic damage of conventional chemotherapy [86]. Trans-resveratrol blocks cancer proliferation by the downregulation of β-catenin expression and executes the inhibition of its transport into the nucleus by interfering with the long non-coding RNA metastasis-associated lung adenocarcinoma transcript-1 (MALAT1) [87]. Additional anti-proliferative action by trans-resveratrol is carried out via its inhibition of transcription factor Snail, inhibition of TGF-β/Smad-stimulated epithelial-mesenchymal transition, the decrease of the expression of (kappa B kinase0) Ikk-induced transforming growth factor-beta (TGF-β), and the downregulation of NF-kB [82, 88]. Further to this, the invasion has been found to be inhibited by trans-resveratrol by way of the inhibition of p-PI3K/p-AKT-mediated (forkhead box-03) FOXO3a nuclear accumulation as well as the inhibition of proto-oncogene tyrosine-protein kinase (Src)-STAT3 phosphorylation and the induction of cancer cell apoptosis [82, 89]. Trans-resveratrol also inhibits AKT/MAPK-induced hypoxia-inducible factor 1-alpha (HIF-1α) activity whilst increasing the degradation rate of HIF-1α protein, inhibiting angiogenesis [82, 90].

4.4 Trans-resveratrol and metabolic disease

Studies investigating the effect of trans-resveratrol supplementation on the management of the systemic metabolic disorder, DMII, which increases the risk for other conditions such as periodontitis [91], heart disease [92], neuropathy [93], hepatic steatosis [94], and obesity [95], have shown that trans-resveratrol has a beneficial effect [91]. For example, a randomized, double-blinded placebo-controlled clinical trial from 2022 reported that 24 days of supplementation with trans-resveratrol (200 mg/day), as an adjunct to hypoglycemics medication, significantly reduced diabetic parameters, fasting plasma glucose, HOMA-IR, TNF-α, IL-6, highly-sensitive c-reactive protein (hs-CRP), Hb1c, and malondialdehyde (MDA), compared to placebo [96]. In 2024, a randomized controlled clinical trial (NCT05172947) explored the effect of 90 days of trans-resveratrol supplementation (500 mg/day) with or without pharmaceutical care on diabetic neuropathy. It was found that the group that received trans-resveratrol with pharmaceutical care demonstrated a significant decrease in hyperglycemia, Doleur Neuropathique 4 (DN4), and Michigan Neuropathy Screening Instrument (MNSI) questionnaire scores. Further to this, the electroneurographic parameters of the trans-resveratrol with pharmaceutical care were significantly improved, identifying trans-resveratrol as a viable adjunct therapy for the amelioration of diabetic neuropathy [97]. Another randomized clinical trial conducted in 2023 (ISRCTN15172592) examined the effect of 6 months of either 1000 mg/day or 500 mg/day of trans-resveratrol supplementation on molecular and oxidative stress markers and SIRT-1 in 124 DMII patients. The study found the most significant increase in antioxidant capacity, antioxidant gap, percentage of subjects without oxidative stress, and SIRT-1, in the 1000 mg/day group ($P < 0.05$) [98].

4.5 Trans-resveratrol and neurodegenerative disease

Alzheimer's Disease (AD) is characterized by the aggregation of amyloid-beta (Aβ) peptides and phosphorylated tau protein, oxidative stress, and inflammation in the CNS. The blood brain barrier is breached in AD patients, which allows for the infiltration of unwanted proteins. Many studies have reported that trans-resveratrol exhibits neuroprotective, anti-inflammatory activity as well as the inhibition of neurodegeneration and support of neurogenesis in AD patients [99]. Moreover, trans-resveratrol has also been found to inhibit the accumulation of Aβ peptides, making it a promising therapeutic for AD. For example, a randomized double-blind clinical trial (CTR20151780X) on patients with mild to moderate AD, which was conducted in 2021, examined the effect over 52 weeks of oral supplementation with 500 mg/day of trans-resveratrol. Interestingly, the investigators found a 46% reduction ($p = 0.033$) in MMP-9 in the CSF, which suggests that trans-resveratrol may be effective in maintaining the integrity of the BBB in AD patients [100].

4.6 Trans-resveratrol and autoimmune disease

The autoimmune disease, rheumatoid arthritis (RA) is a chronic inflammatory condition presenting with synovitis, formation of a pannus, destruction of bone, and the deformation and loss of function of the involved joints [101, 102]. Trans-resveratrol may mitigate cartilage destruction in RA via the activation of SIRT1 resulting in the downregulation of NF-kB, MMP-1, and MMP-13, leading to the reduction of pro-inflammatory cytokines. Moreover, since trans-resveratrol has been found to trigger apoptosis in deregulated and destructive fibroblast-like synovial cells, it may be effective in the alleviation of synovitis [102].

4.7 Trans-resveratrol and pulmonary disease

Chronic obstructive pulmonary disease (COPD), such as chronic bronchitis and emphysema, is a progressive disease presenting with compromised lung structure and function, which is often accompanied by extrapulmonary complications [103]. The oxidative stress and systemic inflammation seen in COPD are partly governed by NF-kB, which provides insight into possible drug targets [103, 104]. Moreover, there have been studies using experimental models that have consistently reported the mitigation of oxidative stress and inflammation in pulmonary tissue following treatment with trans-resveratrol, which exerts anti-inflammatory via the downregulation of NF-kB, SIRT1 activation [105–107]. Further to this, the cardioprotective and metabolic optimization features of trans-resveratrol are also of interest, since COPD patients frequently present with extrapulmonary conditions such as cardiovascular disease and cachexia. Fortunately, trans-resveratrol activates AMPK, which in turn activates SIRT1, which may promote mitochondrial biogenesis and function in the muscular and pulmonary tissues of COPD patients. Additionally, trans-resveratrol activates Nrf2, which ultimately results in a decrease in pro-inflammatory cytokines, an increase in antioxidant enzymes, and the inhibition of oxidative stress in the pulmonary tissues. Trans-resveratrol is a promising candidate for the treatment of COPD due to its ability to diminish damage to the lungs whilst enhancing the mitochondrial activity in skeletal muscle. However, further human studies must be conducted to confirm the dosage and duration of treatment [105].

4.8 Trans-resveratrol and adverse pregnancy outcomes

Some common adverse pregnancy outcomes include preeclampsia, gestational diabetes, restricted foetal growth, and preterm birth [108, 109]. The effect of trans-resveratrol supplementation on oxidative stress inflammation and other metabolic deregulation associated with common adverse pregnancy outcomes has been examined extensively using animal models [110–113]. Trans-resveratrol was reported to inhibit DNA damage, activate antioxidant enzymes, and modulate intracellular redox signaling. Further to this, trans-resveratrol crosses the placental barrier providing antioxidant action to the fetus and placenta [114]. Overall, research indicates that trans-resveratrol has a positive effect on the mother and fetus and has been reported as safe. However, further studies are required to ensure safety as some reports expressed concerns of toxicity at high doses [114].

5. Curcumin and trans-resveratrol: improving drug profiles

There have been thousands of papers published on the therapeutic potential of curcumin and trans-resveratrol over a few decades, including many pre-clinical trials. However, the reports have been inconsistent as both polyphenols have tissue-specific effects which combined with their biphasic dose response increase the complexity involved in dosing for specific ailments [11, 115].

Additionally, in crude form, both curcumin and trans-resveratrol demonstrate low water solubility, poor bioavailability, rapid metabolism, and clearance [11, 115–117]. Further to this, trans-resveratrol is also photosensitive and stable within a narrow optimal pH range (pH 6–8), making stability an issue. The disappointing pharmacological profile of trans-resveratrol and curcumin has motivated researchers to harness their potential by finding novel ways to improve the pharmacokinetics/dynamics of both molecules to unlock their potential as viable therapeutics [117].

One natural way to improve the pharmacological profile of curcumin and trans-resveratrol is via combinations that encourage synergy. For example, trans-resveratrol and curcumin have been found to have a synergistic effect when combined with each other [118–120]. Further to this, curcumin has been found to be synergistic when combined with the polyphenol, piperine, a combination already existing in Indian cuisine and traditional medicine (i.e., turmeric and pepper) [121].

One of the most significant areas that has led researchers to more potentized curcumin and trans-resveratrol involves the integration of nanotechnology. Nanotechnology entails the exploitation of the unique properties of matter at the nanoscale (i.e., one nanometer (nm) is 1×10^{-9} m). A nanomaterial is defined as any material with at least one dimension that is 100 nm or less [122].

5.1 Nano-formulations of curcumin and trans-resveratrol

There are many ways that a drug delivery system can be engineered using nanotechnology and many nanotechnology-enhanced formulas have been reported to improve the drug profile of hydrophobic therapeutics, including both curcumin and trans-resveratrol [123, 124]. For example, orally administered nano-enhanced formulas of curcumin have demonstrated a 60-fold increase in bioavailability in animal models [125].

However, there are many different nano-formulation types, each engineered to enhance therapeutic action. For example, liposomes, which are phospholipid-derived vesicles resembling the cell membrane, have many benefits including high stability, biocompatibility, biodegradability as well as low toxicity [13, 126]. Moreover, liposomal curcumin has been reported to have potent anticancer activity *in vitro* and *in vivo*. For example, a study on PC-3 human prostate cancer cells concluded that cell survival was much lower compared to curcumin in its crude form [127].

Nanoparticles (NPs), which are 1–100 nm in size, represent another viable nano-formulation for the enhancement of the activity of curcumin [13]. For example, curcumin solid lipid nanoparticles (CURC-SLN) were found to display greater stability and dispersibility whilst activating greater apoptosis in adenocarcinoma breast cancer cells (MDA-MB-231 cell line) *in vitro* compared to crude curcumin [128]. Nanoparticles can be configured in a myriad of ways, as evidenced by the *in vivo* animal model (xenograft) study on the effect of human serum albumin nanoparticles loaded with curcumin (CURC-HSA-NPs) on antitumor activity. The study showed that the CURC-HSA-NPs demonstrated higher antitumor action than crude curcumin [129]. Another NP type includes the formation of conjugates via chemical bonding. Interestingly, a study using an NP conjugate of PVP, gold, and curcumin (PVP-CURC-Au) presented with high bioavailability and loading efficiency and was found to prevent the formation of amyloid beta protein aggregates, making it a promising therapeutic for the treatment and prevention of AD [130].

Some nano-formulations can be engineered to assemble once in the body. For example, the application of specific surfactant-oil-co-surfactant ratios can produce self-nanoemulsifying drug delivery systems (SNEDDS) loaded with the hydrophobic phytochemical. Since SNEDDS are engineered to spontaneously emulsify into easily absorbable nanoparticles once they enter the body, they have been found to enhance the bioavailability of the therapeutic agent whilst decreasing its clearance. Both curcumin and trans-resveratrol have been designed as SNEDDS with successful enhancement of their bioavailability [131, 132].

Polymeric nanoparticles (PNPs) are polymer-coated nanocarriers that have been used to assess the effect of enhanced curcumin on the experimental autoimmune encephalomyelitis (EAE) murine model, 12.5 mg/Kg nano-curcumin polymer had a significant effect on myelin repair [133].

Dendrimers, which are complex, extensively branched polymeric nanospheres with special properties, are designed to target specific tissues and have been found to increase stability and render resveratrol water-soluble resulting in its enhanced bioavailability [134].

Nanocarriers have also been designed using non-metallic inorganic materials such as mesoporous silica. A 2022 animal study employing a murine model and MGF-7 human breast cancer cells showed that resveratrol-loaded mesoporous silica nanoparticles (MSN-RES) were able to impede the progress of breast cancer development to a greater degree than crude Trans-resveratrol [135].

Cyclodextrin encapsulation is also an effective approach to nano-formulations that increase polyphenol stability and bioavailability. A 2021 study testing the biofilm attenuating effect of a pediatric oral spray containing hydroxypropyl-beta-cyclodextrin trans-resveratrol (RV-HPβCD) reported a significant reduction after 2 weeks of treatment in clinical parameters (oral biofilm, bleeding gingiva, and salivary pH) [136].

Functional foods have been enriched, enhanced, fortified, and/or altered with the intention of optimizing their nutritional profile. Nanotechnology allows for the fortification of food phytonutrients like trans-resveratrol, which would normally breakdown during processing and lose bioactivity. Stable nano scaled powders of trans-resveratrol have been produced by encapsulating them with biological macromolecules like starch, casein, or chitin and nanoencapsulation allows for designing foods with desired qualities such as time-release [137].

6. Conclusion

From an ethnobotanical perspective, *Curcumin longa* (Haldi in Ayurvedic medicine), which contains curcumin, and *Polygonum cuspidatum* (Hu Zhang in traditional Chinese medicine), which contains a substantial amount of resveratrol in its roots, have been used to treat many ailments for hundreds or in the case of Haldi, thousands of years [138, 139]. **Figure 3** depicts an overview of the actions of curcumin and trans-resveratrol. Regarding conventional medicine, several studies have shown that the polyphenols curcumin and resveratrol have the potential to improve the quality of life for many humans via the prevention, management, and/or treatment of a myriad of conditions that are mediated by chronic inflammation, immune deregulation, and tissue destruction. Unfortunately, there has been a delay in their clinical application due to the inconsistency in results which has in part been attributed to the complexity of their biphasic pharmacokinetics and tissue-specific actions, making dosing difficult, as well as their extensively reported low bioavailability, rapid metabolism, and rapid clearance in crude form. Fortunately, recent advances in nanotechnology indicate that the poor clinical translation of many promising *in vitro* and pre-clinical studies exploring the efficacy of these polyphenols in their crude form, may indeed be an idea from the past. With the application of nanotechnology, which offers the opportunity for seemingly endless designs, an array of new safe and effective precise medicines could emerge on the market. However, since nano-formulations alter the pharmacokinetics and pharmacodynamics of these molecules, a standard posology needs to be established for each design to ensure their safety and efficacy.

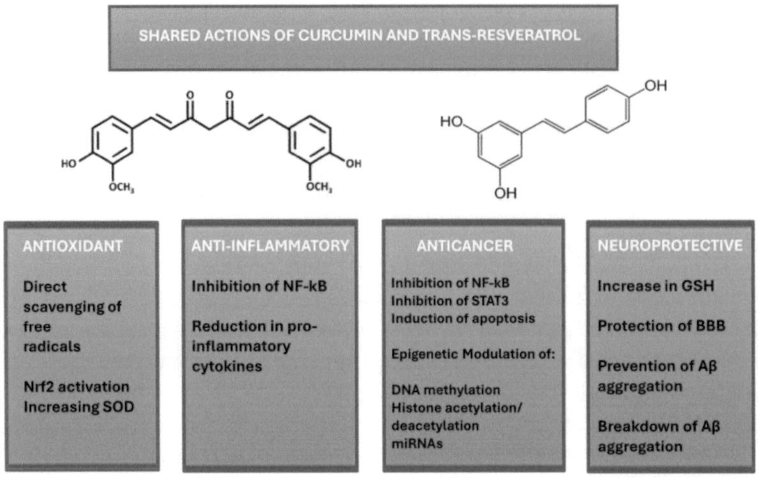

Figure 3.
A general overview of action shared by curcumin and trans-resveratrol.

Author details

Tracey Lynn Harney
Bermuda College, Paget, Bermuda

*Address all correspondence to: tharney@college.bm

References

[1] de Almeida Roediger M et al. Inflammation and quality of life in later life: Findings from the health, well-being and aging study (SABE). Health and Quality of Life Outcomes. 2019;**17**(1):1-7. DOI: 10.1186/s12955-019-1092-2

[2] Holmstrup P et al. Comorbidity of periodontal disease: Two sides of the same coin? An introduction for the clinician. Journal of Oral Microbiology. 2017;**9**(1):1332710. DOI: 10.1080/20002297.2017.1332710

[3] Teles F et al. Viruses, periodontitis, and comorbidities. Periodontology 2000. 2022;**89**(1):190-206. DOI: 10.1111/prd.12435

[4] Hobbins S et al. Is periodontitis a comorbidity of COPD or can associations be explained by shared risk factors/behaviors? International Journal of Chronic Obstructive Pulmonary Disease. 2017;**12**:1339-1349. DOI: 10.2147/copd.s127802

[5] Hajishengallis G, Chavakis T. Local and systemic mechanisms linking periodontal disease and inflammatory comorbidities. Nature Reviews Immunology. 2021;**21**(7):426-440. DOI: 10.1038/s41577-020-00488-6

[6] Soares CL et al. Biochemical aspects of the inflammatory process: A narrative review. Biomedicine & Pharmacotherapy. 2023;**168**:115764. DOI: 10.1016/j.biopha.2023.115764

[7] Nisar A et al. Phytochemicals in the treatment of inflammation-associated diseases: The journey from preclinical trials to clinical practice. Frontiers in Pharmacology. 2023;**14**:1-25. DOI: 10.3389/fphar.2023.1177050

[8] Huang X et al. Brief literature review and comprehensive bioinformatics analytics unravel the potential mechanism of curcumin in the treatment of periodontitis. BMC Oral Health. 2023;**23**(1):1-13. DOI: 10.1186/s12903-023-03181-x

[9] Solomon SM et al. Curcumin as a natural approach of periodontal adjunctive treatment and its immunological implications: A narrative review. Pharmaceutics. 2022;**14**(5):982. DOI: 10.3390/pharmaceutics14050982

[10] Nikniaz S, Vaziri F, Mansouri R. Impact of resveratrol supplementation on clinical parameters and inflammatory markers in patients with chronic periodontitis: A randomized clinical trail. BMC Oral Health. 2023;**23**(1):1-7. DOI: 10.1186/s12903-023-02877-4

[11] Nelson KM et al. The essential medicinal chemistry of curcumin. Journal of Medicinal Chemistry. 2017;**60**(5):1620-1637. DOI: 10.1021/acs.jmedchem.6b00975

[12] Almeida L et al. Pharmacokinetic and safety profile of *trans*-resveratrol in a rising multiple-dose study in healthy volunteers. Molecular Nutrition & Food Research. 2009;**53**(S1):S7-S15. DOI: 10.1002/mnfr.200800177

[13] Karthikeyan A, Senthil N, Min T. Nanocurcumin: A promising candidate for therapeutic applications. Frontiers in Pharmacology. 2020;**11**:1-24. DOI: 10.3389/fphar.2020.00487

[14] Robinson K, Mock C, Liang D. Pre-formulation studies of resveratrol. Drug Development and Industrial Pharmacy. 2014;**41**(9):1464-1469. DOI: 10.3109/03639045.2014.958753

[15] Bohara RA et al. Recent overview of Resveratrol's beneficial effects and its nano-delivery systems. Molecules. 2022;**27**(16):5154. DOI: 10.3390/molecules27165154

[16] Jodynis-Liebert J, Kujawska M. Biphasic dose-response induced by phytochemicals: Experimental evidence. Journal of Clinical Medicine. 2020;**9**(3): 1-28. Available from: https://www.ncbi.nlm.nih.gov/pmc/articles/PMC7141213/

[17] Calabrese EJ. Should hormesis be the default model in risk assessment? Human & Experimental Toxicology. 2005;**24**(5):243. DOI: 10.1191/0960327105ht518ed

[18] Hajishengallis G, Chavakis T, Lambris JD. Current understanding of periodontal disease pathogenesis and targets for host-modulation therapy. Periodontology 2000. 2020;**84**(1):14-34. Available from: https://www.ncbi.nlm.nih.gov/pmc/articles/PMC7457922/

[19] Abdulkareem AA, Al-Taweel FBH, Al-Sharqi AJ, Gul SS, Sha AM, Chapple C. Current concepts in the pathogenesis of periodontitis: From symbiosis to dysbiosis. Journal of Oral Microbiology. 2023;**15**(1):1-19

[20] Salvi GE, Roccuzzo A, Imber J, Stähli A, Klinge B, Lang NP. Clinical periodontal diagnosis. Periodontology 2000. 2023:1-19. DOI: 10.1111/prd.12487

[21] Bhanji S, Williams B, Sheller B, Elwood T, Mancl L. Transient bacteremia induced by toothbrushing a comparison of the sonicare toothbrush with a conventional toothbrush. PubMed. 2002;**24**(4):295-299

[22] Maharaj B, Coovadia Y, Vayej AC. An investigation of the frequency of bacteraemia following dental extraction, tooth brushing and chewing. Cardiovascular Journal of Africa. 2012;**23**(6):340-344

[23] Yucel-Lindberg T, Båge T. Inflammatory mediators in the pathogenesis of periodontitis. Expert Reviews in Molecular Medicine. 2013;**15**:1-22

[24] Madi M, Abuohashish HM, Attia D, AlQahtani N, Alrayes N, Pavlic V, et al. Association between periodontal disease and comorbidities in Saudi's Eastern Province. BioMed Research International. 2021;**2021**:1-9

[25] Păunică I, Giurgiu M, Dumitriu AS, Păunică S, Pantea Stoian AM, Martu MA, et al. The bidirectional relationship between periodontal disease and diabetes mellitus—A review. Diagnostics. 2023;**13**(4):681

[26] Barutta F, Bellini S, Durazzo M, Gruden G. Novel insight into the mechanisms of the bidirectional relationship between diabetes and periodontitis. Biomedicine. 2022;**10**(1):178

[27] Okamura H, Hirota K, Yoshida K, Weng Y, He Y, Shiotsu N, et al. Outer membrane vesicles of *Porphyromonas gingivalis*: Novel communication tool and strategy. Japanese Dental Science Review. 2021;**57**:138-146. Available from: https://www.sciencedirect.com/science/article/pii/S1882761621000168 [Accessed: August 28, 2022]

[28] Ryder MI. The link between periodontitis and Alzheimer's disease: Reality or yet another association. Current Oral Health Reports. 2022;**9**:157-166. DOI: 10.1007/s40496-022-00319-8

[29] Czerniuk MR, Surma S, Romańczyk M, Nowak JM, Wojtowicz A, Filipiak KJ. Unexpected relationships: Periodontal diseases:

Atherosclerosis–plaque destabilization? From the teeth to a coronary event. Biology. 2022;**11**(2):272. Available from: https://www.ncbi.nlm.nih.gov/pmc/articles/PMC8869674/#:~:text=Observational%20studies%20found%20that%20patients

[30] Zepeda-Rivera M, Minot SS, Bouzek H, Wu H, Blanco-Míguez A, Manghi P, et al. A distinct Fusobacterium nucleatum clade dominates the colorectal cancer niche. Nature. 2024;**628**:1-9. Available from: https://www.nature.com/articles/s41586-024-07182-w

[31] Martínez-García M, Hernández-Lemus E. Periodontal inflammation and systemic diseases: An overview. Frontiers in Physiology. 2021;**12**:709438. Available from: https://www.ncbi.nlm.nih.gov/pmc/articles/PMC8578868/

[32] Ramanauskaite E, Machiulskiene V. Antiseptics as adjuncts to scaling and root planing in the treatment of periodontitis: A systematic literature review. BMC Oral Health. 2020;**20**(1):1-19

[33] Golub LM, Lee H. Periodontal therapeutics: Current host-modulation agents and future directions. Periodontology 2000. 2019;**82**(1):186-204

[34] Ganesh PR, Karthikeyan R, Malathi K. Perio-scopy: A new paradigm in periodontal therapy. International Journal of Dental and Medical Research. 2015;**1**(6):168-171

[35] Kwan JY. Enhanced periodontal debridement with the use of micro ultrasonic, periodontal endoscopy. Journal of the California Dental Association. 2005;**33**(3):241-248

[36] Ribeiro FV, Mehta JJ, Monteiro MF, Moore J, Casati MZ, Nibali L. Minimal invasiveness in nonsurgical periodontal therapy. Periodontology 2000. 2023;**91**(1):1-13

[37] Mahajan A, Chandel N, Asi KS, Walhe MS. Managing periodontitis with host modulation therapy: Current concept and future perspective. Dental Journal of Advance Studies. 2024;**12**(1):29-33

[38] Attia MS, Alblowi JA. Effect of subantimicrobial dose doxycycline treatment on gingival crevicular fluid levels of MMP-9 and MMP-13 in periodontitis stage 2, grade B in subjects with type 2 diabetes mellitus. Journal of Immunology Research. 2020;**2020**:1-8

[39] Fu YS, Chen TH, Weng L, Huang L, Lai D, Weng CF. Pharmacological properties and underlying mechanisms of curcumin and prospects in medicinal potential. Biomedicine & Pharmacotherapy. 2021;**141**:111888

[40] Ahsan R, Arshad M, Khushtar M, Ahmad MA, Muazzam M, Akhter MS, et al. A comprehensive review on physiological effects of curcumin. Drug Research. 2020;**70**(10):441-447

[41] Al-Kattan R. The role of curcumin in periodontal therapy: An update. Functional Foods in Health and Disease. 2024;**14**(5):290-298. DOI: 10.31989/ffhd.v14i5.1327

[42] Zeng L, Yang T, Yang K, Yu G, Li J, Xiang W, et al. Curcumin and Curcuma longa extract in the treatment of 10 types of autoimmune diseases: A systematic review and meta-analysis of 31 randomized controlled trials. Frontiers in Immunology. 2022;**13**:896476. Available from: https://www.ncbi.nlm.nih.gov/pmc/articles/PMC9376628/

[43] Mohammad CA, Ali KM, Al-Rawi RAR, Gul SS. Effects of

curcumin and tetracycline gel on experimental induced periodontitis as an anti-inflammatory, osteogenesis promoter and enhanced bone density through altered iron levels: Histopathological study. Antibiotics. 2022;**11**(4):521-521

[44] Kumbar V, Peram MR, Kugaji M, Shah T, Patil SP, Muddapur UM, et al. Effect of curcumin on growth, biofilm formation and virulence factor gene expression of *Porphyromonas gingivalis*. Odontology. 2020;**109**(1):18-28

[45] Hugar SS, Patil S, Metgud R, Nanjwade B, Hugar SM. Influence of application of chlorhexidine gel and curcumin gel as an adjunct to scaling and root planing: A interventional study. Journal of Natural Science, Biology, and Medicine. 2016;**7**(2):149-149

[46] Cox FF, Misiou A, Vierkant A, Ale-Agha N, Grandoch M, Haendeler J, et al. Protective effects of curcumin in cardiovascular diseases—Impact on oxidative stress and mitochondria. Cells. 2022;**11**(3):342

[47] Yang C, Zhu Q, Chen Y, Ji K, Li S, Wu Q, et al. Review of the protective mechanism of curcumin on cardiovascular disease. Drug Design Development and Therapy. 2024;**18**:165-192

[48] Pourbagher-Shahri AM, Farkhondeh T, Ashrafizadeh M, Talebi M, Samargahndian S. Curcumin and cardiovascular diseases: Focus on cellular targets and cascades. Biomedicine & Pharmacotherapy. 2021;**136**:111214

[49] Salehi B, Del Prado-Audelo ML, Cortés H, Leyva-Gómez G, Stojanović-Radić Z, Singh YD, et al. Therapeutic applications of curcumin nanomedicine formulations in cardiovascular diseases. Journal of Clinical Medicine. 2020;**9**(3): 746. Available from: https://www.mdpi.com/2077-0383/9/3/746/htm

[50] Hao M, Chu Y, Lei J, Yao Z, Wang P, Chen Z, et al. Pharmacological mechanisms and clinical applications of curcumin: Update. Aging and Disease. 2023;**14**(3):716-749. Available from: https://www.ncbi.nlm.nih.gov/pmc/articles/PMC10187702/

[51] Yang ZJ, Huang SY, Zhou DD, Xiong RG, Zhao CN, Fang AP, et al. Effects and mechanisms of curcumin for the prevention and management of cancers: An updated review. Antioxidants. 2022;**11**(8):1481

[52] Hassan FU, Rehman MSU, Khan MS, Ali MA, Javed A, Nawaz A, et al. Curcumin as an alternative epigenetic modulator: Mechanism of action and potential effects. Frontiers in Genetics. 2019;**10**:514. Available from: https://www.ncbi.nlm.nih.gov/pubmed/31214247

[53] Ming T, Tao Q, Tang S, Zhao H, Yang H, Liu M, et al. Curcumin: An epigenetic regulator and its application in cancer. Biomedicine & Pharmacotherapy. 2022;**156**:113956. Available from: https://www.sciencedirect.com/science/article/pii/S0753332222013452?via%3Dihub

[54] Ngu MH, Norhayati MN, Rosnani Z, Zulkifli MM. Curcumin as adjuvant treatment in patients with non-alcoholic fatty liver (NAFLD) disease: A systematic review and meta-analysis. Complementary Therapies in Medicine. 2022;**68**:102843

[55] Marton LT, Pescinini-e-Salzedas LM, Camargo MEC, Barbalho SM, dos Santos Haber JF, Sinatora RV, et al. The effects of curcumin on diabetes mellitus: A systematic review. Frontiers in Endocrinology. 2021;**12**:1-12

[56] Zhang T, He Q, Liu Y, Chen Z, Hu H. Efficacy and safety of curcumin supplement on improvement of insulin resistance in people with type 2 diabetes mellitus: A systematic review and meta-analysis of randomized controlled trials. Evidence-Based Complementary and Alternative Medicine. 2021;**2021**:1-19

[57] Zeng Y, Luo Y, Wang L, Zhang K, Peng J, Zhang Y. Therapeutic effect of curcumin on metabolic diseases: Evidence from clinical studies. International Journal of Molecular Sciences. 2023;**24**(4):3323-3323. Available from: https://www.ncbi.nlm.nih.gov/pmc/articles/PMC9959718/

[58] Perales-Salinas V, Purushotham SS, Buskila Y. Curcumin as a potential therapeutic agent for treating neurodegenerative diseases. Neurochemistry International. 2024;**178**:105790

[59] Benameur T, Giacomucci G, Panaro MA, Ruggiero M, Trotta T, Monda V, et al. New promising therapeutic avenues of curcumin in brain diseases. Molecules. 2021;**27**(1):236

[60] Genchi G, Lauria G, Catalano A, Carocci A, Sinicropi MS. Neuroprotective effects of curcumin in neurodegenerative diseases. Food. 2024;**13**(11):1774-1774

[61] Cheng J, Zhou Y, Qiao H, Jiang H, Fan Y. Curcumin protects from LPS-induced activation of astrocytes via AMPK pathway. NeuroReport/Neuroreport. 2023;**34**(15):748-758

[62] Kou H, Huang L, Jin M, He Q, Zhang R, Ma J. Effect of curcumin on rheumatoid arthritis: A systematic review and meta-analysis. Frontiers in Immunology. 2023;**14**:1-11. Available from: https://www.ncbi.nlm.nih.gov/pmc/articles/PMC10264675/

[63] Dent EL, Taylor EB, Turbeville HR, Ryan MJ. Curcumin attenuates autoimmunity and renal injury in an experimental model of systemic lupus erythematosus. Physiological Reports. 2020;**8**(13):1-13. Available from: https://www.ncbi.nlm.nih.gov/pmc/articles/PMC7354090/ [Accessed: January 31, 2021]

[64] Safari S, Davoodi P, Soltani A, Fadavipour M, Rezaeian AR, Heydari F, et al. Curcumin effects on chronic obstructive pulmonary disease: A systematic review. Health Science Reports. 2023;**6**(3):1-9. Available from: https://www.ncbi.nlm.nih.gov/pmc/articles/PMC9987200

[65] Ghaneifar Z, Yousefi Z, Tajik F, Nikfar B, Ghalibafan F, Abdollahi E, et al. The potential therapeutic effects of curcumin on pregnancy complications: Novel insights into reproductive medicine. IUBMB Life. 2020;**72**(12):2572-2583

[66] Filardi T, Varì R, Ferretti E, Zicari A, Morano S, Santangelo C. Curcumin: Could this compound be useful in pregnancy and pregnancy-related complications? Nutrients. 2020;**12**(10):3179

[67] Tossetta G, Fantone S, Giannubilo SR, Marzioni D. The multifaced actions of curcumin in pregnancy outcome. Antioxidants. 2021;**10**(1):126

[68] Zhang LX, Li CX, Kakar MU, Khan MS, Wu PF, Amir RM, et al. Resveratrol (RV): A pharmacological review and call for further research. Biomedicine & Pharmacotherapy. 2021;**143**:112164. Available from: https://www.sciencedirect.com/science/article/pii/S0753332221009483

[69] Malviya V, Tawar M, Burange P, Jodh R. A brief review on resveratrol.

Asian Journal of Research in Pharmaceutical Sciences. 2022;**112**(2): 157-162

[70] Bejenaru LE, Biță A, Belu I, Segneanu AE, Radu A, Dumitru A, et al. Resveratrol: A review on the biological activity and applications. Applied Sciences. 2024;**14**(11):4534. Available from: https://www.mdpi.com/2076-3417/14/11/4534 [Accessed: June 13, 2024]

[71] Corrêa MG, Pires PR, Ribeiro FV, Pimentel SZ, Casarin RCV, Cirano FR, et al. Systemic treatment with resveratrol and/or curcumin reduces the progression of experimental periodontitis in rats. Journal of Periodontal Research. 2016;**52**(2):201-209. Available from: https://www.mountsinai.on.ca/care/dentistry/centre-for-advanced-dental-research-and-care/research/resveratrol-curumin2-corr-a-et-al-2016.pdf [Accessed: January 14, 2020]

[72] Tamaki N, Orihuela-Campos RC, Inagaki Y, Fukui M, Nagata T, Itô H. Resveratrol improves oxidative stress and prevents the progression of periodontitis via the activation of the Sirt1/AMPK and the Nrf2/antioxidant defense pathways in a rat periodontitis model. Free Radical Biology and Medicine. 2014;**75**:222-229

[73] Casati MZ, Algayer C, Cardoso da Cruz G, Ribeiro FV, Casarin RCV, Pimentel SP, et al. Resveratrol decreases periodontal breakdown and modulates local levels of cytokines during periodontitis in rats. Journal of Periodontology. 2013;**84**(10):e58-e64

[74] Bhattarai G, Poudel SB, Kook SH, Lee JC. Resveratrol prevents alveolar bone loss in an experimental rat model of periodontitis. Acta Biomaterialia. 2016;**29**:398-408

[75] Jiang H, Ni J, Hu L, Xiang Z, Zeng J, Shi J, et al. Resveratrol may reduce the degree of periodontitis by regulating ERK pathway in gingival-derived MSCs. International Journal of Molecular Sciences. 2023;**24**(14):11294-11294

[76] Izzo C, Vitillo P, Di Pietro P, Visco V, Strianese A, Virtuoso N, et al. The role of oxidative stress in cardiovascular aging and cardiovascular diseases. Life. 2021;**11**(1):60

[77] Fan S, Hu Y, You Y, Xue W, Chai R, Zhang X, et al. Role of resveratrol in inhibiting pathological cardiac remodeling. Frontiers in Pharmacology. 2022;**13**:1-19

[78] Hoseini A, Namazi G, Farrokhian A, Reiner Ž, Aghadavod E, Bahmani F, et al. The effects of resveratrol on metabolic status in patients with type 2 diabetes mellitus and coronary heart disease. Food & Function. 2019;**10**(9):6042-6051

[79] Ji W, Sun J, Hu Z, Sun B. Resveratrol protects against atherosclerosis by downregulating the PI3K/AKT/mTOR signaling pathway in atherosclerosis model mice. Experimental and Therapeutic Medicine. 2022;**23**(6):1-9

[80] Guo S, Zhou Y, Xie X. Resveratrol inhibiting TGF/ERK signaling pathway can improve atherosclerosis: Backgrounds, mechanisms and effects. Biomedicine & Pharmacotherapy. 2022;**155**:113775-113775

[81] Cheng CK, Luo J, Lau CW, Chen Z, Tian XY, Huang Y. Pharmacological basis and new insights of resveratrol action in the cardiovascular system. British Journal of Pharmacology. 2019;**177**(6):1258-1277

[82] Ren B, Kwah MXY, Liu C, Ma Z, Shanmugam MK, Ding L, et al. Resveratrol for cancer therapy: Challenges and future perspectives. Cancer Letters. 2021;**515**:63-72

[83] Song B, Wang W, Tang X, Goh RMWJ, Thuya WL, Ho PCL, et al. Inhibitory potential of resveratrol in cancer metastasis: From biology to therapy. Cancers. 2023;**15**(10):2758. Available from: https://www.mdpi.com/2072-6694/15/10/2758 [Accessed: June 11, 2023]

[84] Ko JH, Sethi G, Um JY, Shanmugam MK, Arfuso F, Kumar AP, et al. The role of resveratrol in cancer therapy. International Journal of Molecular Sciences. 2017;**18**(12):1-36. Available from: https://www.ncbi.nlm.nih.gov/pubmed/29194365

[85] Yuan L, Zhou M, Huang D, Wasan H, Zhang K, Sun L, et al. Resveratrol inhibits the invasion and metastasis of colon cancer through reversal of epithelial- mesenchymal transition via the AKT/GSK-3β/snail signalling pathway. Molecular Medicine Reports. 2019;**20**:2783-2795

[86] Cotino-Nájera S, Herrera LA, Domínguez-Gómez G, Díaz-Chávez J. Molecular mechanisms of resveratrol as chemo and radiosensitizer in cancer. Frontiers in Pharmacology. 2023;**14**:1-24

[87] Ji Q, Liu X, Fu X, Zhang L, Sui H, Zhou L, et al. Resveratrol inhibits invasion and metastasis of colorectal cancer cells via MALAT1 mediated Wnt/β-catenin signal pathway. PLoS One. 2013;**8**(11):e78700

[88] Ashrafizadeh M, Najafi M, Orouei S, Zabolian A, Saleki H, Azami N, et al. Resveratrol modulates transforming growth factor-Beta (TGF-β) signaling pathway for disease therapy: A new insight into its pharmacological activities. Biomedicines. 2020;**8**(8):261

[89] Jang JY, Im E, Kim ND. Mechanism of resveratrol-induced programmed cell death and new drug discovery against cancer: A review. International Journal of Molecular Sciences. 2022;**23**(22):13689. Available from: https://www.mdpi.com/1422-0067/23/22/13689

[90] Kamaleddin MA. The paradoxical pro- and antiangiogenic actions of resveratrol: Therapeutic applications in cancer and diabetes. Annals of the New York Academy of Sciences. 2016;**1386**(1):3-15

[91] Casanova L, Hughes FJ, Preshaw PM. Diabetes and periodontal disease. BDJ Team. 2015;**1**:1

[92] Leon BM, Maddox TM. Diabetes and cardiovascular disease: Epidemiology, biological mechanisms, treatment recommendations and future research. World Journal of Diabetes. 2015;**6**(13):1246. Available from: https://www.ncbi.nlm.nih.gov/pmc/articles/PMC4600176/

[93] Osmanlıoğlu HÖ, Nazıroğlu M. Resveratrol modulates diabetes-induced neuropathic pain, apoptosis, and oxidative neurotoxicity in mice through TRPV4 channel inhibition. Molecular Neurobiology. 2024;**61**:7269-7286

[94] Cusi K. Nonalcoholic fatty liver disease in diabetes: A call to action. Diabetes Spectrum. 2024;**37**(1):5-7

[95] Klein S, Gastaldelli A, Yki-Järvinen H, Scherer PE. Why does obesity cause diabetes? Cell Metabolism. 2022;**34**(1):11-20. Available from: https://www.ncbi.nlm.nih.gov/pmc/articles/PMC8740746/#:~:text=Obesity%2C%20particularly%20when%20associated%20with,resistance%20and%20%CE%B2%2Dcell%20dysfunction

[96] Mahjabeen W, Khan DA, Mirza SA. Role of resveratrol supplementation in regulation of glucose hemostasis, inflammation and oxidative stress in

patients with diabetes mellitus type 2: A randomized, placebo-controlled trial. Complementary Therapies in Medicine. 2022;**66**:102819

[97] Sabir G, Marouf BH, Namiq HS, Salih JM. Impact of resveratrol and pharmaceutical care on type 2 diabetes mellitus and its neuropathic complication: A randomized placebo controlled clinical trial. Journal of Clinical Pharmacy and Therapeutics. 2024;**2024**:1-18

[98] García-Martínez BI, Ruíz-Ramos M, Pedraza-Chaverri J, Santiago-Osorio E, Víctor Manuel Mendoza-Núñez. Effect of resveratrol on markers of oxidative stress and sirtuin 1 in elderly adults with type 2 diabetes. International Journal of Molecular Sciences. 2023;**24**(8):7422-7422

[99] Arbo BD, André-Miral C, Nasre-Nasser RG, Schimith LE, Santos MG, Costa-Silva D, et al. Resveratrol derivatives as potential treatments for Alzheimer's and Parkinson's disease. Frontiers in Aging Neuroscience. 2020;**12**:1-15. Available from: https://www.ncbi.nlm.nih.gov/pmc/articles/PMC7180342/

[100] Gu J, Li Z, Chen H, Xu X, Li Y, Gui Y. Neuroprotective effect of trans-resveratrol in mild to moderate Alzheimer disease: A randomized, double-blind trial. Neurology and Therapy. 2021;**10**(2):905-917. Available from: https://pubmed.ncbi.nlm.nih.gov/34402024/ [Accessed: November 8, 2021]

[101] McInnes IB, Schett G. The pathogenesis of rheumatoid arthritis. New England Journal of Medicine. 2011;**365**(23):2205-2219

[102] Sheng S, Wang X, Liu X, Hu X, Shao Y, Wang G, et al. The role of resveratrol on rheumatoid arthritis: From bench to bedside. Frontiers in Pharmacology. 2022;**13**:1-12. Available from: https://www.ncbi.nlm.nih.gov/pmc/articles/PMC9465647/ [Accessed: August 7, 2023]

[103] MacNee W. Pathology, pathogenesis, and pathophysiology. BMJ. 2006;**332**(7551):1202-1204

[104] Edwards MR, Bartlett NW, Clarke D, Birrell M, Belvisi M, Johnston SL. Targeting the NF-κB pathway in asthma and chronic obstructive pulmonary disease. Pharmacology & Therapeutics. 2009;**121**(1):1-13

[105] Beijers RJHCG, Gosker HR, Schols AMWJ. Resveratrol for patients with chronic obstructive pulmonary disease. Current Opinion in Clinical Nutrition & Metabolic Care. 2018;**21**(2):138-144

[106] Wang XL, Li T, Li JH, Miao SY, Xiao XZ. The effects of resveratrol on inflammation and oxidative stress in a rat model of chronic obstructive pulmonary disease. Molecules. 2017;**22**(9):1529

[107] Ma B, Li X. Resveratrol extracted from Chinese herbal medicines: A novel therapeutic strategy for lung diseases. Chinese Herbal Medicines. 2020;**12**:349-358

[108] Chen J, Yang X, Zhang W, Peng D, Xia Y, Lu Y, et al. Therapeutic effects of resveratrol in a mouse model of LPS and cigarette smoke-induced COPD. Inflammation. 2016;**39**(6):1949-1959

[109] Lewey J, Beckie TM, Brown HL, Brown SD, Garovic VD, Khan SS, et al. Opportunities in the postpartum period to reduce cardiovascular disease risk after adverse pregnancy outcomes: A scientific statement from the American

Heart Association. Circulation. 2024;**149**(7):1-31

[110] Yao L, Wan J, Li H, Ding J, Wang Y, Wang X, et al. Resveratrol relieves gestational diabetes mellitus in mice through activating AMPK. Reproductive Biology and Endocrinology. 2015;**13**(1):1-7

[111] Bourque SL, Dolinsky VW, Dyck JRB, Davidge ST. Maternal resveratrol treatment during pregnancy improves adverse fetal outcomes in a rat model of severe hypoxia. Placenta. 2012;**33**(5):449-452

[112] Singh CK, Kumar A, LaVoie HA, DiPette DJ, Singh US. Diabetic complications in pregnancy: Is resveratrol a solution? Experimental Biology and Medicine. 2013;**238**(5):482-490

[113] Habiburrahman M, Rakasiwi M, Putra A. Promising benefit of resveratrol in preventing preterm birth: A systematic review. World Academy of Sciences Journal. 2024;**6**(2):1-18

[114] Ramli I, Posadino AM, Giordo R, Fenu G, Fardoun M, Iratni R, et al. Effect of resveratrol on pregnancy, prenatal complications and pregnancy-associated structure alterations. Antioxidants. 2023;**12**(2):341

[115] Sharma RA, Steward WP, Gescher AJ. Pharmacokinetics and pharmacodynamics of curcumin. Advances in Experimental Medicine and Biology. 2007;**595**:453-470

[116] Anand P, Kunnumakkara AB, Newman RA, Aggarwal BB. Bioavailability of curcumin: Problems and promises. Molecular Pharmaceutics. 2007;**4**(6):807-818. Available from: https://www.ncbi.nlm.nih.gov/pubmed/17999464

[117] Wang Y, Liang L, Zhao Y. Curcumin delivery systems: How far from clinical application in tumor therapy? Natural Product Communications. 2024;**19**(2):1-13

[118] Patra S, Pradhan B, Nayak R, Behera C, Rout L, Jena M, et al. Chemotherapeutic efficacy of curcumin and resveratrol against cancer: Chemoprevention, chemoprotection, drug synergism and clinical pharmacokinetics. Seminars in Cancer Biology. 2021;**73**:310-320. Available from: https://www.sciencedirect.com/science/article/pii/S1044579X20302157

[119] Hesarooeyeh ZG, Basham A, Sheybani-Arani MH, Abbaszadeh M, Asl AS, Moghbeli M, et al. Effect of resveratrol and curcumin and the potential synergism on hypertension: A mini-review of human and animal model studies. PTR Phytotherapy Research/Phytotherapy Research. 2023;**38**:42-58

[120] Ochoa-Sanchez A, Sahare P, Pathak S, Banerjee A, Estevez M, Duttaroy AK, et al. Evaluation of the synergistic effects of curcumin-resveratrol co-loaded biogenic silica on colorectal cancer cells. Frontiers in Pharmacology. 2024;**15**:1-18

[121] Boonrueng P, Wasana PWD, Hasriadi OV, Rojsitthisak P, Towiwat P. Combination of curcumin and piperine synergistically improves pain-like behaviors in mouse models of pain with no potential CNS side effects. Chinese Medicine. 2022;**17**(1):1-21. Available from: https://www.ncbi.nlm.nih.gov/pmc/articles/PMC9590184 [Accessed: October 11, 2023]

[122] Satalkar P, Elger BS, Shaw DM. Defining Nano, nanotechnology and nanomedicine: Why should it matter? Science and Engineering Ethics. 2015;**22**(5):1255-1276

[123] Tagde P, Tagde P, Islam F, Tagde S, Shah M, Hussain ZD, et al.

The multifaceted role of curcumin in advanced nanocurcumin form in the treatment and management of chronic disorders. Molecules. 2021;**26**(23):7109

[124] Sharifi-Rad J, Quispe C, Mukazhanova Z, Knut E, Turgumbayeva A, Kipchakbayeva A, et al. Resveratrol-based nanoformulations as an emerging therapeutic strategy for cancer. Frontiers in Molecular Biosciences. 2021;**8**:1-22

[125] Ma Z, Shayeganpour A, Brocks DR, Lavasanifar A, Samuel J. High-performance liquid chromatography analysis of curcumin in rat plasma: Application to pharmacokinetics of polymeric micellar formulation of curcumin. Biomedical Chromatography. 2007;**21**(5):546-552

[126] Moballegh Nasery M, Abadi B, Poormoghadam D, Zarrabi A, Keyhanvar P, Khanbabaei H, et al. Curcumin delivery mediated by bio-based nanoparticles: A review. Molecules. 2020;**25**(3):689

[127] Tian Y. Inhibitory effect of curcumin liposome on PC-3 human prostate cancer cells. Zhonghua shiyan waike zazhi. 2014;**31**(5):1075-1078

[128] Bhatt H, Rompicharla SVK, Komanduri N, Aashma S, Paradkar S, Ghosh B, et al. Development of curcumin-loaded solid lipid nanoparticles utilizing glyceryl monostearate as single lipid using QbD approach: Characterization and evaluation of anticancer activity against human breast cancer cell line. Current Drug Delivery. 2018;**15**(9):1271-1283

[129] Kim TH, Jiang HH, Youn YS, Park CW, Tak KK, Lee S, et al. Preparation and characterization of water-soluble albumin-bound curcumin nanoparticles with improved antitumor activity. International Journal of Pharmaceutics. 2011;**403**(1-2):285-291

[130] Brahmkhatri VP, Sharma N, Sunanda P, D'Souza A, Raghothama S, Atreya HS. Curcumin nanoconjugate inhibits aggregation of N-terminal region (Aβ-16) of an amyloid beta peptide. New Journal of Chemistry. 2018;**42**(24):19881-19892

[131] Khursheed R, Singh SK, Kumar B, Wadhwa S, Gulati MAA, et al. Self-nanoemulsifying composition containing curcumin, quercetin, ganoderma lucidum extract powder and probiotics for effective treatment of type 2 diabetes mellitus in streptozotocin induced rats. International Journal of Pharmaceutics. 2022;**612**:121306

[132] Józsa L, Vasvári G, Sinka D, Nemes D, Ujhelyi Z, Vecsernyés M, et al. Enhanced antioxidant and anti-inflammatory effects of self-nano and microemulsifying drug delivery systems containing curcumin. Molecules/Molecules Online/Molecules Annual. 2022;**27**(19):6652-6652

[133] Mohajeri M, Sadeghizadeh M, Najafi F, Javan M. Polymerized nano-curcumin attenuates neurological symptoms in EAE model of multiple sclerosis through down regulation of inflammatory and oxidative processes and enhancing neuroprotection and myelin repair. Neuropharmacology. 2015;**99**:156-167

[134] Chauhan AS. Dendrimer nanotechnology for enhanced formulation and controlled delivery of resveratrol. Annals of the New York Academy of Sciences. 2015;**1348**(1):134-140

[135] Gu Y, Fei Z. Mesoporous silica nanoparticles loaded with resveratrol are used for targeted breast cancer therapy. Journal of Oncology. 2022;**2022**:1-11

[136] Berta GN, Romano F, Vallone R, Abbadessa G, Di Scipio F, Defabianis P. An innovative strategy for oral biofilm control in early childhood based on a resveratrol-cyclodextrin nanotechnology approach. Materials. 2021;**14**(14):3801

[137] Wang X, Chen C, Bao Y, Wang Y, Strakh YL. Encapsulation of three different types of polyphenols in casein using a customized pH-driven method: Preparation and characterization. Food Research International. 2024;**189**:114547-114547

[138] Prasad S, Aggarwal BB. Turmeric, the golden spice: From traditional medicine to modern medicine. In: Benzie IFF, Wachtel-Galor S, editors. Herbal Medicine: Biomolecular and Clinical Aspects. 2nd ed. Boca Raton (FL): CRC Press/Taylor & Francis; 2011. Available from: https://www.ncbi.nlm.nih.gov/books/NBK92752/

[139] Zhang H, Li C, Kwok ST, Zhang QW, Chan SW. A review of the pharmacological effects of the dried root of *polygonum cuspidatum* (Hu Zhang) and its constituents. Evidence-based Complementary and Alternative Medicine. 2013;**2013**:1-13

Section 2

Exploration of Functional Properties

Chapter 3

An Overview of Medicinal Plant Species Used in Treating and Managing Diarrhea by Zimbabwean Traditional Healers: A Toxicological Assessment

Elliot Nyagumbo, Trust Nyirenda, Cephas Mawere, Alfred Mutaramutswa, Godwins Ngorima, Donald T. Kapanga, Leroy Nhari, Marvellous Matsheza, Christine Midzi, William Pote, Fabian Maunganidze, Lucy Mabaya and Michael Bhebhe

Abstract

Inadequate sanitation and water infrastructure in Zimbabwe have led to rising endemicity of gastrointestinal tract infections such as diarrhea. Traditional medicine remains the primary treatment approach for diarrhea in Zimbabwe due to affordability and accessibility. This study aimed to document medicinal plants traditionally used for treating diarrhea in Zimbabwe over the past four decades. A comprehensive literature review was conducted based on published papers, books, book chapters, scientific reports and theses. A total of 129 medicinal plants belonging to 52 plant families used for diarrhoeal treatments were identified. Fabaceae emerged as the most abundant family with 26 plant species. The study also documented plant distribution across Zimbabwe and their traditional preparation. The most common method of preparing plants was infusions of about 45%. Toxicity assays were evaluated revealing 53.5% toxicological evaluation studies of the documented medicinal plants. With a concerning toxicity of approximately 46.5% from the aforementioned plant population, which is presently in use without any documented toxicity evaluation, this analysis revealed promising medicinal plant candidates for further investigation and development of future gastrointestinal management strategies.

Keywords: Ethnomedicinal plants, gastrointestinal diseases, diarrhea, cholera, dysentery, toxicity, pharmacology, Zimbabwe

1. Introduction

Diarrhea is a symptom of infections caused by various bacterial, viral and parasitic organisms, many of which are transmitted through water contaminated with fecal matter [1]. Common pathogens that cause diarrhea include rotaviruses, *Escherichia coli, Salmonella spp., Shigella spp., Vibrio cholerae* and *Campylobacter spp*. [2]. Rotaviruses are the most predominant pathogen globally and, in sub-Saharan Africa, contributing to approximately 40% of deaths in children under 5 [3, 4]. *Escherichia coli* is the second important pathogen responsible for childhood diarrhea in developing nations and is an increasingly antimicrobial-resistant entero-pathogen in the developed countries [5]. Diarrheal diseases are prevalent in all age groups, causing morbidity and mortality globally, and they are the leading cause of hospitalizations [6]. Despite advancements in healthcare, diarrhea continues to be a leading cause of death in young children under the age of 5 worldwide, resulting in around 443,832 deaths in children under 5 and an additional 50,851 deaths in children aged 5 to 9 years [1]. It is estimated that approximately 1.6 million people around the world die of diarrhea with the highest burden occurring in the developing countries [3, 4].

Diarrheal diseases have a significant impact on public health in Africa. In 2020, there were an estimated 1.008 billion cases of diarrhea and approximately 515,031 deaths attributed to diarrhoeal diseases in the African region [2]. In sub-Saharan Africa, diarrhea contributes significantly to child mortality and morbidity [7]. In Zimbabwe, diarrhea continues to be a notable health concern, especially among children under the age of five. Deaths from diarrhoeal diseases have declined over time, but they still pose a significant burden. The prevalence was at 15% in 2019, a reduction from the 25% recorded in 2015 and 30% in 1995 [8]. The contributing factors to the high prevalence of diarrhea in Zimbabwe and other developing countries include inadequate access to clean water, limited health care services, poor sanitation and malnutrition [1]. Inadequate sanitation and water infrastructure in Zimbabwe have led to a notable surge in the number of diarrhoeal disease cases recently [9]. With the emergence of antibiotic-resistant strains, current efforts to control diarrhoeal diseases may face obstacles.

Over the recent decades, Zimbabwe has experienced numerous outbreaks of antibiotic-resistant strains of both cholera and typhoid, both characterized by symptoms of acute diarrhea. Between 2017 and 2018, there was an outbreak of antibiotic (ciprofloxacin)-resistant strain in Zimbabwe, mainly in Harare province [10, 11]. Between 2018 and 2019, Zimbabwe faced a significant cholera outbreak that was resistant to antibiotics. The outbreak was caused by the *Vibrio cholera* strain, which showed resistance to nearly all antibiotics typically used to treat cholera [10]. The 2019 isolates carried 14 additional antimicrobial resistance genes on an approximately 160-kb IncA/C2 plasmid, resulting in a broader resistance profile compared to the T13 isolates, which were isolated in 2018 [12]. The 2019 isolates showed 100% sensitivity to azithromycin. To contain the outbreak, the treatment was switched from the standard recommended ciprofloxacin to azithromycin [11].

Herbal medicine refers to the utilization of natural substances as therapeutic agents for the prevention or treatment of various medical conditions [13]. They contain bioactive constituents, such as alkaloids, flavonoids, terpenes, lycopene, anthocyanidins, omega-3 fatty acids, phytoestrogens, glucosinolates and polyphenols that can interact with the body giving therapeutic benefits [14]. Herbal medicines are the most frequently used traditional and complementary medicines worldwide. Developed and developing countries are experiencing a remarkable increase in acceptance and public interest towards natural therapies. This surge has made herbal remedies widely available even in food stores and supermarkets [15]. The surge in recognizing medicinal plants as a source of drugs and other products is mainly due to their effectiveness, with little to no side effects associated with their application. As the global use of herbal medicines continues to increase and more new products are on the market, the need for standardization and safety concerns is increasing [16].

Implementing rigorous testing and quality assurance protocols can eliminate the potential risks associated with herbal medication products, such as contamination, high/low dosage, adulteration and the presence of harmful substances. This ensures the safety of these products for consumption [17]. In Zimbabwe, traditional medicine persists as the primary and readily available form of treatment within the primary healthcare system of poor communities due to its affordability and accessibility. It is therefore critical to fast tract regulatory measures on herbal medicines in Zimbabwe. To date, there has been a lack of comprehensive research examining the utilization of medicinal plants for the treatment of digestive system disorders in Zimbabwe. Digestive system disorders, particularly those associated with poor sanitation, lack of sewage control and inadequate water treatment, are endemic in Zimbabwe. This study aims to document the traditional medicinal plants utilized by the population of Zimbabwe for treating gastrointestinal disorders. The importance of this study is to safeguard the local indigenous knowledge of the plants used to treat gastrointestinal disorders, conserve the biological diversity of our local medicinal plants and provide the ethnopharmacological basis for drug research.

2. Materials and methods

This overview was conducted to compile data on medicinal plants traditionally used for the management of diarrhoeal disorders in Zimbabwe. Peer-reviewed publications and abstracts were retrieved from recognized online scientific databases, and relevant information was searched from electronically accessible books, book chapters, scientific reports and project theses originating from universities across Zimbabwe up to 31 December 2020. Other sources utilized include the National Herbarium and Botanic Gardens libraries. A comprehensive search strategy was implemented using a combination of controlled vocabulary and keyword terms in the online databases. These terms encompassed, herbal medicines used to treat diarrhea, gastrointestinal diseases, cholera or dysentery, “Ethnomedicinal plants for the treatment of diarrhoea, gastrointestinal disorders, cholera and dysentery”, “Traditional remedies, gastrointestinal disorders, Zimbabwe”, “Toxicity of plant” and “biological activities or properties of plant species”. This approach ensured the identification and incorporation of relevant and reliable scientific data on medicinal plants used in the treatment of diarrhea within the Zimbabwean context.

Plant species’ scientific/botanical names and local and/or common names were verified using https://www.zimbabweflora.co.zw and http://www.theplantlist.org websites. Plants having reported traditional use against diarrhea were selected and collated using the information provided. **Table 1** contains a master list of medicinal plants used in Zimbabwe for the treatment and management of diarrhea. A search of the above-mentioned databases was also conducted for toxicological properties, which could provide scientific evidence of the medicinal usage of these plants, in line with their ethnopharmacological use. A summary of all the information was compiled into

Scientific name [Family]	Growth habit [Distribution]	Parts used and its use(s)	Reported toxicological evaluations
Acacia karroo Hayne [Fabaceae]	Tree [N, W, C, E, S]	Bark, gum and leaves: Concoctions and infusions are used to treat diarrhea and dysentery [18].	Weak or low toxicity or mildly toxic—LD50 < 1600 mg/kg [19].
Acalypha brachiata C. Krauss [Euphorbiaceae]	Shrub, bush perennial [N, W, C, E, S]	Root: Decoction to treat diarrhea with blood [20].	No records found
Adenia gummifera (Harv.) Harms [Passifloraceae]	Climber or liane. [N, W, C, E, S]	Root: Decoction taken orally to treat diarrhea [20].	Safe or nontoxic—LD50–4000 mg/kg [21].
Albizia amara (Roxb) Biov. Subsp. *sericocephala* (Benth.) Brenan [Fabaceae]	Tree [N, W, C, E, S]	Leaves: Leaf infusion taken to treat diarrhea [20].	Safe or nontoxic—LD50–2000 mg/kg [22].
Albizia antunesiana Harms [Fabaceae]	Tree [N, W, C, E, S]	Roots: Root crushed and extract drunk as diarrhea (hot) [20].	No records found
Alepidea amatymbica Eckl. & Zeyh. [Apiaceae]	Herb [E]	Tuberous root: Infusion taken by mouth or powder taken in porridge to treat diarrhea [20].	No records found
Aloe spp. [Asphodelaceae]	Shrub-like, succulent. [N, W, C, E, S]	Leaves: Infusion of leaves taken for diarrhea [20].	Safe or non-toxic—LD50–2000 mg/kg [23].
Amaranthus spp. [Amakanthaceae]	Herb [N, W, C, E, S]	Root: Diarrhea [20].	No records found
Ampelocissus africana (Lour.) Merr. [Vitaceae]	Climber, shrub under 2 m. [N, W, C, E, S]	Roots: Extract drunk as diarrhea medicine [24].	No records found
Ampelocissus obtusata (Welw. ex Baker) Planch. [Vitaceae]	Climber, shrub under 2 m [N, W, C, E, S]	Roots: Extract drunk as diarrhea medicine [24, 25]	No records found
Annona stenophylla Engl & Diels subsp. *nana* (Exell) N. Robson [Annonacea]	Shrub [N, W, C, E, S]	Root: Root infusion taken to treat diarrhea with blood [20, 26].	Safe or non-toxic: LC50 μg/ml—leaves 1190 ± 212 μg/ml and roots 2300 ± 276 μg/ml; LD50 > 2000 mg/kg [27].
Ansellia africana Lindl. [Orchidaceae]	Epiphyte. [N, W, C, E, S]	Pseudobulbs: Diarrhea [28].	Safe or non-toxic—LD50–12,589.25 mg/ml [29].

Scientific name [Family]	**Growth habit [Distribution]**	**Parts used and its use(s)**	**Reported toxicological evaluations**
Aristolochia heppi Merxm. [Aristolochiaceae]	Herb [N, C, E, S]	Root: Root infusion used to treat diarrhea with blood [20].	No records found
Asparagus africanus Lam. [Asparagaceae]	Climber [N, W, C, E, S]	Roots: Crushed root hot extract drunk as diarrhea [24]. Roots and tubers: Diarrhea [25].	Safe or non-toxic—LD50 > 5000 mg/kg in rats [30].
Asparagus aspergillus Jessop. [Asparagaceae]	Shrub [N, W, C, S]	Roots and tubers: Diarrhea [28].	No records found
Asparagus spp except *A. asparagoides* [Asparagaceae]	Climber, tree, liane, [N, W, C, E, S]	Root: Root infusion or decoction taken for diarrhea [20].	No records found
Asparagus virgatus Bak [Asparagaceae]	Stiff, erect herbaceous subshrub up to 1 m [C, E, S]	Roots and tubers: Diarrhea [28].	No records found
Aspilia pluriseta Schweinf. subsp. *pluriseta* [Asteraceae]	Herb [N, C, E]	Root: Decoction is used to treat diarrhea [20].	No records found
Bobgunnia madagascariensis (Desv.) J.H. Kirkbr. & Wiersama [Fabaceae]	Tree, shrub over 2 m. [N, W, C, E, S]	Root: Ground into powder and added to porridge to treat diarrhea. Treating dysentery [20].	Unsafe/Toxic—LD50 of 288.5 mg/kg [31].
Bridelia cathartica G. Bertol *subsp. melanthesoides* (Baill.) J. Léonard [Phyllanthaceae]	Scrambling shrub or small tree [N, W, C, E, S]	Root: Diarrhea medicine [28].	Safe or nontoxic—LC50 > 1000 μg/ml [32].
Bridelia mollis Hutch [Phyllanthaceae]	Shrub or small tree [N, W, C, E, S]	Root: Diarrhea medicine [28, 33].	No records found
Burkea africana Hook [Fabaceae]	Tree [N, W, C, E, S]	Root: Decoction taken orally to treat diarrhea with blood [20].	Safe or non-toxic—LD50 > 5000 mg /kg [34].
Capparis tomentosa Lam [Capparaceae]	Climber, liane, shrub over 2 m. [N, W, C, E, S]	Root: Diarrhea treatment [28].	Safe or non-toxic—LD50 > 5000 mg/kg [35].

Scientific name [Family]	Growth habit [Distribution]	Parts used and its use(s)	Reported toxicological evaluations
Carissa bispinosa (L.) Desf. ex Brenan [Apocynaceae]	Shrub [E]	Roots: Extract drunk as diarrhea medicine [25].	No records found
Carissa spinarum L. [Apocynaceae]	Tree [N, W, C, E, S]	Roots: Hot extract drunk as diarrhea medicine [24, 25]	Safe or non-toxic—LD50 > 5000 mg/kg [36].
Cassia abbreviata Oliv. [Fabaceae]	Tree [N, W, C, E, S]	Root: Root infusion or root dried and ground to powder taken to treat diarrhea [20, 37].	Safe or non-toxic—LC50 > 1319.37 ± 356.63 μg/ml [38].
Catunaregam swynnertonii (S. Moore) Bridson [Rubiaceae]	Tree, shrub over 2 m. [E, S]	Root: Diarrhea medicine [28].	Safe or non-toxic—LD50 > 2000 mg/kg [39].
Cissampelos mucronata A. Rich. [Menispermaceae]	Liane [N, W, C, E, S]	Root: Root infusion used to treat diarrhea [20, 40].	Safe or non-toxic—LD50 > 5000 mg/kg [41].
Colophospermum mopane (Benth.) J. Leonard [Fabaceae]	Tree, shrub over 2 m. [N, W, C, E, S]	Roots: Diarrhea medicine [28].	No records found
Combretum apiculatum Sond. *subsp. apiculatum* [Combretaceae]	Tree [N, W, C, E, S]	No information: Diarrhea [42].	No records found
Combretum imberbe Wawra [Combretaceae]	Tree [N, W, C, E, S]	Root: Decoction taken orally to treat diarrhea [20, 42].	Highly toxic—LC50–168.6 μg/ml [43].
Combretum molle R.Br ex G. Don [Combretaceae]	Tree [N, W, C, E, S]	Root infusion taken orally to treat diarrhea and diarrhea with blood [20].	Safe or non-toxic—LD50–8000 mg/kg [44].
Combretum platypetalum Laws. subsp. *oatesii* (Rolfe) Exell [Combretaceae]	Shrub [N, W, C, E, S]	Root infusion or decoction taken to treat diarrhea [20].	No records found
Combretum zeyheri Sond. [Combretaceae]	Tree [N, W, C, E, S]	Root infusion taken orally to treat diarrhea in blood. Leaves: Diarrhea [20].	No records found

Scientific name [Family]	**Growth habit [Distribution]**	**Parts used and its use(s)**	**Reported toxicological evaluations**
Combretum elaeagnoides Klotzsch [Combretaceae]	Tree [N, W, C, E]	Root: Diarrhea medicine [28].	No records found
Commiphora angolensis Engl. [Burseraceae]	Shrub or small deciduous tree [N, W, E, S]	Root: Diarrhea medicine [28].	No records found
Crossopteryx febrifuga (Afzel. ex G. Don) Benth [Rubiaceae]	Shrub [N, W, C, E, S]	Bark: Powder added to porridge as remedy for cholera, diarrhea and dysentery [20, 25, 45, 46]	Safe or non-toxic—LD50–5000 mg/kg [47].
Cussonia natalensis (Sond) [Araliaceae]	Tree. [W, C, E, S]	No information: Diarrhea [48].	No records found
Cyphostemma junceum (Webb) Desc. ex Wild & R.B. Drumm. [Vitaceae]	Herb [N, C, S]	Tuberous root: Infusion taken to treat diarrhea [20].	No records found
Cyphostemma rhodesiae (Gilg & M. Brandt) Desc. ex Wild & R.B. Drumm [Vitaceae]	Herb [N, C, S]	Tuberous root: Ground into powder and added to porridge to treat diarrhea [20].	No records found
Dichrostachys cinerea (L.) Wight. & Arn. [Fabaceae]	Tree, shrub over 2 m. [N, W, C, E, S]	Root: Infusion to treat diarrhea with blood. Infusion and powder of root to treat diarrhea caused by a suckling pregnant mother. [20, 28].	Safe or non-toxic—LD50 > 3500 mg/kg [49].
Dicoma anomala Sond subsp. *anomala* [Asteraceae]	Herb [N, W, C, E, S]	Root: Decoction used to treat diarrhea and dysentery. Tuber: Crushed and mixed with water for broad spectrum [20, 27, 50].	Safe or non-toxic—LD50 > 2000 mg/kg [51].
Diplolophium zambesianum Hiern [Apiaceae]	Shrub [N, W, C, E, S]	Root: Body washed with infusion which is then taken by mouth to treat diarrhea [20].	No records found
Dolichos kilimandscharicus Harms ex Taub. [Fabaceae]	Herb [N, C, E, S]	Tuber: Ground powder taken in porridge to treat diarrhea [20].	Highly toxic—LC50 values 58.06–0.63 µg/ml [52].

Scientific name [Family]	Growth habit [Distribution]	Parts used and its use(s)	Reported toxicological evaluations
Ectadiopsis oblongifolia (Meisn.) Bullock [Asclepiadaceae]	Shrub [N, W, C, E, S]	Root: Decoction taken to treat diarrhea [20].	No records found
Ekebergia benguelensis C.DC. [Meliaceae]	Tree [N, C, E, S]	Root: Infusion taken for diarrhea (in porridge) [20].	No records found
Elaedendron matabelicum Loes. [Celastraceae]	Tree [N, W, C, E, S]	Roots: used to treat diarrhea and dysentery [53].	Safe or non-toxic—LC50 value of 1012.31 ± 217.69 μg/ml [38, 53].
Elephantorrhiza elephantina (Burch.) Skeels [Fabaceae]	Shrub under 2 m. [N, W, C, E, S]	Root: Infusion to treat diarrhea [20, 54, 55].	Weak or low toxicity or mildly toxic—LD50 > 1600 mg/kg [56].
Elephantorrhiza goetzei (Harms) Harms [Fabaceae]	Shrub [N, W, C, E, S]	Roots: Extract drunk as a diarrhea medicine. Root infusion to treat diarrhea [20, 25, 57]	Moderately toxic—LC 50–356.55 μg/ml [57].
Elephantorrhiza suffruticosa Schinz [Fabaceae]	Shrub over 2 m. [C, E, S]	Root: Infusion or root ground to powder and added to porridge to treat diarrhea with blood [20, 34, 37].	No records found
Erythrina abyssinica DC. [Fabaceae]	Tree [N, C, E, S]	Bark: Infusion to treat diarrhea [20]	Safe or non-toxic—LC50–5440 μg/ml [27].
Euclea divinorum Hiern [Ebenaceae]	Shrub [N, W, C, E, S]	Roots: Extract drunk as diarrhea medicine. Ground into powder and mixed with porridge used to treat diarrhea [20, 25]	Safe or non-toxic—LD50–2000 mg/kg [58].
Euphorbia matabelensis Pax [Euphorbiaceae]	Tree, shrub over 2 m. [N, W, C, E, S]	Root: To cure diarrhea, however, if taken orally it may cause abortion, severe diarrhea and vomiting [20].	No records found
Faurea saligna Harv. [Proteaceae]	Tree [N, W, C, E, S]	Root: Infusion of the root taken to treat diarrhea [20, 48].	No records found
Ficus sur Forssk. *Ficus capensis* Thunb. [Moraceae]	Tree [N, W, C, E, S]	Roots: Extract drunk as diarrhea medicine [59].	Safe or non-toxic—LD 50 of 2154 mg/kg [60].

Scientific name [Family]	Growth habit [Distribution]	Parts used and its use(s)	Reported toxicological evaluations
Flacourtia indica (Burm.f.) Merr [Flacourtiaceae]	Tree, shrub over 2 m. [N, W, C, E, S]	Root: Infusion taken orally or leaves browsed and chewed and juice swallowed to treat diarrhea [20, 24, 25].	Moderately toxic—LC50–467.31 ± 39.01 μg/ml [61].
Flemingia grahamiana Wight & Arry [Fabaceae]	Shrub over 2 m. [N, C, E, S]	Root: Decoction taken for diarrhea [20].	No records found
Flueggea virosa (Roxb. ex Willd.) Voigt [Phyllanthaceae]	Shrub or small tree [N, W, C, E, S]	Root: Powder taken orally in porridge or infusion to treat diarrhea [20].	Safe or non-toxic—LD50 > 5000 mg/kg [62].
Garcinia buchananii Bak [Clusiaceae]	Tree [N, C, E, S]	Bark or root: Infusion taken orally to treat diarrhea [20].	Highly toxic—LC 50 values - 60.6 - 207.0 μg/ml [27].
Grewia bicolor Juss. [Malvaceae]	Shrub [N, W, C, E, S]	Roots: Hot extract drunk as diarrhea [24, 25].	Safe or non-toxic—LD50 value - 2663.92 mg/kg [63].
Grewia flavescens Juss. [Malvaceae]	Shrub [N, W, C, E, S]	Root: Infusion to treat diarrhea in infants [20].	No records found
Grewia monticola Sond. [Malvaceae]	Tree [N, W, C, E, S]	Roots: Hot extract drunk as diarrhea medicine [20, 24, 25].	No records found
Grewia subspathulata N.E. Br. [Malvaceae]	Shrub or small tree [N, W, C, E, S]	Root: Diarrhea medicine [28]	No records found
Gymnosporia senegalensis Loes [Celastraceae]	Tree, shrub over 2 m. [N, W, C, E, S]	Root: Infusion and decoction to treat diarrhea [20].	Safe or non-toxic—LC50 value of 2185.61 ± 872. LD50 > 1600 mg/kg in mice [64].
Hoslundia opposita Vahl [Lamiaceae]	Shrub over 2 m, shrub under 2 m. [N, W, C, E, S]	Root: Infusion to treat diarrhea in infants [20].	Safe or non-toxic—LD50 > 5000 mg/kg [65, 66].
Hydnora abyssinica A. Braun ex Schweinf. [Hydnoraceae]	Root parasite [W, C, S]	Swollen underground stem: Infusion is taken to treat diarrhea with blood [20].	No records found

Scientific name [Family]	Growth habit [Distribution]	Parts used and its use(s)	Reported toxicological evaluations
Indigofera setiflora Baker [Fabaceae]	Herb [N, W, C, E, S]	Roots: extract drunk as diarrhea medicine. Crushed roots are used to prepare a decoction to treat diarrhea, cholera and dysentery [25].	No records found
Kigelia africana (Lam.) Benth. [Bignoniaceae]	Tree [N, W, C, E, S]	Bark, fruit, root and seeds: Diarrhea [53].	Moderately toxic—LC50 < 300 μg/ml [38].
Kirkia acuminata Oliv. [Kirkiaceae]	Tree [N, W, C, E, S]	Bark: bark decoction drunk or bark powder mixed with food as cholera, broad spectrum, diarrhea and dysentery medicine [20, 24, 25, 67, 68]	No records found
Lannea discolor (Sond.) Engl. [Anacardiaceae]	Tree [N, W, C, E, S]	Bark: Ground into powder and mixed with porridge to treat diarrhea with blood. Bark, fruit pulp, root and stem bark: decoctions taken orally for diarrhea [20, 69].	No records found
Lannea edulis (Sond.) Engl [Anacardiaceae]	Shrub under 2 m. [N, W, C, E, S]	Root: Infusion taken to treat diarrhea [20, 24, 70].	Safe or non-toxic—LD50 > 6000 mg/kg [71].
Lannea schweinfurthii (Engl.) Engl. Var. *stuhlmanni* (Engl.) Kokwaro [Anacardiaceae]	Tree [N, W, E, S]	Root: Infusion taken to treat diarrhea. Stems, leaves, bark and roots: amoebic dysentery, diarrhea and dysentery [20].	Safe or non-toxic—LD50 > 5000 mg/kg [72].
Loranthus spp parasitizing *Prunus africana* [Loranthaceae]	Mistletoe [N, W, C, E, S]	Whole plant: Whole plant is ground into powder and mixed with milk and drank for treating diarrhea [20].	No records found
Mangifera indica L. [Anacardiaceae]	Tree [Cultivated]	Bark: Extract drunk as diarrhea medicine [25].	Safe or non-toxic—LD50 > 2000 mg/kg [73].
Manilkara mochisia (Bak.) Dubard [Sapotaceae]	Shrub or small tree [N, W, C, E, S]	Root: Diarrhea medicine [28].	No records found
Moringa oleifera Lour [Moringaceae]	Tree [N]	Leaves: Extract drunk as diarrhea medicine [24, 25].	Safe or non-toxic—LD50 value 3458.3 mg/kg [74].
Musa spp. [Musaceae]	Tree [Cultivated]	Root: Roots are boiled and the strained liquid taken by mouth, if diarrhea accompanies abdominal pain [28].	Safe or non-toxic—LD50 > 5000 mg/kg [75].

Scientific name [Family]	**Growth habit [Distribution]**	**Parts used and its use(s)**	**Reported toxicological evaluations**
Nymphaea nouchali Burm. f. var. *caerulea* (Savigny) Verdc. [Nymphaeaceae]	Aquatic [N, W, C, E, S]	Root: Root infusion taken to treat diarrhea in infants [20].	Weak or low toxicity—LD50–681 mg/kg [76].
Ochna pulchra Hook. subsp. *pulchra* [Ochanaceae]	Tree [N, W, C, E, S]	Root: cooked with beans and soup eaten to treat diarrhea with blood [20, 25].	No records found
Ocimum angustifolium Benth. [Lamiaceae]	Herb [N, W, C, S]	Root: boiled together with meat and decoction is taken orally to treat diarrhea with blood in stool [20].	No records found
Oldenlandia herbacea (L.) Roxb. [Rubiaceae]	Herb [N, W, C, E, S]	Stem and leaves: Infusion used to treat diarrhea [20].	Safe or non-toxic—LD50 > 2000 mg/kg [77].
Opilia amentacea Roxb. [Opiliaceae]	Climber, liane, shrub over 2 m. [N, E, S]	Roots: Diarrhea [28].	No records found
Ozoroa reticulata (Baker f.) R. Fern. & A. Fern. [Anacardiaceae]	Tree [N, W, C, E, S]	Root: Infusion or decoction taken to treat diarrhea [20, 25].	Highly toxic—LC50–2.21–10.63 μg/ml [78].
Paederia bojeriana (A.Rich.) Drake subsp. *foetens* (Hiern) Verdc. [Rubicaeae]	Climber, liane. [N, W, C, E, S]	Root: Diarrhea medicine [28].	No records found
Parinari curatellifolia (Planch.) Benth [Chrysobalanaceae]	Tree [N, W, C, E, S]	Root and leaves: Chronic diarrhea treatment [20, 28].	Safe or non-toxic—LC50 > 1000 μg/ml [79].
Pavetta schumanniana F. Hoffm. ex K. Schum. [Rubiaceae]	Shrub or small semi-deciduous tree. [N, W, C, E, S]	Leaves: Infusion to treat diarrhea [20].	No records found
Pelargonium luridium (Andr.) Sweet [Geraniaceae]	Herb [W, C, E]	Root: Infusion taken to treat diarrhea [20].	No records found
Peltophorum africanum Sond. [Fabaceae]	Tree, shrub over 2 m. [N, W, C, E, S]	Root: Decoction or infusion taken to treat dysentery and diarrhea [20, 24, 25].	Weak or low toxicity or mildly toxic LC 50—ranges 913 ± 7.32–1060 ± 106 μg/ml [80].

Scientific name [Family]	Growth habit [Distribution]	Parts used and its use(s)	Reported toxicological evaluations
Pericopsis angolensis (Bak.) van Meeuwen [Fabaceae]	Tree [N, C, E]	Root: Decoction to treat diarrhea. Bark: Infusion used to treat diarrhea with blood. Leaves: Diarrhea medicine [20, 28].	No records found
Philenoptera violacea (Klotzsch) Schrire [Fabaceae]	Tree [N, W, C, E, S]	Roots: Diarrhea medicine [28].	No records found
Piliostigma thonningii (Schumach.) Milne-Redh. [Fabaceae]	Tree [N, W, C, E, S]	Root and Leaves: Infusion taken to treat diarrhea [20].	Safe or non-toxic—LD50 > 5000 mg/kg [81].
Protea angolensis Welw. [Proteaceae]	Shrub [N, C, E]	Root: Root ground into powder and mixed with porridge to treat diarrhea [20].	No records found
Prunus persica L. [Rosaceae]	Tree [Cultivated]	Leaves: Extract drunk as diarrhea medicine [25].	Safe or non-toxic—LD50 up to 2000 mg/kg [82].
Pseudarthria hookeri Wight & Arn [Fabaceae]	Herb [N, W, C, E, S]	Root: Mixed with ground nuts and decoction taken for diarrhea. Root powder taken for diarrhea in infants [20].	No records found
Pseudolachnostylis marouneifolia Pax [Phyllanthaceae]	Tree [N, W, C, E, S]	Root: Infusion taken to treat diarrhea [20].	No records found
Psorospermum febrifugum Spach [Clusiaceae]	Tree, shrub over 2 m. [N, C, E, S]	Root: Ground into powder and added to porridge to treat diarrhea [20].	Safe or non-toxic—LD 50 > 2000 mg/kg body weight [83].
Pterocarpus angolensis DC. [Fabaceae]	Tree, shrub over 2 m. [N, W, C, E, S]	Bark or root: Infusion taken to treat diarrhea. Root: Infusion taken to treat diarrhea with blood [20, 28, 84].	Weak or low toxicity or mildly toxic—roots LC 50–1320 ± 266, bark LC 50–478 ± 29.7 [27].
Rhynchosia insignis (O. Hoffm.) R.E. Fr. [Fabaceae]	Herb [N, C, E]	Leaves: Treatment of diarrhea [20].	No records found
Rhynchosia resinosa (Hochst. ex A. Rich.) Baker [Fabaceae]	Climber, perennial, shrub over 2 m. [N, W, C, E, S]	Root: Infusion taken to treat diarrhea [20].	Highly toxic—LC50–222.43 μg/ml [78].

Scientific name [Family]	**Growth habit [Distribution]**	**Parts used and its use(s)**	**Reported toxicological evaluations**
Ricinus communis L. [Euphorbiaceae]	Tree, annual, perennial, shrub over 2 m, shrub under 2 m. [N, W, C, E, S]	Seed: Pulverized and infusion taken to treat diarrhea [20].	Safe or non-toxic—LD50–8000 mg/kg [85].
Rubia cordifolia L. [Rubicaeae]	Climber [E, C]	Root: Diarrhea medicine [28].	Weak or low toxicity or mildly toxic—LD50 > 1000 mg/kg body weight [86, 87].
Sansevieria hyacinthoides (L.) Druce [Asparagaceae]	Herb [N, C, E, S]	Leaves, rhizomes, roots and whole plant for treating diarrhea [25, 88, 89].	No records found
Sclerocarya birrea (A. Rich.) Hochst. [Anacardiaceae]	Tree [N, W, C, E, S]	Bark and stem: Decoction of stem, bark taken as remedy for cholera, dysentery and diarrhea. Bark: treating diarrhea [20, 24, 25, 90].	Safe or non-toxic—LD50 > 1000 mg/kg [91].
Searsia dentata (Thunb.) F.A. Barkley [Anacardiaceae]	Tree, shrub over 2 m. [W, C, E]	Leaves: Leaf sap taken as remedy for diarrhea. Juice from leaves is swallowed to treat diarrhea [25].	No records found
Searsia lancea (L.f.) F.A. Barkley *Rhus lancea* L.f. [Anacardiaceae]	Tree [N, W, C, E, S]	Root: Infusion taken to treat diarrhea with blood [20].	Weak or low toxicity or mildly toxic—LC 50–600 μg/ml [92].
Searsia longipes (Engl.) Moffett var. *longipes* [Anacardiaceae]	Tree, shrub over 2 m. [N, C, E]	Root: Infusion taken to treat diarrhea [20].	Safe or non-toxic—LD50 > 5000 mg/kg [93, 94].
Securidaca longipedunculata Fresen [Polygalaceae]	Tree, shrub over 2 m. [N, W, C, E, S]	Root: Infusion used to treat diarrhea [20].	Safe or non-toxic—LD50 > 5000 mg/kg [95].
Solanum campylacanthum [Solanaceae]	Shrub [N, W, C, E, S]	Root: Infusion taken orally to treat diarrhea [20].	Safe or non-toxic—LD50 > 2000 mg/kg [96].
Solanum nigrum L. [Solanaceae]	Herb or shrub [N, E, S]	Root: Diarrhea medicine [28].	Weak or low toxicity or mildly toxic—LD50–510 mg/kg [97].
Solanum tettense Klotzsch var. *renschii* (Vatke) A.E. Gonç. [Solanaceae]	Shrub [N, W, C, E, S]	Root: Diarrhea medicine [28]	No records found

Scientific name [Family]	Growth habit [Distribution]	Parts used and its use(s)	Reported toxicological evaluations
Sphenostylis erecta (Baker f.) Hutch. ex Baker f. [Fabaceae]	Subshrub [N, C, E, S]	Root: Diarrhea medicine [28].	No records found
Tamarindus indica L [Fabaceae]	Tree [N, W, E]	Gastro-intestinal problems including diarrhea and dysentery [20].	Safe or non-toxic—LD50 > 5000 mg/kg [98].
Terminalia brachystemma Welw. [Combretaceae]	Shrub or small tree [N, W, C]	Bark: Infusion taken by mouth to treat diarrhea [20].	No records found
Terminalia prunioides M.A. Lawson [Combretaceae]	Shrub or small tree [N, W, C, E, S]	No information: Diarrhea [41].	No records found
Terminalia sericea Burch. ex DC. [Combretaceae]	Tree [N, W, C, E, S]	Root or Bark: Ground into powder and taken to treat diarrhea. Root: Powder added to porridge to treat diarrhea [20, 28].	Toxic—LC50 < 300 μg/ml [38, 99].
Tetradenia riparia (Hochst.) Codd sensu lato [Lamiaceae]	Shrub or small tree [N, W, C, E, S]	Leaves: Ground into powder and mixed with porridge to treat diarrhea [20].	No records found
Thunbergia oblongifolia Oliv. [Acanthaceae]	Herb [N, C, E]	Root: Powder mixed with porridge to treat diarrhea [20].	Safe or non-toxic—LD50 > 2000 mg/kg [100].
Triumfetta welwitschii Mast [Malvaceae]	Herb [N, W, C, E, S]	Tuber: Ground into powder and added to porridge to treat diarrhea.	No records found
Turraea nilotica Kotschy & Peyr. [Meliaceae]	Tree, shrub over 2 m. [N, W, C, E, S]	Root: Infusion taken to treat diarrhea (in porridge) [20, 37].	Weak or low toxicity—LC50 - roots 701 ± 25.650 μg/ml [27, 101].
Tylosema fassoglense (Kotschy ex Schweinf.) Torre & Hillc. [Fabaceae]	Climber [N, W, C, E, S]	Tuber: Porridge prepared with infusion to treat diarrhea [20].	No records found
Vangueria infausta Burch. [Rubiaceae]	Tree [N, W, C, E, S]	Roots: Hot extract drunk as diarrhea medicine. Bark, leaf, root: decoction taken orally to treat diarrhea [20].	Moderately toxic—LC50 values of 338 ± 23.4 μg/mL and 416 ± 28.3 μg/mL [102].

DOI: http://dx.doi.org/10.5772/intechopen.1006302

Scientific name [Family]	Growth habit [Distribution]	Parts used and its use(s)	Reported toxicological evaluations
Vernonia amygdalina Del. [Asteraceae]	Tree, shrub over 2 m. [N, W, C, E, S]	Root: Infusion taken orally to treat diarrhea [20]	Safe or non-toxic—LD50 of 4808.33 mg/kg [103].
Waltheria indica L. [Malvaceae]	Shrub [N, W, C, E, S]	Root: Infusion taken orally to treat diarrhea [20].	Safe or non-toxic—LD50–3000 mg/kg weight [104].
Warburgia sulcata [Canellaceae]	no information	No information: Diarrhea [105].	No records found
Ximenia caffra Sond. [Olacaeceae]	Tree, shrub over 2 m. [N, W, C, E, S]	Leaves and roots: Diarrhea. Roots: extract drunk as diarrhea [20, 24, 25].	Safe or non-toxic—LC50 > 1020752.7 mg/ml [106].
Zanha africana (Radlk) Excell. [Sapindaceae]	Tree, shrub over 2 m. [N, W, C, E, S]	Bark, leaves, root, bark and roots: Gastro-intestinal problems including diarrhea and dysentery [20, 107].	Highly toxic—LC50 values ranging from 41.1 μg/mL and 240.0 μg/mL [107].
Zanthoxylum chalybeum Engl. *Fagara chalybea* (Engl.) [Rutaceae]	Tree, shrub over 2 m. [N, W, C]	Root: Infusion taken to treat diarrhea [20].	Safe or non-toxic—LD50 > 5000 mg/kg [108].
Zanthoxylum humile (E.A. Bruce) P. G. Waterman [Rutaceae]	Shrub [W, S]	Roots: Roots are fused to make a decoction that is taken orally to treat conditions diarrhea [109].	No records found
Ziziphus mucronata Willd. [Rhamnaceae]	Tree [N, W, C, E, S]	Root: Infusion used to treat diarrhea and cholera [20, 24, 25].	Safe or non-toxic—LD50 > 5000 mg/kg [110].

Table 1.
Medicinal plant species used in the treatment and management of diarrhea by Zimbabwean traditional healers.

Toxicological profile	No of plants	Names of the plant species
Safe or nontoxic LC50 ≥ 1000 µg/ml 2000 ≤ LD50 ≤ 5000 mg/kg body weight	47	*Adenia gummifera, Albizia amara, Aloe spp., Annona stenophylla, Ansellia africana, Asparagus africanus, Bridelia cathartica, Burkea africana, Capparis tomentosa, Carissa spinarum, Cassia abbreviata, Catunaregam swynnertonii, Cissampelos mucronata, Combretum molle, Crossopteryx febrifuga, Dichrostachys cinerea, Dicoma anomala, Elaedendron matabelicum, Erythrina abyssinica, Euclea divinorum, Ficus sur, Grewia bicolor, Flueggea virosa, Gymnosporia senegalensis, Holarrhena pubescens, Lannea edulis, Lannea schweinfurthii, Mangifera indica, Moringa oleifera, Musa spp., Oldenlandia herbacea, Parinari curatellifolia, Piliostigma thonningii, Prunus persica, Psorospernum febrifugum, Ricinus communis, Sclerocarya birrea, Searsia longipes, Securidaca longipedunculata, Solanum campylacanthum, Tamarindus indica, Thunbergia oblongifolia, Vernonia amygdalina, Waltheria indica, Ximenia caffra, Zanthoxylum chalybeum, Ziziphus mucronata.*
Weak or low toxicity or mildly toxic 1000 ≤ LD50 ≤ 2000 mg/kg body weight 500 ≤ LC50 ≤ 999 µg/ml	9	*Acacia karoo, Elephantorrhiza elephantina, Nymphaea nouchali, Peltophorum africanum Rubia cordifolia, Searsia lancea, Solanum nigrum, Pterocarpus angolensis, Turraea nilotica.*
Moderately toxic 250 ≤ LC50 ≤ 499 µg/ml 300 ≤ LD50 ≤ 1000 mg/kg body weight	4	*Elephantorrhiza goetzei, Flacourtia indica, Kigelia africana, Vangueria infausta.*
Toxic 50 ≤ LD50 ≤ 300 mg/kg body weight	2	*Bobgunnia madagascariensis, Terminalia sericea* (**Figure** 7).
Highly toxic LC50 ≤ 249 µg/ml 0 ≤ LD50 ≤ 50 mg/kg body weight	6	*Combretum imberbe, Dolichos kilimandscharicus, Garnia buchananii, Ozoroa reticulata, Rhynchosia resinosa, Zanha africana.*
No records found	61	*Acalypha brachiata, Albizia antunesiana, Alepidea amatymbica, Amaranthus spp, Ampelocissus africana, Ampelocissus obtusata, Aristolochia heppi, Asparagus spp except A. asparagoides, Asparagus aspergillus, Asparagus uirgatus, Aspilia pluriseta, Bridelia mollis, Carissa bispinosa, Colophospermum mopane, Combretum apiculatum, Combretum platypetalum, Combretum elaeagnoides, Combretum zeyheri, Commiphora angolensis, Cussonia natalensis, Cyphostemma junceum, Cyphostemma rhodesiae, Diplolophium zambesianum, Ectadiopsis oblongifolia, Ekebergia benguelensis, Elephantorrhiza suffruticosa, Euphorbia matabelensis, Faurea saligna, Flemingia grahamiana, Grewia flavescens, Grewia monticola, Grewia subspathulata, Hydnora abyssinica, Indigofera setiflora, Kirkia acuminata, Lannea discolor, Loranthus spp parasitizing Prunus africana, Manilkara mochisia, Ochna pulchra, Ocimum angustifolium, Opilia amentacea, Paederia bojeriana, Pavetta schumanniana, Pelargonium luridium, Pericopsis angolensis, Philenoptera violacea, Protea angolensis, Pseudarthria hookeri, Pseudolachnostylis marouneifolia, Rhynchosia insignis, Sansevieria hyacinthoides, Searsia dentata, Solanum tettense, Sphenostylis erecta, Terminalia brachystemma, Terminalia prunioides, Tetradenia riparia, Triumfetta welwitschia, Tylosema fassoglense, Warburgia sulcata, Zanthoxylum humile.*

Table 2.
Toxicological evaluation of medicinal plants plant species used in the treatment and management of diarrhea by Zimbabwean traditional healers.

two tables (**Tables 1** and **2**) and seven figures (**Figures 1–7**). The overview excluded medicinal plants for abdominal pain and veterinary use, limiting the plants to those used only to treat and control diarrhea in humans.

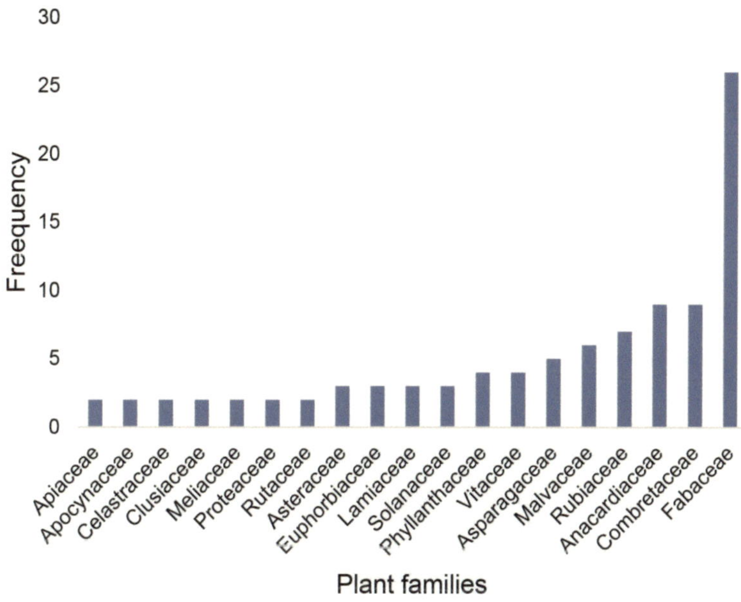

Figure 1.
Families of medicinal plant species used to treat and manage diarrhea in Zimbabwe.

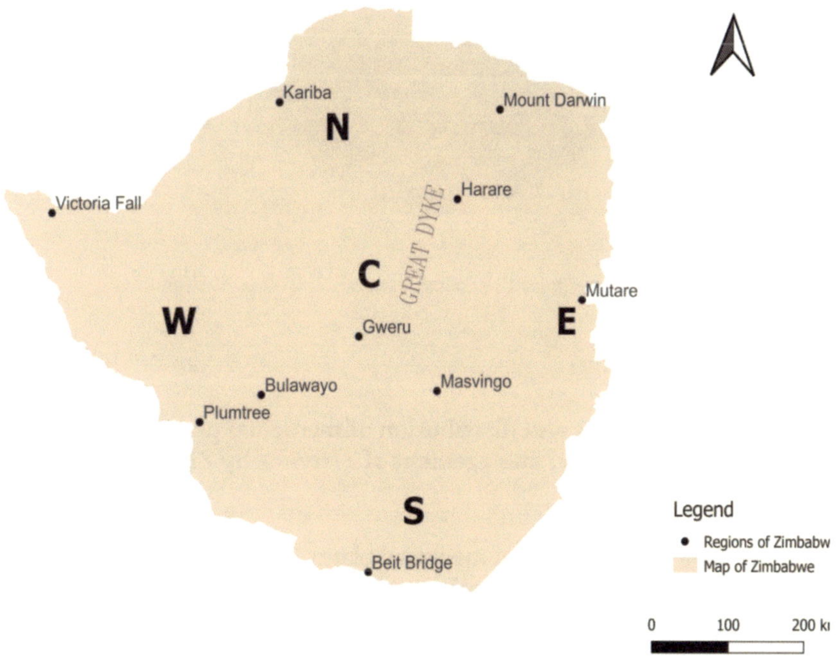

Figure 2.
The general distribution of medicinal plants throughout Zimbabwe's floristic zones.

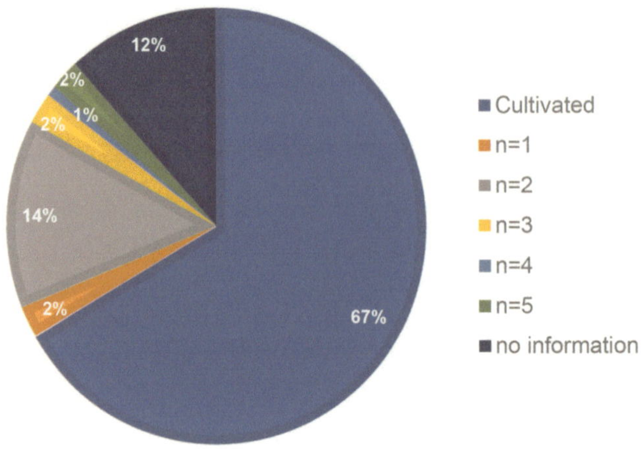

Figure 3.
Status of the medicinal plants with numbers (1, 2, 3, 4 and 5) representing the number of floristic regions (N, W, E, C and S).

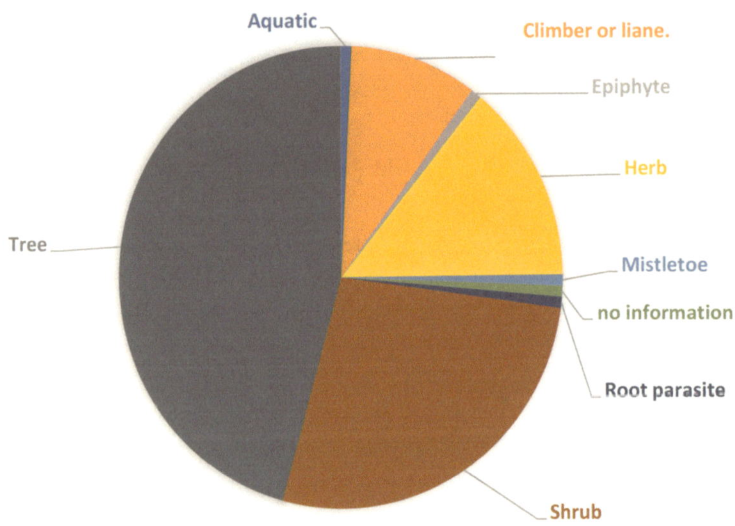

Figure 4.
Growth habit of plants used for the treatment and management of diarrhea in Zimbabwe.

3. Results and discussion

3.1 Ethnobotanical surveys and distribution of medicinal plants plant species used in the treatment and management of diarrhea by Zimbabwean traditional healers

The study highlighted the use of medicinal plants to treat and manage diarrhea which is a symptom of gastro-intestinal disorders, which also includes abdominal pains, amoebic dysentery, dysentery, stomach problems and stomach aches. The review's primary goal was to focus on targeting the treatment and management of diarrhea. A key symptom of dysentery which is bloody diarrhea was also noted. Shopo et al. [112], cited at least 60 out of 127 medicinal plants being responsible for treating

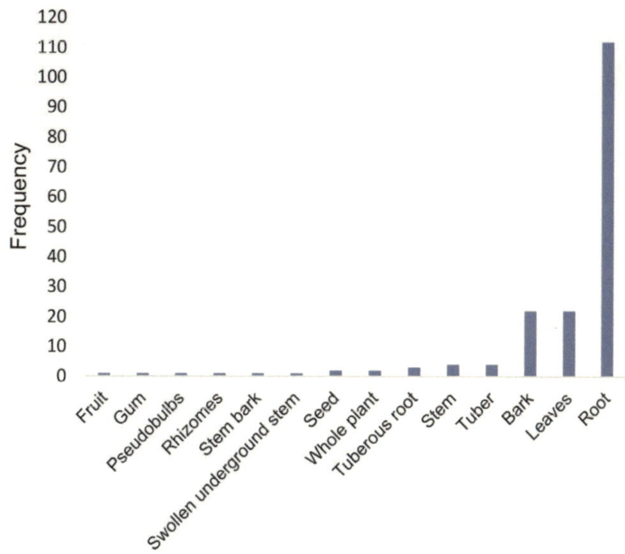

Figure 5.
Plant parts used for medicinal preparations used for the management of diarrhea in Zimbabwe.

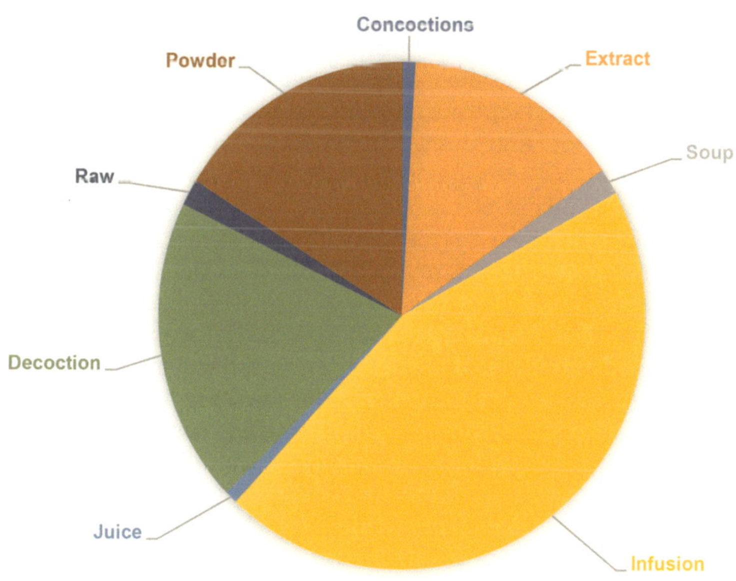

Figure 6.
Mode of preparation of plants used for the treatment and management of diarrhea in Zimbabwe.

and managing gastrointestinal disorders in Gokwe-South, Zimbabwe. The knowledge of frequently reported illnesses and/or diseases can provide an indication of health care concerns in Zimbabwean communities, and health care organizations and government should take an active interest in this information.

A total of 52 (129 plant species) plant families were reported with 33 plant families reporting single plant species (**Table 1**). At least seven plant families exhibited more than two plant species. According to **Figure 1** above, Fabaceae [n = 26] plant family

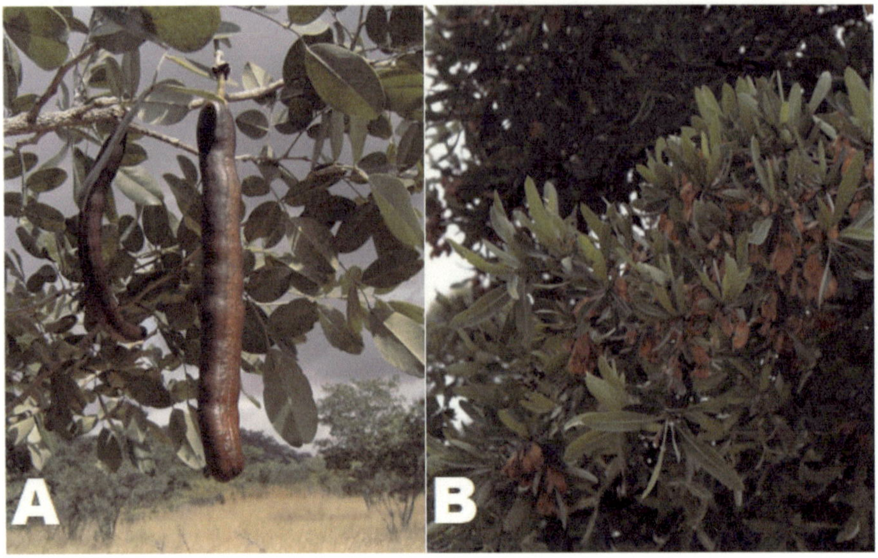

Figure 7.
The two medicinal plants classified as toxic A: Bobgunnia madagascariensis; *B:* Terminalia sericea *[111].*

dominates in terms of species diversity. Anacardiaceae and Combreaceae plant families both with [n = 9] species. Ethnobotanical surveys by Maroyi [24]; Shopo et al. [112]; and Nyasvisvo et al. [113] have reported Fabaceae species as the most common and dominant herbal plant family used in Zimbabwe, and reviews by Nyagumbo et al. [114, 115] and Maroyi [116] also support the fact. There is a tendency for the most readily accessible and available plants to be better known and hence more frequently used. The Fabaceae family holds a significant ethnomedicinal importance due to its richness in medicinal properties. Maroyi [116] reported plant species from the Fabaceae family addressing at least 134 medical conditions, including gastrointestinal disorders such as diarrhea. According to Van Wyk [117], inventory and analysis of medicinal plants used as traditional medicine reported the dominant Fabaceae plant family with 567 plant species and 156 genera. This overview highlights the Asteraceae and Rubiceae as the second and third placed plant family contenders, which concurs with Van Wyk [117] analysis with the two highly ranked. Van Wyk [117] highlighted Fabaceae and Apocynaceae as the dominant commercially used plant families in sub-Saharan countries. With notable plant families, Rubiaceae (n = 7) and Malvaceae (n = 6) exhibit a narrow gap between them. One feature of this study is the fact that each family represented had at least a plant that can be used to deal with diarrhoeal diseases. The overview findings show a wide diversity and plethora of plant species in Zimbabwe. According to Maroyi [118], *Sclerocarya birrea* was the highly cited medicinal plant species in South Africa and Zimbabwe as an antidiarrhoeal remedy.

Zimbabwe is divided into various floristic regions according to **Figure 2** influenced by varying climatic conditions. Medicinal plant species distribution is important on the basis of conservation and propagation of these plants. Hotspots of crucial medicinal plants can be found all over the country. As a result of the varying climate, there are excellent growing conditions for diverse kinds of plants. Several climatic factors enhance secondary metabolites, while other abiotic factors reduce the growth of plants. As shown in **Table 1**, there were plants found in all the five floristic regions of the country: Northern, Eastern, Central, Western and Southern (N, W, E, C and S) (**Figure 2**).

Figure 3 reveals the medicinal plant's diversity across the five floristic distribution regions of Zimbabwe are defined by influencing factors that may include soil texture and rainfall patterns. Data show 86 plant species were found widely distributed across all floristic regions (N, W, E, C and S) of Zimbabwe. Therefore, at least 66.7% of the medicinal plant species are evenly distributed across the country. The remaining plant species were distributed in certain regions across the country with (n = 15) plant species distributed in four regions, mostly distributed in the N, C, E and S regions. Plant species (n = 18) were located in three regions, (n = 3) in two regions and (n = 3) in one region. Single regions were specifically notable from the E and N regions. Data also revealed that three of the plant species are cultivated, suggesting the potential for targeted cultivation practices within specific regions that offer suitable environmental conditions. No information was found from one plant species therefore requiring an insight and further research on its distribution. Taking the whole distribution patterns into account, the Eastern region seems to harbor most of the plant species.

Native trees and herbs that have been used by generations are well adapted to the local environment. The fact that most of the plants are native to Zimbabwe further cements the role and integration of traditional medicine in Zimbabwean healthcare systems as complementary and alternative medicine. Indigenous plants are well documented as slow growing and tough to propagate in the laboratory. As a result, any unsustainable use can result in the extinction certain plant species. Conservation of medicinal plants and biodiversity in general can be achieved through an integrated approach that balances *in situ* with *ex situ* strategies [113]. This is common for the roots being used. As with all living organisms in the biosphere, medicinal and aromatic plants (MAPs) are affected by climate change. Climate change may have particularly devastating effects on MAPs, due to their importance as alternative and complementary medicine and as beneficial plants for the economy [119].
The following plant species namely *Mangifera indica, Prunus persica* and *Musa spp.* were also found to be effective in treating and managing diarrhea. An advantage for using them is that they can be cultivated anywhere as they are exotic to the country's flora. This provides easy access to them for anyone in any of the regions of the country.

3.2 Growth habit of medicinal plants plant species used in the treatment and management of diarrhea by Zimbabwean traditional healers

Medicinal plants used to treat and manage diarrhea had a tree growth habit represented with 45.7% of the 129 plants studied. Several factors contribute to the high frequency of the use of trees in Zimbabwe as sources of herbal treatments. These factors include their abundance and ease of availability throughout the year. Shrubs (suffrutex or subshrub) were second in line at 27.1%, followed by herbs, at 14%. A notable number of climber or lianes we recorded, representing close to 10% of the growth habit. Growth forms such as epiphyte, root parasite, mistletoe and aquatic were the less prevalent growth forms as reflected in **Figure 4**. Considering the differences in distribution among plant growth forms, the review concluded that not all plant growth forms were equally used as remedies.

3.3 Parts used of medicinal plants plant species used in the treatment and management of diarrhea by Zimbabwean traditional healers

As shown in **Figure 5**, the roots have been predominantly used at 86.8% of the time, followed by leaves and bark with similar usage at 17.1%. The major parts used are a bone of contention among conservationists especially roots and the bark. In most cases, the root extraction process results in the plant being damaged or killed. Roots are the plant's ground anchoring component that contains numerous bioactive chemicals that have healing properties for many human illnesses. Scientific investigations have already contributed to the discovery of many phytochemicals from plant roots, some of which are presently in therapeutic use [120, 121]. The use of leaves is highly likely as these are more conservative to the plant.

The whole plant usage was at 1.6%, while the other ones were used partially as reflected by their low percentages. The use of whole plant may be attributed to the reported plant growth forms that include herbs as the second highest plant growth habit. Other growth habits used as whole plants also include root parasite, mistletoe and climber or liane. Plant parts such as the gum, pseudobulbs, stem bark, rhizomes and fruit were also found useful in the treatment and management of diarrhoeal diseases. Plant parts that include fruit, seeds and flowers are, however, seasonal and this directly influences accessibility and availability of these plant parts. Notably, the low percentages are also attributed to the rare plant parts in the category, for instance fewer plant species exhibit gum, rhizomes and pseudobulbs as plant parts.

3.4 Methods of preparation used of medicinal plants plant species used in the treatment and management of diarrhea by Zimbabwean traditional healers

The methods used to prepare herbal medicines may differ depending on the cost, location and culture. Plant materials may be used fresh or dried. With experience, a certain procedure is chosen to improve efficacy while at the same time reducing toxicity [122]. Extracts include highly concentrated cold and hot infusions. **Figure 6** shows the preferred methods used for preparing medicinal plants used to treat diarrhea in Zimbabwe. Among the investigated plants, infusion, a technique that involves steeping plant material in hot water below boiling point or cold water is the dominant preparation method, accounting for 44.9% of the medicinal plants. Decoction, a method involving boiling plant parts in water, represents the second most used preparation method, accounting for at most 20% of the listed plants. Powder (some were reported to be mixed in porridge) and medicinal extracts were reported to be 16.1% and 14.4%, respectively. Lower cases of mode of preparation such as raw form, concotions (mixtures with other plants), juice and soup (prepared with beans, groundnuts and/or meat) were also cited in their use. Mode of preparation also depends on the clinical condition of the disease as this directly influences administration of the medication. The most common method of administering medicinal plants and herbal medicine is through oral administration, but inhalation, intraperitoneal and dermal methods are also available [123].

3.5 Pharmacological evaluation of medicinal plants plant species used in the treatment and management of diarrhea by Zimbabwean traditional healers

Bioactive compounds from plants have emerged as promising antimicrobial agents in the fight against pathogenic microorganisms. Pharmacological studies have been conducted on most of the identified medicinal plants. The majority of the identified plants possess anti-inflammatory, antimicrobial, antioxidant, gastro-protective, anti-spasmodic, anti-diarrhoeal and prokinetic activities. Antioxidative properties of these medicinal plants help to protect the gut from oxidative stress and damage through modulating gut microbiota [124]. These pharmacological findings corroborate the traditional use of the identified plants as herbal medicine for diarrhea in Zimbabwe.

A variety of clinical diseases (cholera, diarrhea and dysentry) have been treated with the use of plant species, so it is vital to use scientific methods in order to gain an understanding of their pharmacological effects. Compounds from medicinal plants may inhibit bacterial, fungi, viral and protozoal growth through different mechanisms than those of currently used antimicrobials and may have therapeutic value in the treatment of resistant microbial strains [125]. Crude extracts exhibiting minimum inhibitory concentration (MIC) values below 1 mg/mL are classified as having significant antibacterial activity, while extracts with MIC values above1mg/mL are classified as non-inhibitors [126]. The findings from these studies suggest that several of the plants tested could be potential sources of novel antibacterial medicines, including those effective against antibiotic-resistant strains. Despite a number of successful studies identifying specific plant species as antimicrobials in *in vitro* models, it is imperative to subject these plants to animal studies as well as human studies to evaluate their efficacy [127].

3.6 Toxicological evaluation of medicinal plants plant species used in the treatment and management of diarrhea by Zimbabwean traditional healers

The science-based approach as described by Aydın et al. [128] indicates that many herbal remedies have a long history of use in traditional medicine, but their safety for humans should be documented by scientific evidence. It is expected that an understanding of the traditional uses of plant materials will be valuable for planning the experimental toxicity studies. According to literature, certain combinations of herbal drugs have been shown in most herbal traditions to reduce toxicity and others to increase it [122, 129, 130]. Toxicity tests have been widely developed to evaluate plant extracts, and among which are the tests using *Artemia salina* L. and *Allium cepa* L. as bioindicators. The acute toxicity test on *A. salina L.* is internationally used due to its great reproductive potential, easy acquisition on the market, easy hatching of specimens and good reproducibility [131]. *A. cepa* L. can be used to monitor the presence of toxic compounds, with the most analysed parameter being phytotoxicity, through determination of root growth inhibition, root weight and weight gain of the bulbs after exposure to a potentially toxic substance [131, 132].

The toxicological analysis revealed that out of 129 medicinal plants, 68 plants have documented toxicological evaluations, while the remaining 61 plants lack documented data. Therefore, further toxicological evaluations are critical for the 61 unvalidated plants as it is a concern as these plants are already being use for ethnomedicinal purposes without toxicity verification. For the 69 plant species with toxicological profiles, toxicity evaluation methods were used to assess these plant extracts activities. As highlighted by Aydın et al. [128], Kumari and Kotecha's [133] toxicity assessment of herbal medicines encompasses a set of techniques, including *in vivo*, *in vitro* and cell line studies, along with advanced microarray analysis. The Brine Shrimp Lethality Test (BSLT) and acute toxicity studies in rodents were the most frequently utilized methods for evaluating the toxicity of the 69 plants with documented profiles. As reported by Munodawafa et al. [27] and Erhabor et al. [134] findings highlight that the

BSLT and rodent acute toxicity tests were the most common methods used to assess the toxicity of herbal extracts. BSLT reported to be relatively cost-effective, quick, high degree of repeatability, simple and accurate toxicity [115, 135, 136].

Acute toxicity testing involves administering a single dosage of the tested product to each test animal. The animals' symptoms of toxicity and mortality are monitored for a period of 14 days in order to calculate parameters such as the maximum tolerated dose and the half-lethal dose [123]. Acute toxicity is evaluated using the half-lethal dose (LD50) according to Munodawafa et al. [27] and Erhabor et al. [134]. The *in vivo* assay half-lethal dose (LD50) relates to the dose of a substance required to cause mortality in 50% of the test population, typically mice or rats [27]. Based on LD50 values, plant extracts are classified into classes of acute toxicity. Those with LD50 values less than 50 mg/kg body weight are considered highly toxic, while those between 50 and 300 mg/kg are classified as toxic. Moderately toxic substances have LD50 values ranging from 300 to 1000 mg/kg, while mildly toxic substances fall within the 1000 to 2000 mg/kg range. Finally, plant extracts with LD50 values exceeding 2000 mg/kg are considered safe or non-toxic [64]. Researches by Loomis and Hayes [137] and Erhirhie et al. [138] have classified practically non-toxic lethal doses at 5000 to 15,000 mg/ml, declaring anything above 15,000 mg/ml to be relatively harmless.

Considering the ethical issues surrounding toxicological tests, alternative models should be substituted for animals whenever possible. The brine shrimp lethality test (BSLT) offers an alternative method for assessing acute toxicity [27, 134]. A significant contribution to the field of brine shrimp lethality bioassay is the maximum working concentration of solvents. Therefore, developing new solvents and detergents as well as carefully designing experiments will also contribute to the improvement of this assay [139]. This *in vitro* assay measures the median lethal concentration (LC50), which is the concentration of a substance causing death in 50% of the brine shrimp [27, 134]. Similar to the LD50 classification, BSLT results are used to categorize acute toxicity based on LC50 values [134]. Plant extracts with LC50 values less than or equal to 249 μg/mL are classified as highly toxic, while those between 250 and 499 μg/mL are considered moderately toxic. LC50 values ranging from 500 to 999 μg/mL indicated weak or low toxicity, and plant extracts with LC50 values over 1000 μg/mL are considered safe [114, 134, 140].

Out of the 68 medicinal plants with toxicological profiles, the results indicated that 47 plants (68.1%) are classified as safe or non-toxic, 9 plants (13.2%) exhibit weak or low toxicity or mild toxicity, 4 plants (5.9%) are moderately toxic, 2 plants (2.9%) are classified as toxic and 6 plants (8.8%) are reported to be highly toxic.

The toxicological evaluation data provide an insight on the need of caution in the use of medicinal plants especially for children, pregnant women and immune-compromised patients. The review has highlighted the ethnomedicinal use of *Grewia flavescens* and *Pseudarthria hookeri* in treating and manging diarrhea in infants; however, there are no studies scientifically evaluating their toxicity. On the other hand, the ethnomedicinal use of *Hoslundia opposite* (safe/non-toxic) and *Nymphaea nouchali* (weak or low toxicity) in treating and managing diarrhea in infants have been evaluated. *Euphorbia matabelensis* has been reported to potentially cause abortion, severe diarrhea and vomiting if administered orally. The presence of existing sesquiterpene lactones, polyacytelenes and thiophenes in *Aspilia pluriseta* may cause dermatitis and allergy. There are various elements that contribute to the toxicity of herbal medicine products which include plant components or metabolites with a toxic potential, adulteration, environmental pollutants (heavy metals, pesticides) or contamination of microorganisms (toxigenic fungi) [123, 127].

4. Conclusions

Zimbabwe has a wide range of medicinal plants that can be used to manage and/or treat diarrhea. This overview investigates on documented traditional knowledge regarding medicinal plants used by the Zimbabwean population for treating diarrhea. It adds valuable insights to the existing body of knowledge on Zimbabwean medicinal plants. Scientific research on medicinal plants for various ailments is on the increase in Zimbabwe. This study suggests that traditional healers are a primary source of herbal remedies knowledge for the management of diarrheal health conditions, inclusive of both mild and severe diarrhea. Understanding this is crucial for defining the appropriate role of herbal medicine in the healthcare system. Scientific evaluation of medicinal plant pharmacology and toxicology is necessary to validate their use in herbal medicine. This evaluation ensures the safety of consumers and paves the way for potential drug development based on these traditional practices.

Conflict of interest

The authors declare no conflict of interest.

Author details

Elliot Nyagumbo[1*], Trust Nyirenda[1], Cephas Mawere[2], Alfred Mutaramutswa[1], Godwins Ngorima[1], Donald T. Kapanga[1], Leroy Nhari[1], Marvellous Matsheza[3], Christine Midzi[3], William Pote[3], Fabian Maunganidze[1], Lucy Mabaya[1] and Michael Bhebhe[1]

1 Midlands State University, Gweru, Zimbabwe

2 Harare Institute of Technology, Harare, Zimbabwe

3 Great Zimbabwe University, Masvingo, Zimbabwe

*Address all correspondence to: nyagumboelliot@gmail.com

References

[1] World Health Organization. Diarrhoeal Disease. Who.Int. World Health Organization: WHO; 2024. Available from: https://www.who.int/news-room/fact-sheets/detail/diarrhoeal-disease [Accessed: August 01, 2024]

[2] Thystrup C, Majowicz SE, Kitila DB, Desta BN, Fayemi OE, Ayolabi CI, et al. Etiology-specific incidence and mortality of diarrhoeal diseases in the African region: A systematic review and meta-analysis. BMC Public Health. 2024; **24**(1):1864

[3] Troeger C, Blacker BF, Khalil IA, Rao PC, Cao S, Zimsen SR, et al. Estimates of the global, regional, and national morbidity, mortality, and aetiologies of diarrhoea in 195 countries: A systematic analysis for the global burden of disease study 2016. The Lancet Infectious Diseases. 2018;**18**(11): 1211-1228

[4] Troeger C, Khalil IA, Rao PC, Cao S, Blacker BF, Ahmed T, et al. Rotavirus vaccination and the global burden of rotavirus diarrhoea among children younger than 5 years. JAMA Pediatrics. 2018;**172**(10):958-965

[5] Zhou Y, Zhu X, Hou H, Lu Y, Yu J, Mao L, Mao L, Sun Z. Characteristics of diarrhoeagenic Escherichia coli among children under 5 years of age with acute diarrhoea: A hospital based study. BMC Infectious Diseases. 2018;**18**:1-10

[6] Wolde D, Tilahun GA, Kotiso KS, Medhin G, Eguale T. The burden of diarrhoeal diseases and its associated factors among under-five children in Welkite town: A community based cross-sectional study. International Journal of Public Health. 2022; **67**:1-9

[7] Tareke AA, Enyew EB, Takele BA. Pooled prevalence and associated factors of diarrhoea among under-five years children in East Africa: A multilevel logistic regression analysis. PLoS One. 2022;**17**(4):1-16

[8] Garatsa C, Mohammadnezhad M, Kostrzynska EB, Nwankwo B, Hagan VM. Risk factors of diarrhoea among under-five children in Zimbabwe: A systematic review. American Journal of Biomedical Science & Research. 2023;**19**(3):334

[9] Moyo TM, Juru TP, Sibanda E, Marape G, Gombe NT, Govha E, et al. Risk factors for contracting watery diarrhoea in Mzilikazi, Bulawayo City, Zimbabwe, 2020: A case control study. Pan African Medical Journal. 2022;**41**(145)

[10] World Health Organization. How Vaccines Can Help to Prevent Antibiotic Resistance - Zimbabwe's Response to Drug-Resistant Outbreaks of Typhoid and Cholera. Who.Int. World Health Organization: WHO; 2021 https://www.who.int/news/item/11-09-2021-stories-from-the-field-how-vaccines-can-help-to-prevent-antibiotic-resistance—zimbabwe-s-response-to-drug-resistant-outbreaks-of-typhoid-and-cholera [Accessed: August 01, 2024]

[11] Mashe T, Chaibva BV, Nair P, Sani KA, Jallow M, Tarupiwa A, et al. Descriptive epidemiology of the cholera outbreak in Zimbabwe 2018–2019: Role of multi-sectorial approach in cholera epidemic control. BMJ Open. 2023;**13**(1): e059134

[12] Mashe T, Domman D, Tarupiwa A, Manangazira P, Phiri I, Masunda K, et al. Highly resistant cholera outbreak strain in Zimbabwe. New England Journal of Medicine. 2020;**383**(7):687-689

[13] Governa P, Baini G, Borgonetti V, Cettolin G, Giachetti D, Magnano AR, et al. Phytotherapy in the management of diabetes: A review. Molecules. 2018; **23**(1):105

[14] Nasim N, Sandeep IS, Mohanty S. Plant-derived natural products for drug discovery: Current approaches and prospects. The Nucleus. 2022;**65**(3): 399-411

[15] Chaughule RS, Barve RS. Role of herbal medicines in the treatment of infectious diseases. Vegetos. 2024;**37**(1): 41-51

[16] Nissen M. Factors responsible for increased use of herbal medicines and self- medication. Advances in Pharmacoepidemiology and Drug Safety. 2022;**11**(3):10-11

[17] Giacometti J, Kovačević DB, Putnik P, Gabrić D, Bilušić T, Krešić G, et al. Extraction of bioactive compounds and essential oils from mediterranean herbs by conventional and green innovative techniques: A review. Food Research International. 2018;**113**:245-262

[18] Maroyi A. Acacia karroo Hayne: Ethnomedicinal uses, phytochemistry and pharmacology of an important medicinal plant in southern Africa. Asian Pacific Journal of Tropical Medicine. 2017;**10**(4):351-360

[19] Adedapo AA, Sofidiya MO, Masika PJ, Afolayan AJ. Safety evaluations of the aqueous extract of Acacia karroo stem bark in rats and mice. Records of Natural Products. 2008;**2**(4):128-134

[20] Gelfand M, Mavi S, Drummond RB, Ndemera B. Zambeziana: A New Series on Culture and Society in Central Africa. 17. The Traditional Medical Practitioner in Zimbabwe: His Principles of Pratice and Pharmacopoeia. Gweru, Zimbabwe: Mambo Press; 1985

[21] Ndhlala AR, Ncube B, Okem A, Mulaudzi RB, Van Staden J. Toxicology of some important medicinal plants in southern Africa. Food and Chemical Toxicology. 2013;**62**:609-621

[22] Gundamaraju R, Hwi KK, Singla RK, Vemuri RC, Mulapalli SB. Antihyperlipidemic potential of Albizia Amara (Roxb) Boiv. Bark against triton X-100 induced hyperlipidemic condition in rats. Pharmacognosy Research. 2014;**6**(4):267

[23] Steenkamp V, Stewart MJ. Medicinal applications and toxicological activities of aloe. Products. Pharmaceutical biology. 2007;**45**(5):411-420

[24] Maroyi A. An ethnobotanical survey of medicinal plants used by the people in Nhema communal area, Zimbabwe. Journal of Ethnopharmacology. 2011; **136**(2):347-354

[25] Maroyi A. Traditional use of medicinal plants in south-Central Zimbabwe: Review and perspectives. Journal of ethnobiology and ethnomedicine. 2013;**9**:1-8

[26] Maroyi A. Annona stenophylla Engl. & Diels: Review of its botany, medicinal uses and biological activities. Journal of Pharmaceutical Sciences and Research. 2019;**11**(10):3385-3390

[27] Munodawafa T, Moyo S, Chipurura B, Chagonda L. Brine shrimp lethality bioassay of some selected Zimbabwean traditional medicinal plants. International Journal of Phytopharmacology. 2016;7(4):229-232

[28] Chinemana F, Drummond RB, Mavi S, De Zoysa I. Indigenous plant remedies in Zimbabwe. Journal of

Ethnopharmacology. 1985;**14**(2–3): 159-172

[29] Oko OO, Agiang EA, Osim EE, Asuquo OR. Toxicological evaluation of Aspilia africana leaf in mice. American Journal of Pharmacology and Toxicology. 2011;**6**(3):96-101

[30] Kebede S, Afework M, Debella A, Ergete W, Makonnen E. Toxicological study of the butanol fractionated root extract of Asparagus africanus Lam., on some blood parameter and histopathology of liver and kidney in mice. BMC Research Notes. 2016;**9**:1-9

[31] Amang AP, Baponwa O, Mezui C, Siwe GT, Vandi LV, Njuh A, et al. Effects of aqueous extract of root barks of Swartzia madagascariensis (Caesalpiniaceae) on acute kidney failure induced with gentamicin in Wistar rats. Journal of Medicinal Plants Studies. 2020;**8**(4):183-197

[32] Shirinda H, Leonard C, Candy G, Van Vuuren S. Antimicrobial activity and toxicity profile of selected southern African medicinal plants against neglected gut pathogens. South African Journal of Science. 2019;**115**(11–12):1

[33] Maroyi A. Utilization of Bridelia mollis as herbal medicine, nutraceutical and functional food in southern Africa: A review. Tropical Journal of Pharmaceutical Research. 2019;**18**(1): 203-209

[34] Namadina MM, Aliyu BS, Haruna H, Sunusi U, Kamal RM, Balarabe S, et al. Pharmacognostic and acute toxicity study of Burkea africana root. Journal of Applied Sciences and Environmental Management. 2020;**24**(4):565-573

[35] Gebrehiwot S. Evaluation of acute and sub-acute toxicity of hydroalcoholic extract of Capparis tomentosa Lam in swiss albino mice. Journal of Scientific and Innovative Research. 2018;7(3): 60-63

[36] Gebrehiwot S. In vivo acute and sub-acute toxicity study of root extract of Carissa spinarum Linn. in swiss albino mice. International Journal of Pharmacy and Pharmaceutical Sciences. 2019; **11**(6):62-65

[37] Gelfand M, Tredgold RC. Medicine and Magic of the MaSh. Cape Town: Juta and Co.; 1956

[38] Viol DI, Chagonda LS, Moyo SR, Mericli AH. Toxicity and antiviral activities of some medicinal plants used by traditional medical practitioners in Zimbabwe. American Journal of Plant Sciences. 2016;7(11):1538

[39] Saini H, Dwivedi J, Paliwal H, Kataria U, Sharma M. An ethno-pharmacological evaluation of Catunaregam spinosa (thumb.) tirveng for antioxidant activity. Journal of Drug Delivery and Therapeutics. 2019;**9**(4-s): 280-284

[40] Maroyi A. A synthesis and review of medicinal uses, phytochemistry and pharmacological properties of Cissampelos mucronata a. Rich. (Menispermaceae). Journal of Pharmacy and Nutrition Sciences. 2020;**10**(5): 213-222

[41] Tanko Y, Yaro AH, Isa AI, Yerima M, Saleh MI, Mohammed A. Toxicological and hypoglycaemic studies on the leaves of Cissampelos mucronata (Menispermaceae) on blood glucose levels of streptozotocin-induced diabetic Wistar rats. Journal of Medicinal Plant Research: Planta Medica. 2007;**1**(5): 113-116

[42] Mangoyi R, Mafukidze W, Marobela K, Mukanganyama S.

Antifungal activities and preliminary phytochemical investigation of Combretum species from Zimbabwe. Microbial and Biochemical Technology. 2012;**4**:037-044

[43] Masoko P, Picard J, Eloff JN. The use of a rat model to evaluate the in vivo toxicity and wound healing activity of selected Combretum and Terminalia (Combretaceae) species extracts. Onderstepoort Journal of Veterinary Research. 2010;**77**(1):1-7

[44] Yeo D, Bouagnon R, Djyh BN, Tuo C, N'guessan JD. Acute and subacute toxic study of aqueous leaf extract of Combretum molle. Tropical Journal of Pharmaceutical Research. 2012;**11**(2):217-223

[45] Masocha M, Kariaga BM. Identification of medicinal plants used in the treatment of human abdominal diseases: The case of Mutirikwi communal area of Masvingo, Zimbabwe. Geographical Journal of Zimbabwe. 2001 (32):1-0.

[46] Chigora P, Masocha R, Mutenheri F. The role of indigenous medicinal knowledge (IMK) in the treatment of ailments in rural Zimbabwe: The case of Mutirikwi communal lands. Journal of sustainable development in Africa. 2007; **9**(2):26-43

[47] Salawu OA, Chindo BA, Tijani AY, Obidike IC, Salawu TA, Akingbasote AJ. Acute and sub-acute toxicological evaluation of the methanolic stem bark extract of Crossopteryx febrifuga in rats. Afr. J. Pharm. and Pharmacol. 2009; **3**(12):621-626

[48] Mangoyi R, Mukanganyama S. In vitro antifungal activities of selected medicinal plants from Zimbabwe against Candida albicans and Candida krusei. The African Journal of Plant Science and Biotechnology. 2011;**5**(1):1-7

[49] Babu PS, Krishna V, Maruthi KR, Shankarmurthy K, Babu RK. Evaluation of acute toxicity and hepatoprotective activity of the methanolic extract of Dichrostachys cinerea (Wight and Arn.) leaves. Pharmacognosy Research. 2011; **3**(1):40

[50] Maroyi A. Dicoma anomala Sond.: A review of its botany, ethnomedicine, phytochemistry and pharmacology. Asian Journal of Pharmaceutical and Clinical Research. 2018;**11**:70-77

[51] Balogun FO, Tom Ashafa AO. Acute and subchronic oral toxicity evaluation of aqueous root extract of Dicoma anomala Sond. in Wistar rats. Evidence-Based Complementary and Alternative Medicine. 2016;**2016**(1):3509323

[52] Munissi J. Cytotoxic and antimicrobial activities of the constituents of ten Plant species from Tanzania. Tanzania Journal of Science. 2019;**45**(1):44-52

[53] Viol DI. Screening of Traditional Medicinal Plants from Zimbabwe for Photochemistry, Antioxidant, Antimicrobial, Antiviral and Toxicological Activities (Doctoral dissertation). Harare, Zimbabwe: University of Zimbabwe; 2009

[54] Wild H, Gelfand M. Some native herbal remedies at present in use in Mashonaland. Central African Journal of Medicine. 1959;**5**(6):292-305

[55] Maroyi A. Elephantorrhiza elephantina: Traditional uses, phytochemistry, and pharmacology of an important medicinal plant species in southern Africa. Evidence-Based Complementary and Alternative Medicine. 2017;**2017**(1):6403905

[56] Maphosa V, Masika PJ, Moyo B. Toxicity evaluation of the aqueous extract of the rhizome of Elephantorrhiza elephantina (Burch.) Skeels.(Fabaceae), in rats. Food and Chemical Toxicology. 2010;**48**(1): 196-201

[57] Maroyi A. Phytochemical and ethnopharmacological review of Elephantorrhiza goetzei (harms) harms. Asian Pacific Journal of Tropical Medicine. 2017;**10**(2):107-113

[58] Woldemedhin B, Nedi T, Shibeshi W, Sisay M. Evaluation of the diuretic activity of the aqueous and 80% methanol extracts of the root of Euclea divinorum Hiern (Ebenaceae) in Sprague Dawley rats. Journal of Ethnopharmacology. 2017;**202**:114-121

[59] Chavunduka GL, Gelfand M, Roberts RS. Traditional Healers and the Shona Patient. Gweru. Zimbabwe: Mambo Press; 1976

[60] Suleiman M, Kio AA. Antidiabetic activity of the leaves of Ficus sur Forssk (Moraceae) on alloxan induced diabetic rats. Saudi Journal of Medical and Pharmaceutical Sciences. 2018;**4**(1): 140-146

[61] Moshi MJ, Innocent E, Magadula JJ, Otieno DF, Weisheit A, Mbabazi PK, et al. Brine shrimp toxicity of some plants used as traditional medicines in Kagera region, north western Tanzania. Tanzania Journal of Health Research. 2010;**12**(1):63-67

[62] Ezeonwumelu JO, Matuki E, Ajayi A, Okoruwa AG, Tanayen J, Adiukwu C, et al. Phytochemical screening, acute toxicity and analgesic properties of aqueous extract of flueggea virosa's root in rats. Ibnosina Journal of Medicine and Biomedical Sciences. 2013;**5**(01):15-21

[63] Ibrahim SM. Toxicological profile of Grewia bicolor root extract. Journal of Pharmacy and Biological Sciences. 2017; **12**(1):52-56

[64] Malebo HM, Wiketye V, Katani SJ, Kitufe NA, Nyigo VA, Imeda CP, et al. In vivo antiplasmodial and toxicological effect of Maytenus senegalensis traditionally used in the treatment of malaria in Tanzania. Malaria Journal. 2015;**14**:1-7

[65] Akah PA, Odo CI. Hepatoprotective effect of the solvent fractions of the stem of Hoslundia opposita Vahl (Lamiaceae) against carbon tetrachloride-and paracetamolinduced liver damage in rats. International Journal of Green Pharmacy (IJGP). 2010;**4**(1):54-58

[66] Regina KM, Adama H, Jeanne M, Odile N. Ethnobotany and Ethnopharmacognosy of Lamiaceae species from Central Burkina Faso: Leucas martinicensis (Jacquin) R. Brown, Hoslundia opposita Vahl and Orthosiphon pallidus Royle ex Benth. American Journal of Ethnomedicine. 2015;**2**(4):219-232

[67] Maroyi A. Ethnomedicinal uses, phytochemistry and pharmacological properties of the genus, Kirkia. Tropical Journal of Pharmaceutical Research. 2016;**15**(11):2507-2516

[68] Maroyi A. Kirkia acuminata Oliv.: A review of its ethnobotany and pharmacology. African Journal of Traditional, Complementary and Alternative Medicines. 2017;**14**(2): 217-226

[69] Maroyi A. Lannea discolor: Its botany, ethnomedicinal uses, phytochemistry, and pharmacological properties. Asian Journal of Pharmaceutical and Clinical Research. 2018;**11**(10):49

[70] Gelfand M. African Background: The Traditional Culture of the Shona Speaking People. First ed. Cape Town, Zimbabwe: Juta & Co.; 1965

[71] Maroyi A. Medicinal uses, biological and chemical properties of wild grape (Lannea edulis): An indigenous fruit plant of tropical Africa. Asian Journal of Pharmaceutical and Clinical Research. 2019;**12**:16-20

[72] Maroyi A. Review of ethnomedicinal, phytochemical and pharmacological properties of Lannea schweinfurthii (Engl.) Engl. Molecules. 2019;**24**(4):732

[73] Reddeman RA, Glávits R, Endres JR, Clewell AE, Hirka G, Vértesi A, et al. A toxicological evaluation of mango leaf extract (Mangifera indica) containing 60% mangiferin. Journal of Toxicology. 2019;**2019**(1):4763015

[74] Hamed MM, Mohamed MA, Ahmed WS. Chemical constituents, in vitro antioxidant activity, oral acute toxicity and LD50 determination of Moringa oleifera leaves. International Journal of Pharmacy and Pharmaceutical Sciences. 2017;**9**(5):240-247

[75] Ugbogu EA, Ude VC, Elekwa I, Arunsi UO, Uche-Ikonne C, Nwakanma C. Toxicological profile of the aqueous-fermented extract of Musa paradisiaca in rats. Avicenna Journal of Phytomedicine. 2018;**8**(6):478

[76] Raja MM, Sethiya NK, Mishra SH. A comprehensive review on Nymphaea stellata: A traditionally used bitter. Journal of Advanced Pharmaceutical Technology & Research. 2010;**1**(3): 311-319

[77] Pandian S, Badami S, Shankar M. Hepatoprotective activity of methanolic extract of Oldenlandia herbacea against D-Galactosamine induced rats. International Journal of Applied Research in Natural Products. 2013;**6**(1): 16-19

[78] Haule EE, Moshi MJ, Nondo RS, Mwangomo DT, Mahunnah RL. A study of antimicrobial activity, acute toxicity and cytoprotective effect of a polyherbal extract in a rat ethanol-HCl gastric ulcer model. BMC Research Notes. 2012;**5**:1-9

[79] Mbunde MV, Innocent E, Mabiki F, Andersson PG. Ethnobotanical survey and toxicity evaluation of medicinal plants used for fungal remedy in the southern highlands of Tanzania. Journal of Intercultural Ethnopharmacology. 2017;**6**(1):84

[80] Mongalo NI. Peltophorum africanum Sond [Mosetlha]: A review of its ethnomedicinal uses, toxicology, phytochemistry and pharmacological activities. Journal of Medicinal Plants Research. 2013;**7**(48):3484-3491

[81] Olela B, Mbaria J, Wachira T, Moriasi G. Acute Oral toxicity and anti-inflammatory and analgesic effects of aqueous and Methanolic stem bark extracts of Piliostigma thonningii (Schumach.). Evidence-Based Complementary and Alternative Medicine. 2020;**2020**(1):5651390

[82] Suh SJ, Koo BS, Jin UH, Hwang MJ, Lee IS, Kim CH. Pharmacological characterization of orally active cholinesterase inhibitory activity of Prunus persica L. Batsch in rats. Journal of Molecular Neuroscience. 2006;**29**:101-107

[83] Agbogba F, Senou M, Tchogou AP, Lokonon JE, Sacramento TI, Medoatinsa E, et al. Ethyl acetate fraction of Psorospermum febrifugum Spach aqueous extract did not exhibit acute or sub-chronic toxicity. Experimental study on Wistar rats.

International Journal of Biology. 2019; **11**(4):123-129

[84] Moura I, Duvane JA, Ribeiro N, Ribeiro-Barros I. Woody species from the Mozambican Miombo woodlands: A review on their ethnomedicinal uses and pharmacological potential. Journal of Medicinal Plants Research. 2018;**12**(2): 15-31

[85] Sadashiv PS. Acute toxicity study for Ricinus communis. Der Pharmacia Lettre. 2011;**3**(5):132-137

[86] Anantharaman A, Priya RR, Hemachandran H, Akella S, Rajasekaran C, Ganesh J, et al. Toxicity study of dibutyl phthalate of Rubia cordifolia fruits: in vivo and in silico analysis. Environmental Toxicology. 2016;**31**(9):1059-1067

[87] Ali A, Aslam M, Chaudhary SS. A review a review on Pharmacognostic and therapeutic uses of Rubia cordifolia. Journal of Drug Delivery and Therapeutics. 2020;**10**(6):195-202

[88] Nyenya RT, Stedje B. Ethnobotanical studies in the genus Sansevieria Thunb. (Asparagaceae) in Zimbabwe. Ethnobotany Research and Applications. 2011;**9**:421-443

[89] Maroyi A. Sansevieria hyacinthoides (L.) Druce: A review of its botany, medicinal uses, phytochemistry, and biological activities. Asian Journal of Pharmaceutical and Clinical Research. 2019;**12**(9):21-26

[90] Maroyi A. Local knowledge and use of Marula [sclerocarya birrea (a. rich.) hochst.] in south-Central Zimbabwe. Indian Journal of Traditional Knowledge. 2013;**12**(3):398-403

[91] Ojewole JA, Mawoza T, Chiwororo WD, Owira PM. Sclerocarya birrea (a. rich) Hochst. ['Marula'] (Anacardiaceae): A review of its phytochemistry, pharmacology and toxicology and its ethnomedicinal uses. Phytotherapy Research: An International Journal Devoted to Pharmacological and Toxicological Evaluation of Natural Product Derivatives. 2010;**24**(5):633-639

[92] McGaw LJ, Van der Merwe D, Eloff JN. In vitro anthelmintic, antibacterial and cytotoxic effects of extracts from plants used in south African ethnoveterinary medicine. The Veterinary Journal. 2007;**173**(2):366-372

[93] Olorunnisola OS, Adetutu A, Owoade AO, Adesina BT, Adegbola P. Toxicity evaluation and protective effect of Rhus longipes Engl. Leaf extract in paracetamol induced oxidative stress in wister rats. Journal of Phytopharmacology. 2017;**6**(2):73-77

[94] Chacha M, Mbugi N. Acute toxicity, brine shrimp lethality and phytochemical screening of Lannea schimperi and searsia longipes. Journal of Chemical Health Risks. 2019;**2**(2):87

[95] Namadina MM, Abdullahi Y, Aliyu BS, Zakari SM, Hayatu M, Saifullahi U, et al. Pharmacognostic and toxicity study of Securidaca longipedunculata root. Jewel Journal of Scientific Research. 2019;**4**(1–2):52-65

[96] Mwonjoria J, Ngeranwa J, Kariuki H, Githinji C, Sagini M, Wambugu S. Ethno medicinal, phytochemical and pharmacological aspects of solanum incanum (lin.). International. Journal of Pharmacology and Toxicology. 2014; **2**(2):17-20

[97] Ganguly P, Gupta AK, Majumder UK, Ghosal S. The chemistry behind the toxicity of black nightshade, Solanum nigrum and the remedy. Pharmacology. 2009;**1**:705-723

[98] Iskandar I, Setiawan F, Sasongko LD, Adnyana IK. Six-month chronic toxicity study of tamarind pulp (Tamarindus indica L.) water extract. Scientia Pharmaceutica. 2017;**85**(1):10

[99] Mongalo NI, McGaw LJ, Segapelo TV, Finnie JF, Van Staden J. Ethnobotany, phytochemistry, toxicology and pharmacological properties of Terminalia sericea Burch. Ex DC.(Combretaceae)–a review. Journal of Ethnopharmacology. 2016; **194**:789-802

[100] Chivapat S, Chavalittumrong P, Attawish A, Bansiddhi J, Padungpat S. Chronic toxicity of Thunbergia laurifolia Lindl. Extract. Journal of Thai Traditional & Alternative Medicine. 2009;**7**(1)

[101] Irungu BN, Adipo N, Orwa JA, Kimani F, Heydenreich M, Midiwo JO, et al. Antiplasmodial and cytotoxic activities of the constituents of Turraea robusta and Turraea nilotica. Journal of Ethnopharmacology. 2015;**174**:419-425

[102] Maroyi A. Nutraceutical and ethnopharmacological properties of Vangueria infausta subsp. infausta. Molecules. 2018;**23**(5):1089

[103] Modirat AA, Akomolafe OS, Alabi OK, Ogundipe L, Omole JG, Olanisoye KP. Protective effect of methanol extract of Vernonia amygdalina (del) leaf on aspirin induced gastric ulceration and oxidative mucosal damage in rat's model of gastric injury. Dose Response. 2018;**16**(3): 1559325818785087

[104] Yougbare-Ziebrou MN, Lompo M, Ouedraogo N, Boubacar YA, Guissoun IP. Antioxidant, analgesic and anti-inflammatory activities of the leafy stems of Waltheria indica L. (Sterculiaceae). Journal of Applied Pharmaceutical Science. 2016;**6**(2): 124-129

[105] Mapfumo P, Mtindi K. Zimbabwe: Country Report to the FAO International Technical Conference on Plant Genetic Resources (Leipzig, 1996). Harare: FAO; 1995

[106] Maroyi A. Ximenia caffra Sond. (Ximeniaceae) in sub-Saharan Africa: A synthesis and review of its medicinal potential. Journal of Ethnopharmacology. 2016;**184**:81-100

[107] Maroyi A. Zanha africana (Radlk.) Exell: Review of its botany, medicinal uses and biological activities. Journal of Pharmaceutical Sciences and Research. 2019;**11**(8):2980-2985

[108] Ngugi DN. Study of Antiplasmodial Activity, Cytotoxicity and Acute Toxicity of Zanthoxylum Chalybeum Engl, and Vernonia Lasiopus o. Hoffman (Doctoral dissertation). Kenya: University of Nairobi; 2014

[109] Pamhidzai D, Isaac G. TLC separation, antibacterial and anti-inflammatory activity of extracts derived from Zanthoxylum humile roots. International Journal of Research in Ayurveda & Pharmacy. 2013;**4**(4): 482-486

[110] Zezi AU, Abdoulaye BB, Danjuma NM, Aliyu IS, Yaro AH, Musa KY. The effects of aqueous stem bark of Ziziphus mucronata on rat kidney functional status after 10 days daily treatment. International Journal of Pharmaceutical Research and Innovation. 2012;**5**:1-6

[111] Hyde MA, Wursten BT, Ballings P & Coates Palgrave M. Flora of Zimbabwe: Species Information. 2024. Available from: https://www.zimbabweflora.co.zw/speciesdata [Accessed: July 17, 2024]

[112] Shopo B, Mapaya RJ, Maroyi A. Ethnobotanical study of medicinal plants traditionally used in Gokwe South District, Zimbabwe. South African Journal of Botany. 2022;**149**:29-48

[113] Nyasvisvo DS, Nhiwatiwa T, Sithole R, Sande S, Chapano C. An ethnobotanical survey of plants used against host-seeking mosquitoes by communities in Mazowe and Shamva districts, Zimbabwe. Ethnobotany Research and Applications. 2024;**28**:1-9

[114] Nyagumbo E, Pote W, Shopo B, Nyirenda T, Chagonda I, Mapaya RJ, et al. Medicinal plants used for the management of respiratory diseases in Zimbabwe: Review and perspectives potential management of COVID-19. Physics and Chemistry of the Earth, Parts A/B/C. 2022;**128**:103232

[115] Nyagumbo E, Nyirenda T, Mawere C, Mutasa I, Kademeteme E, Mutaramutswa AM, et al. Medicinal plants used for the treatment and Management of Bilharziasis and Other Parasitic Infections Affecting Humans in Zimbabwe: A systematic review. Medicinal Plants-Chemical, Biochemical, and Pharmacological Approaches. IntechOpen; 2023

[116] Maroyi A. Medicinal uses of the Fabaceae family in Zimbabwe: A review. Plants. 2023;**12**(6):1255

[117] Van Wyk BE. A family-level floristic inventory and analysis of medicinal plants used in traditional African medicine. Journal of Ethnopharmacology. 2020;**249**:112351

[118] Maroyi A. Treatment of diarrhoea using traditional medicines: Contemporary research in South Africa and Zimbabwe. African Journal of Traditional, Complementary and Alternative Medicines. 2016;**13**(6):5-10

[119] El Gendy AN, Fouad R, Omer EA, Cock IE. Effects of climate change on medicinal plants and their active constituents. In: Climate-Resilient Agriculture, Vol 1: Crop Responses and Agroecological Perspectives. Cham: Springer International Publishing; 2023. pp. 125-156

[120] Das A, Dan VM, Varughese G, Varma A. Roots of medicinal importance. Root Engineering: Basic and Applied Concepts. 2014;**40**:443-467

[121] Chaachouay N, Zidane L. Plant-derived natural products: A source for drug discovery and development. Drugs and Drug Candidates. 2024;**3**(1):184-207

[122] Ozioma EO, Chinwe OA. Herbal medicines in African traditional medicine. Herbal Medicine. 2019;**10**: 191-214

[123] Jităreanu A, Trifan A, Vieriu M, Caba IC, Mârțu I, Agoroaei L. Current trends in toxicity assessment of herbal medicines: A narrative review. PRO. 2022;**11**(1):83

[124] Riaz Rajoka MS, Thirumdas R, Mehwish HM, Umair M, Khurshid M, Hayat HF, et al. Role of food antioxidants in modulating gut microbial communities: Novel understandings in intestinal oxidative stress damage and their impact on host health. Antioxidants. 2021;**10**(10):1563

[125] Vaou N, Stavropoulou E, Voidarou C, Tsigalou C, Bezirtzoglou E. Towards advances in medicinal plant antimicrobial activity: A review study on challenges and future perspectives. Microorganisms. 2021;**9**(10):2041

[126] Makuwa SC, Serepa-Dlamini MH. The antibacterial activity of crude extracts of secondary metabolites from bacterial endophytes associated with

Dicoma anomala. International Journal of Microbiology. 2021;**2021**(1):8812043

[127] Van Vuuren SF. Antimicrobial activity of south African medicinal plants. Journal of Ethnopharmacology. 2008;**119**(3):462-472

[128] Aydın A, Aktay G, Yesilada E. A guidance manual for the toxicity assessment of traditional herbal medicines. Natural Product Communications. 2016;**11**(11): 1763-1773

[129] Che CT, Wang ZJ, Chow MS, Lam CW. Herb-herb combination for therapeutic enhancement and advancement: Theory, practice and future perspectives. Molecules. 2013; **18**(5):5125-5141

[130] Williamson EM, Chan K, Xu Q, Nachtergael A, Burnel V, Zhang L, et al. Evaluating the safety of herbal medicines: Integrated toxicological approaches. 2015;**347**:47-49

[131] Coêlho MD, Maciel LT, de Fátima Kieko Ozaki T, Silva ME, Bozo LS, Consoli YA, et al. Ovicidal and toxicological effect of hydroalcoholic extracts of euphorbia milli var splendens, Synadenium carinatum Boiss and Tagetes minuta L. against Ancylostoma spp.: In vitro study. Journal of Parasitic Diseases. 2021;**45**:252-257

[132] Vujčić Bok V, Gerić M, Gajski G, Gagić S, Domijan AM. Phytotoxicity of bisphenol a to allium cepa root cells is mediated through growth hormone gibberellic acid and reactive oxygen species. Molecules. 2023;**28**(5):2046

[133] Kumari R, Kotecha M. A review on the standardization of herbal medicines. International Journal of Pharma Sciences and Research. 2016;**7**(2):97-106

[134] Erhabor JO, Komakech R, Kang Y, Tang M, Matsabisa MG. Ethnopharmacological importance and medical applications of Myrothamnus flabellifolius Welw. (Myrothamnaceae)- a review. Journal of Ethnopharmacology. 2020;**252**:112576

[135] Hamidi MR, Jovanova B, Panovska TK. Toxicological evaluation of the plant products using brine shrimp (Artemia salina L.) model. Macedonian Pharmaceutical Bulletin/Makedonsko Farmacevtski Bilten. 2014;**60**(1):9-18

[136] Pohan DJ, Marantuan RS, Djojosaputro M. Toxicity test of strong drug using the BSLT (brine shrimp lethality test) method. International Journal of Health Sciences and Research. 2023;**13**(2):203-209

[137] Loomis TA, Hayes AW. Toxicologic testing methods. In: Loomis's Essentials of Toxicology. San Diego, CA: Academic Press, Inc.; 1996. pp. 205-248

[138] Erhirhie EO, Ihekwereme CP, Ilodigwe EE. Advances in acute toxicity testing: Strengths, weaknesses and regulatory acceptance. Interdisciplinary Toxicology. 2018;**11**(1):5-12

[139] Wu C. An important player in brine shrimp lethality bioassay: The solvent. Journal of Advanced Pharmaceutical Technology & Research. 2014;**5**(1):57

[140] Bussmann RW, Malca G, Glenn A, Sharon D, Nilsen B, Parris B, et al. Toxicity of medicinal plants used in traditional medicine in northern Peru. Journal of Ethnopharmacology. 2011; **137**(1):121-140

Chapter 4

Emerging Role of Medicinal Herbs on Alzheimer's Disease and Memory Deficits

Sadaf Naeem, Saira Saeed Khan, Yousra Shafiq and Sadia Suri Kashif

Abstract

Alzheimer's disease (AD) is an age-related neurodegenerative disorder characterized by memory deficits. It is associated with the presence of intracellular neurofibrillary tangles (NFTs) and extracellular amyloid beta plaques, loss of neuronal subpopulations, cholinergic fibers, and microglial inactivation. According to studies, from the year 2000–2020, the death toll attributed to AD increased by 146.2%, and its major causes are neurodegeneration and oxidative stress (OS). Currently, available treatment options are limited, and there is no cure for Alzheimer's disease. In Asia, such as in China and India, herbal medicines have been used in the treatment of neurodegenerative diseases for thousands of years, which has recently attracted considerable attention due to the development of curative drugs for AD. In this chapter, we first summarized the pathogenic factors of AD and secondly, we summarized herbal medicines that have been extensively investigated in both AD models and clinical trials. Also, we specified the potential targets of the herbs in view of the signaling pathways that are implicated in oxidative and inflammatory stress in AD pathogenesis. We consider that this knowledge of herbal medicines can be favorable for the development of disease-modifying drugs for AD.

Keywords: Alzheimer's disease, neurofibrillary tangles, herbal medicine, neuroinflammation, memory enhancer

1. Introduction

Alzheimer's disease is a type of dementia that progressively destroys memory, logical ability, and cognitive abilities that make our lives difficult. Approximately 60–80% of patients with dementia have Alzheimer's disease. The global number of patients having AD was approximated to be nearly 50 million in 2019, with predictions indicating that this might increase to 110 million by 2050 [1]. The risk of Alzheimer's disease begins in the early thirties, and rarely in the mid-sixties, however, it is primarily caused in older people because risk factors increase with age, and the majority of people with Alzheimer's disease are over the age of 65 years [2]. Alzheimer's disease manifests as a progressive decline in cognitive abilities, driven by the presence of senile plaques in the hippocampal region of the brain, that leads to the decline in dendritic arborization as well as neurotransmitter levels, resulting in progressive neuron loss and brain volume [3]. Neuronal loss generates abnormal deposition of hyperphosphorylated tau proteins and amyloid-β (Aβ), increased oxidative stress, and genetic susceptibility. Eventually, with the progression of AD, a significant change detected in the brains of patients involves a decline in the cortical and hippocampal levels of acetylcholine (ACh). Behaviorally, this substantial acetylcholine level decline results in impaired cognitive function [4]. Individuals may experience irritability, hostility, and frustration. In extreme cases, Alzheimer's results in complete incontinence, a disconnection from time and place, and total memory loss, rendering patients totally dependent on others and in need of intensive care. The enzyme, acetylcholinesterase plays a key role in terminating impulse transmission by quickly hydrolyzing the neurotransmitter acetylcholine in various cholinergic pathways centrally and peripherally. The enzyme inactivation by various inhibitors results in acetylcholine accumulation, overstimulation of muscarinic and nicotinic receptors as well as disrupted neurotransmission. Therefore, acetylcholinesterase inhibitors, which interact with the enzyme, are used as significant drugs and toxins [5].

Medicinal Herbs can provide neuroprotection, implying that their bioactive compounds may affect the underlying pathological Alzheimer's disease pathways by diminishing oxidative stress and limiting inflammation [6]. Medicinal herbs serve several potential strategies for diminishing Alzheimer's disease progression and managing symptoms. The production and commercialization of medicines derived from medicinal plants have gained momentum, enhancing their financial and scientific significance in the healthcare sector [7]. In this chapter, our goal is to highlight the significance of medicinal plants in the context of treating Alzheimer's disease, prevention, and challenges to herbal remedies in treating AD. Furthermore, by integrating traditional knowledge with modern scientific research, our aim is to shed light on the potential therapeutic benefits of medicinal plants, providing a holistic perspective of their relevance in Alzheimer's disease treatment. Moreover, we focus on explaining the mechanisms by which these plants act in Alzheimer's disease treatment, bridging gaps and exploring the precise pathways by which their effects are generated.

2. Pathogenesis of Alzheimer's disease progression

Alzheimer's disease is an advanced neurodegenerative illness characterized by dementia. It is an irreversible and progressive disorder affecting the aging population worldwide. Several factors like tau hyperphosphorylation, Aβ peptide abnormal metabolism, oxidative stress, cholinergic neuron damage, and other pathological events may contribute to AD [8]. In addition, demographic factors, like age, are a main risk factor, since the prevalence of AD rises exponentially between 65 and 85 years, and doubles every 5 years. Similarly, the APOE-ε4 allele is a genetic, prevalent risk factor for AD [9]. Other factors like hypertension, physical activity, educational level, diabetes mellitus, increased cholesterol, and homocysteine levels may also contribute to AD. During the middle stages of AD, neuropsychiatric and behavioral symptoms like depression, anxiety, and sleep problems are usually developed [10].

AD pathogenesis involves the amyloid events theory based on amyloid beta (Aβ) plaque deposition and the presence of abnormal tau tangles within the brain.

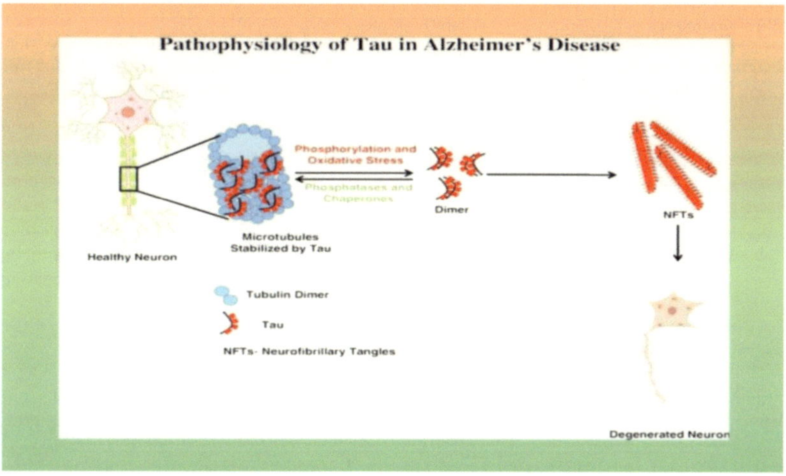

Figure 1.
Schematic diagram displaying pathophysiology of Alzheimer's disease [11].

The pathological AD hallmarks include NFTs (neurofibrillary tangles present intracellularly) and extracellular Aβ plaques (formed from Aβ peptides). Aβ lies consequently to APP (amyloid precursor protein), which is a bulky protein, generates Aβ after cleavage in the presence of proteases including α, β and γ secretase (**Figure 1**) [12, 13].

3. Available treatment options for Alzheimer's disease

Currently, known available drugs for AD treatment are acetylcholine-esterase inhibitors (donepezil, rivastigmine, and galantamine), N-methyl-D-aspartate (NMDA) receptor antagonist (Memantine), and Aβ plaques inhibitors (Lecanemab, Donanemab) are the FDA-approved drugs. The selective serotonin reuptake inhibitors are also used to treat anxiety and depression which is a comorbid symptom called behavioral and psychotic symptoms of dementia. The drugs with less anticholinergic effect (citalopram, sertraline, and escitalopram) is useful to overcome this anxiety. Antipsychotic drugs should be given to the patients as per risk-based assessment. Recently γ-secretase enzyme inhibitor (semagacestat) has been used as a target option because it blocks the cleavage of APP and reduces the production of amyloid β-42, but γ-secretase is also used as a vital agent for normal cell differentiation and communication. This is the reason it is not pursued in further clinical trials. Bapineuzumab, Aducanumab, and solanezumab are IGI antibodies that combine with soluble and fibrillar Aβ, activate the cytokines, and promote clearance by microglial phagocytosis. But they also cause cerebral hemorrhage and vasogenic edema, which is why they were stopped in a phase-2 trial [14].

3.1 Adverse drug reaction of anti-Alzheimer drugs

There are a number of adverse effects of the existing treatment of AD, Ach-E inhibitors, NMDA receptor antagonists, and other drugs that have shown the following ADRs (**Table 1**).

Several studies have shown that the adverse effects are higher with acetylcholine-esterase inhibitors (donepezil-10 mg and galantamine-24 mg) than with the NMDA

Available treatments	Related adverse effect
Ach-E inhibitors (Tacrine, Donepezil, Rivastigmine, Galantamine)	Nausea, vomiting, diarrhea, muscle cramps, fatigue, and weight loss, indigestion, muscle weakness, decreased appetite, dizziness, and headache
NMDA receptor antagonist (phencyclidine, methoxetamine, Memantine)	Constipation, dizziness, headache, diarrhea, and confusion
IGI antibodies (Aducanumab)	Amyloid-related imaging abnormalities (ARIA) can cause fluid rise-up or damage to blood vessels in the brain, as well as headache, dizziness, falls, diarrhea, and confusion

Table 1.
Table displaying available treatments and related adverse effects.

receptor antagonist (memantine). The above-discussed available treatments for AD are also not continued for long-term use due to safety issues and adverse effects [15].

4. Role of medicinal herbs for Alzheimer disease

The current existing therapeutic options are ineffective, have a high number of adverse drug events, and due to high costs have reduced patient adherence. Medicinal herbs are rich in polyphenols, flavonoids, tannins, glycosides, and other therapeutic agents that play a crucial role in diseases. In modern pharmacological research, the major components of herbal medicines (such as *Curcuma longa*, *Ginkgo Biloba*, *Withania somnifera*, and *Anisodus tanguticus*) indeed have been demonstrated to exhibit continuous and considerable effects on the models of AD [16, 17]. Over the past decades, the potential molecular targets of herbal medicine extracts have been extensively discovered, which will facilitate the identification of the bioactive compounds of the pharmacodynamic mechanisms of these herbs. Recent research explained medicinal herbs exert their therapeutic effects through several mechanisms, including antiapoptotic, anti-oxidative, anti-amyloidogenic, anti-Tau, anti-inflammatory, and free radical scavenging pathways, all of which aid in the prevention and treatment of AD Alzheimer's disease (**Figure 2**).

Different biomolecules, extracted from herbal plants display the key characteristics and properties to treat and prevent Alzheimer's disease. These include the fact that their metabolites can cross the blood brain barrier (BBB), exhibit a hydrophobic functional character, and associate with protein. Polyphenols are powerful anti-amyloidogenic, due to physicochemical features such as the presence of aromatic rings, molecular planarity, the capacity to form hydrogen bonds, and the presence of an internal double bond that allows potential inhibition of Tau formation and APP pathways, e.g., reducing amyloid load [18]. Phenolic molecules such as flavonoids, non-flavonoids, gallotannins, ellagitannins, etc., have the potential to modulate AD neuropathology and cognitive dysfunction through multiple mechanisms, including modulating oxidation and inflammation, modulating Aβ metabolism, catabolism, and oligomerization, and directly influencing brain activities [19]. Some of the polyphenol-rich herbs have been investigated for their neuroprotective role against Alzheimer's disease, like *Curcuma longa* (Turmeric) which has antioxidant, anti-amyloidogenic, and anti-inflammatory properties that make it useful in the therapy of Alzheimer's disease. *Curcuma longa* plant extracts have been shown in animal studies to inhibit the formation of tangles and plaque aggregation [20].

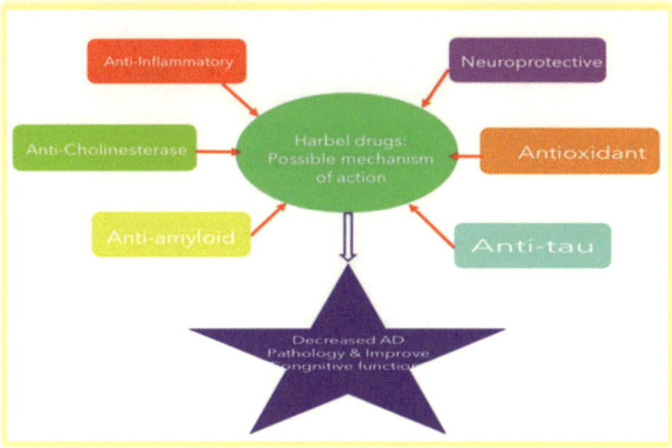

Figure 2.
Schematic diagram displaying possible mechanism of action of herbal medicines in the treatment of AD.

Similarly, *Ginkgo biloba* leaves are used to treat cognitive impairment in Alzheimer's patients. Flavone glycosides (24%) and terpene lactones (6%) are found in the plant extracts [16]. It was reported that it may protect neurons from senile plaque-induced neuronal death by inhibiting apoptosis, oxidative stress, glucose homeostasis, mitochondrial dysfunction, and activation of the extracellular signal-regulated kinase, and c-JUN N-terminal kinase pathways via glutathione, catalase, and SOD activity [21].

Similarly, Cascella et al. reported *Nigella sativa* extract contains thymoquinone that exerts significant antioxidant and anti-inflammatory properties, and could represent an effective neuroprotective agent against Alzheimer's disease [22]. A recent study reported that *Glycyrrhiza glabra* L. contains Glycyrrhizin, which is a natural inhibitor of HMGB1 and is reported with neuroprotective effects through oral administration against Alzheimer's disease [23]. Additionally, the species of *Salvia officinalis* (*S. officinalis*) and its constituent's activity was determined in mice, and memory improvement was observed due to a significant inhibitory effect of acetylcholine esterase [24]. It was reported that *Rosmarinus officinalis* contains a polyphenolic compound called rosmarinic acid, which reduces the accumulation of amyloid- β in mice and enhances the levels of monoamines in the cerebral cortex. Furthermore, *Ficus racemosa*, *Ginkgo biloba*, and *Tinospora cordifolia* have been reported to cause improved acetylcholine levels and mitigate memory deficits (**Table 2**) [31].

4.1 Herbs for anti-amyloid-beta plaque

There are several studies suggesting herbs as an ideal candidate to improve memory and slow down the pathological neurodegenerative cascades of AD [32]. Among them, *Centella asiatica* and *Camellia chinensis* are well-known herbal plants, abundant in alkaloids, triterpenes, flavonoids, and essential oils. *C. asiatica* is already considered for its memory-boosting benefits in traditional medicine. It has potent qualities to lessen oxidative stress, anti-inflammatory effect, capacity to regenerate neurons, ability to inhibit neurotoxicity, ability to inhibit Ach-E, and the capacity to decrease the amyloid plaques [33–35]. Moreover, leaves of *Ginkgo biloba* are reported to inhibit the formation of Aβ fibrillogenesis and guard against various insults that might harm neurons due to its rich phytochemistry, containing neuroprotective Ginkgolides, lactones, and terpenes (**Figure 3**) [36].

Plant extract	Year	Type of study/model	Findings	References
Effect of *Glycyrrhiza glabra* L. extract	2022	The water extract was assayed to determine antioxidant, cell viability against *in-vitro* glutamate toxicity model.	*Glycyrrhiza glabra* L. extract reduced glutamate toxicity with an antioxidant effect and provided neuroprotective effect.	[17]
Effect of *Cinnamomum zeylanicum* L.	2017	The aqueous extract of the cinnamon plant was evaluated using a monosodium glutamate-induced non-transgenic rat model of Alzheimer's.	Results revealed that plants show potent antioxidant activity. Significantly inhibited cholinesterase activity, and improved the learning ability in non-transgenic rats.	[25]
Effect of curcumin and *Ginkgo biloba* extract combination	2023	Evaluation of the beneficial effects of curcumin and *Ginkgo biloba* extract combination on a modified experimental model of AD.	Result indicates that the combination of both extracts successfully attenuates cholinesterase activity, and enhances its anti-inflammatory and antioxidant properties in preventing AD.	[26]
Effect of Green tea and its bioactive component (−)-epigallocatechin-3-gallate	2016	Prospective interventional study, 30 patients with severe AD were recruited and patients were treated with 2 g/day green tea pills in two divided doses	Results of the trial indicate that consumption of green tea for 2 months significantly improves antioxidant system and exerts a beneficial effect on cognitive function.	[27]
Effect of *Withania somnifera* L.	2020	Drosophila melanogaster AD model was used to study the effect of Ashwagandha on the toxicity of beta-amyloid.	Results indicate *W. sominifera* promotes longevity in AD as well as wild-type Drosophila.	[28]
Effect of ginger (*Zingiber officinale*) extract	2018	Molecular docking dynamic simulations of ginger extract as active inhibitors of human acetylcholinesterase enzyme.	Result indicates ginger components could be natural inhibitors of HssACh-E and can be used in the AD treatment, with a similar capacity of transposing the BBB.	[29]
Effect of *Gingko Biloba* extract	2006	Protective effect of *Ginkgo biloba* leaf extract on learning and memory deficit induced by aluminum in model rats.	The result revealed that Gingko extract can ameliorate learning and memory deficits induced by Aluminum, which may be due to inhibition of the Ach-E expression in the hippocampus.	[30]

Table 2.
Table displaying plant extracts and their reported findings.

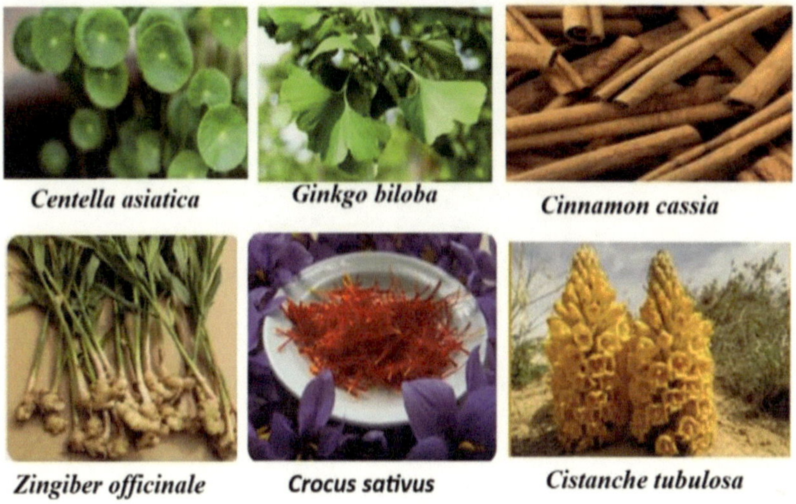

Figure 3.
Schematic diagram displaying herbs used for amyloid-beta plaque.

A natural compound called Cinnamophilin extracted from cinnamon extract considerably lessens the toxicity of poisonous β-amyloid polypeptide (Aβ) oligomers and shields neurons from their harmful effects [37]. It has been observed that the alkaloid piperine found in *Piper nigrum* has anti-amyloid and anti-Ach-E properties and has the ability to replenish antioxidant enzyme levels [38]. Similarly, in China, *Cistanche tubulosa* is already used as a botanical prescription medication for dementia treatment. A recent study suggested the phenylethanoid glycosides in *C. tubulosa* inhibit the deposition and aggregation of amyloid β peptide (Aβ), hence improving AD [39].

4.2 Herbs for anti-neurofibrillary tangles

Curcuma longa has curcumin, which is the most important active ingredient of the turmeric plant. Curcumin targets, Tau and Aβ, are the two histological markers of AD. Research has revealed that curcumin disintegrated neurofibrillary tangles, blocked Aβ aggregation inside the brain, and stopped the formation of Aβ oligomers [40]. Similarly, *Withania somnifera* is a highly valued herb in the Indian Ayurvedic medical system. It swiftly eradicates neurofibrillary tangles in the brain, which ultimately causes the reversal of behavioral abnormalities in AD transgenic mice (**Figure 4**) [41].

Lastly, leaves of *Ginkgo biloba*, worldwide potentially a known neuroprotectant showed inhibition of Aβ aggregation and amyloidogenesis and possess protective effects against tau pathology and neurofibrillary tangle formation [42].

4.3 Herbs for neurotransmitter modulation

Current pharmacological methods produce little impact on disease progression and treatment. Over the last decade, more than 200 intriguing therapeutic candidates have failed clinical trials, indicating that the disease and its causes may be exceedingly complicated [18]. Several scientific investigations have detailed the use of medicinal

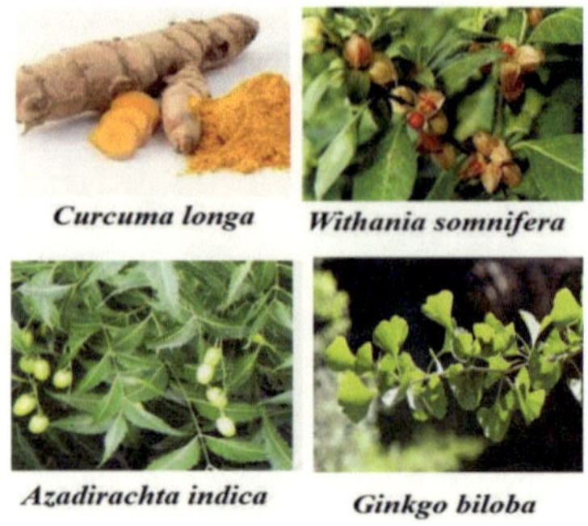

Figure 4.
Schematic diagram displaying herbs used for neurofibrillary tangles.

plants and herbs in the treatment of Alzheimer's disease. It is now envisaged that plants and herbs will be employed in drug development initiatives to identify safe and effective molecules for AD [43].

4.3.1 Glutamatergic system

The well-known traditional Chinese herb *Huperzia serrata* have the capacity to regulate both the glutamatergic and cholinergic systems. Researchers have shown that by inhibiting NMDA ion channels and the ensuing Ca^{2+} mobilization, plants can reduce the excitotoxicity caused by glutamate or NMDA [44]. Similarly, Panax Noto-ginseng and *Panax ginseng* have a potent protective impact on cholinergic and glutamatergic neurons as well as the ability to downregulate the expression of the APP gene in the brain and decrease tau protein hyperphosphorylation, and regulate glutamate release (**Figure 5**) [45].

4.3.2 Cholinergic system

Cassia species has a historic use in many traditional medical systems across the world. Several investigational studies reported that these plants have the ability to disassemble preformed fibrils inhibit Ach-E, and modulate the cholinergic system [46]. Similarly, plants and herbs in the Apiaceae family (e.g., *Angelica*

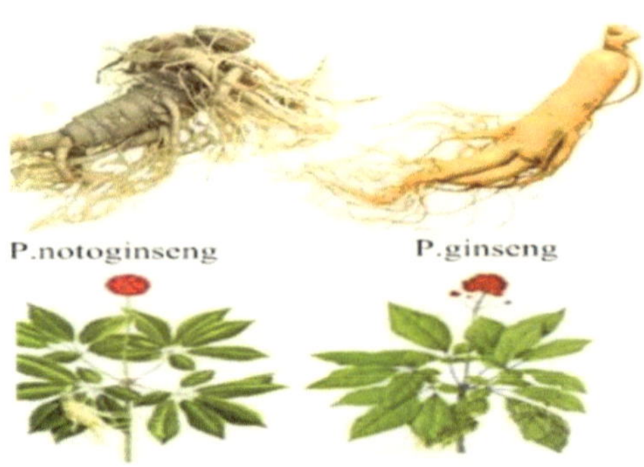

Figure 5.
Schematic diagram showing herbs modulating glutamatergic system.

archangelica, *Anethum graveolens*, *Carum carvi*, *Cuminum cyminum*, *Ferula asafetida*) are abundant in alkaloids, phenols, terpenes, flavonoids, furanocoumarin (i.e., xanthotoxin), essential oil, and α-pinene. Moreover, *Salvia officinalis* species and their constituents have also been shown to significantly suppress Ach-E and enhance memory. These herbs have the ability to inhibit acetylcholinesterase activities. Consequently, memory consolidation helps to prevent memory degradation (**Figure 6**) [47].

4.4 Herbs as anti-tau therapy

Many anti-tau natural products made by plants are polyphenols such as curcumin acts as an antioxidant and significantly increases the production of the anti-inflammatory cytokine IL-4 and reduces Aβ and tau levels in Aβ-overexpressing mice [48]. Furthermore, Sayad-Fathi et al., reported cinnamon (*Cinnamomum zeylanicum*) extract have the ability to inhibit aggregation of human tau *in vitro* leading to an inhibitory activity attributable to the cinnamaldehyde compound. Their study concluded that cinnamon improved cognitive performance in formaldehyde-induced dementia model rats by eliminating tau hyperphosphorylation, limiting inflammatory cytokines, and nuclear damage [49]. Zhang et al. demonstrated that *R. crenulata* extract effectively ameliorates p-tau expression partly by increasing the p-GSK-3β ratio in the hippocampus at 28 days after the Aβ1–42-induced AD model [50]. Similar procyanidins identified from grape seed (*Vitis vinifera*)-derived polyphenolic extracts were found to prevent tau fibrillization into neurotoxic aggregates [51].

The green tea (*Camellia sinensis*) derived (−)-epicatechin-3-gallate showing potent antioxidant and anti-inflammatory effects thereby reducing tau hyperphosphorylation and aggregation, thus preventing the formation of Aβ and its subsequent accumulation [52]. Further, Zhang et al. conducted a clinical trial on green tea and reported regular green tea consumption is associated with better cognitive function among Chinese middle-aged and elderly people, mainly reflected in memory and executive function (**Figure 7**) [53].

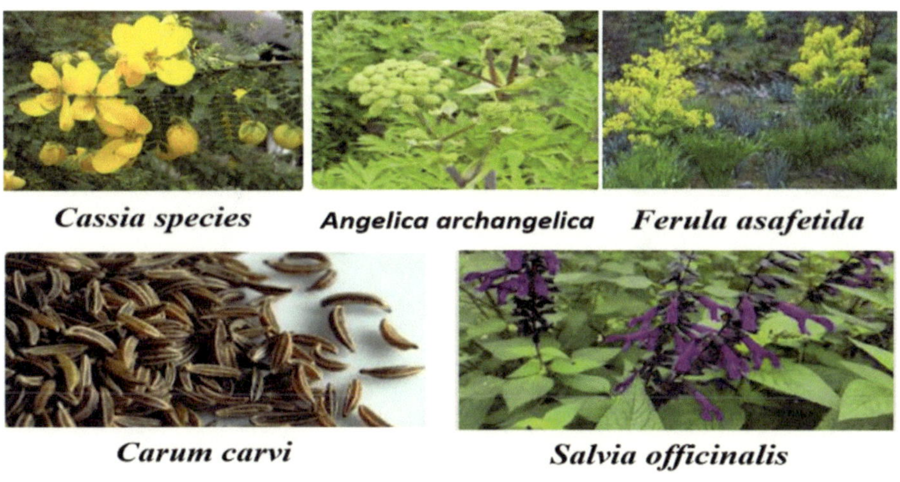

Figure 6.
Schematic diagram displaying herbs modulating cholinergic system.

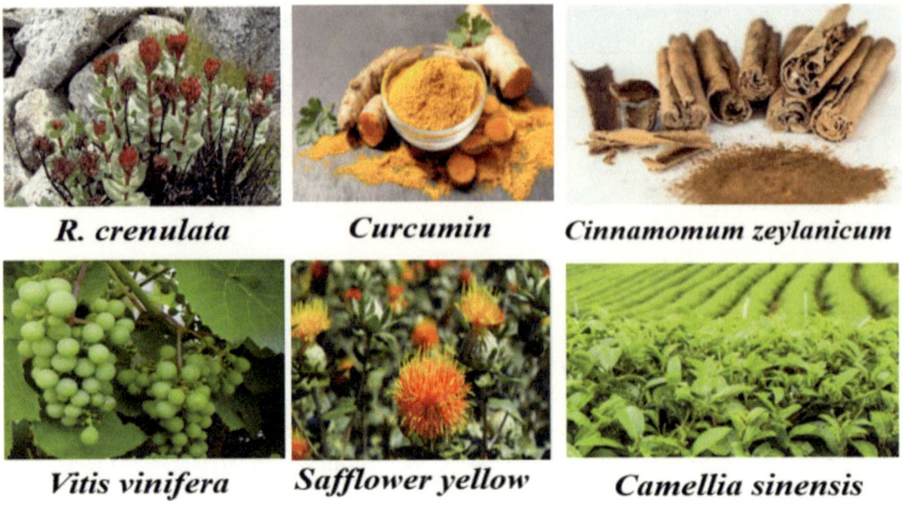

Figure 7.
Schematic diagram displaying herbs used as anti-Tau therapy.

4.5 Herbs for antioxidant effect

It has been discovered that the extract of the plant *Curcuma longa* enhanced the activity of antioxidant enzymes and prevented neurons from mortality. Likewise, garlic extract, which has been shown to inhibit ROS, caspase-3, and DNA fragmentation while shielding cells from programmed cell death [54]. *Vitis vinifera* and, *Arachis hypogaea* are plants rich in compound resveratrol, which shielded cells from reactive oxygen species and avoided DNA fragmentation. Similarly, it has been shown that the plant *Polygonum cuspidatum* inhibits the generation of ROS and DNA fragmentation [55]. Furthermore, Studies have shown that in normal rats, *C. asiatica* exhibits antioxidant and cognitive-improving effects (**Figure 8**) [56].

Moreover, numerous studies have shown that two compounds, quercetin and kaempferol are well recognized to increase resistance to acute oxidative and thermal stress in the central nervous system and to attenuate age-related buildup of ROS. These chemicals are majorly abundant in plant naming, Malus species, *Foeniculum*

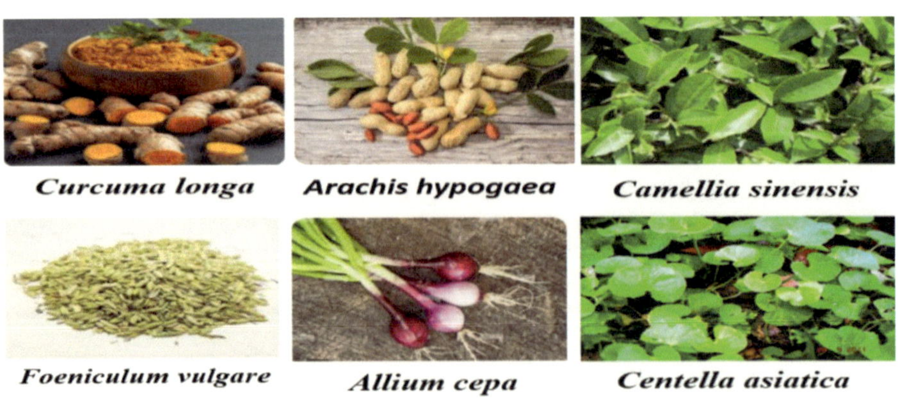

Figure 8.
Schematic diagram displaying antioxidant herbs.

vulgare, *Allium schoenoprasum*, *Asparagus officinalis*, *Brassica oleracea*, and *Allium cepa*. The majority of herbs and plants have also been clinically demonstrated to be effective in the treatment of memory impairments and Alzheimer's disease [57].

4.6 Herbs for limiting neuroinflammation

Several medicinal molecules have been identified from plants and herbal medicinal systems. Among them, *Coffea arabica*, *Tinospora cordifolia*, Cola species (i.e., *Cola acuminata* and *Cola nitida*), *Paullinia cupana*, *Ilex paraguariensis* are the plants that contain the chemicals caffeine and berberine, which are known to have protective effects on the blood-brain barrier. Experimental studies suggesting that caffeine may play a part in maintaining the integrity of the BBB, reduces the synthesis of pro-inflammatory cytokines, regulating microglia, astrocytes, and neurons, thus influencing neuroinflammation [57]. Similarly, *Bacopa monnieri* is a herb that has been shown to have anti-inflammatory properties in rats' brains via inhibiting cyclooxygenase (COX), downregulating TNF-α, inhibiting ROS, and reducing DNA damage in rat astrocytes (**Figure 9**) [58].

Numerous other herbs and plants might be significant therapeutic targets for reducing neuroinflammation. Among them are Magnolia obovata, *Cannabis sativa*, *Linum usitatissimum*, and *Zingiber officinale*, but enough mechanisms or cognitive assessment trials are unavailable and not reported [59].

5. Future perspectives

Recent developments at the interface of green chemistry and nanotechnology indicate significant potential in the biomedical sciences from theragnostic perspectives. Metal nanoparticles have received the utmost attention as anti-inflammatory agents owing to their capability of inhibiting NF-kB expression and following inflammatory reactions. Recently Zhang et al. experimented on aqueous extract of *N. khasiana* leaf silver nanoparticles and concluded these AgNPs could be considered as a potential candidate for the treatment of Alzheimer's disease [60]. Further, the conjugation of the drug-targeting approach with a nano-delivery system would allow the nutraceuticals to be in the proper place at the correct time, increasing the beneficial

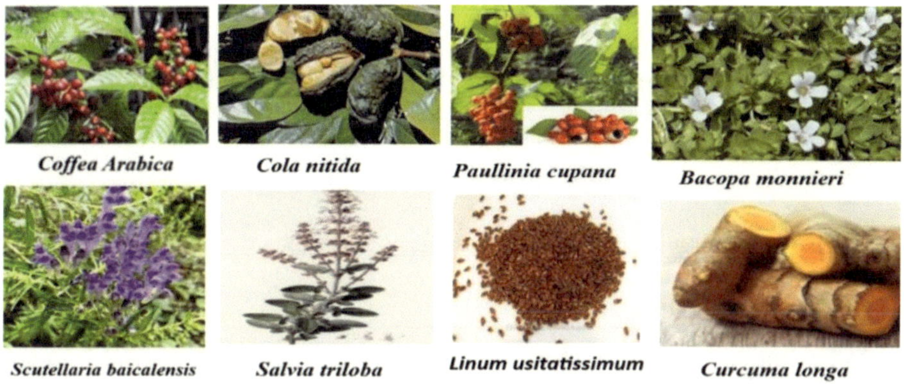

Figure 9.
Schematic diagrams showing herbs used for neuroinflammation.

effects, decreasing undesirable toxic effects, limiting nutraceuticals metabolism, and boosting their bioavailability. However, extensive clinical investigations (trials) are required to validate the efficacy of the herbal extract.

6. Conclusion

In this paper, we have reviewed more details about the management of AD and the medicinal plants with potential therapeutic values. Despite the bulk of knowledge regarding this complex disease, there is no complete cure except symptomatic treatment. So, herbal therapy is now anticipated to control AD progression help to enhance memory, and relieve other symptoms related to AD. Herbal therapy is relatively less toxic and can improve the quality of life of patients with AD and memory deficits. Current research must increasingly focus on the active compounds identified in crude extracts, to enhance precision therapy and to identify compounds that have different but synergistic targets and actions.

Acknowledgements

Sadaf Naeem gratefully acknowledges the support provided by Maheen Zahidi and Rashid Zaib during the course of preparation of this manuscript.

Conflict of interest

The author declares that the research was conducted in the absence of any commercial or financial relationships that could be construed as a potential conflict of interest.

Author details

Sadaf Naeem[1]*, Saira Saeed Khan[2], Yousra Shafiq[1] and Sadia Suri Kashif[3]

1 Institute of Pharmaceutical Sciences, Jinnah Sindh Medical University, Karachi, Pakistan

2 Faculty of Pharmacy and Pharmaceutical Sciences, Department of Pharmacology, University of Karachi, Pakistan

3 Faculty of Pharmacy, Ziauddin University, Karachi, Pakistan

*Address all correspondence to: sadaf.naeem@jsmu.edu.pk

References

[1] Ozgun DO, Gul HI, Yamali C, Sakagami H, Gulcin I, Sukuroglu M, et al. Synthesis and bioactivities of pyrazoline benzensulfonamides as carbonic anhydrase and acetylcholinesterase inhibitors with low cytotoxicity. Bioorganic Chemistry. 2019;**84**:511-517

[2] (NIA), NNIoA. What Is Alzheimer's Disease? 2021. Available from: https://www.nia.nih.gov/health/alzheimers-and-dementia/what-alzheimers-disease#:

[3] Farihi A, Bouhrim M, Chigr F, Elbouzidi A, Bencheikh N, Zrouri H, et al. Exploring medicinal herbs' therapeutic potential and molecular docking analysis for compounds as potential inhibitors of human acetylcholinesterase in Alzheimer's disease treatment. Medicina. 2023;**59**(10):1812

[4] Wynn ZJ, Cummings JL. Cholinesterase inhibitor therapies and neuropsychiatric manifestations of Alzheimer's disease. Dementia and Geriatric Cognitive Disorders. 2003;**17**(1-2):100-108

[5] Colovic MB, Krstic DZ, Lazarevic-Pasti TD, Bondzic AM, Vasic VM. Acetylcholinesterase inhibitors: Pharmacology and toxicology. Current Neuropharmacology. 2013;**11**(3):315-335

[6] Esfandiary E, Karimipour M, Mardani M, Ghanadian M, Alaei HA, Mohammadnejad D, et al. Neuroprotective effects of *Rosa damascena* extract on learning and memory in a rat model of amyloid-β-induced Alzheimer's disease. Advanced Biomedical Research. 2015;**4**(1):131

[7] Hassan NA, Alshamari AK, Hassan AA, Elharrif MG, Alhajri AM, Sattam M, et al. Advances on therapeutic strategies for Alzheimer's disease: From medicinal plant to nanotechnology. Molecules. 2022;**27**(15):4839

[8] Ullah R, Park TJ, Huang X, Kim MO. Abnormal amyloid beta metabolism in systemic abnormalities and Alzheimer's pathology: Insights and therapeutic approaches from periphery. Ageing Research Reviews. 2021;**71**:101451

[9] Kulminski AM, Shu L, Loika Y, He L, Nazarian A, Arbeev K, et al. Genetic and regulatory architecture of Alzheimer's disease in the APOE region. Alzheimer's and Dementia: Diagnosis, Assessment and Disease Monitoring. 2020;**12**(1):e12008

[10] Jeremic D, Jiménez-Díaz L, Navarro-López JD. Past, present and future of therapeutic strategies against amyloid-β peptides in Alzheimer's disease: A systematic review. Ageing Research Reviews. 2021;**72**:101496

[11] Gorantla NV, Chinnathambi S. Tau protein squired by molecular chaperones during Alzheimer's disease. Journal of Molecular Neuroscience. 2018;**66**(3):356-368

[12] Kamble SM, Patil KR, Upaganlawar AB. Etiology, pathogenesis of Alzheimer's disease and amyloid beta hypothesis. In: Alzheimer's Disease and Advanced Drug Delivery Strategies. Amsterdam: Elsevier; 2024. pp. 1-11

[13] Bhatia V, Sharma S. Role of mitochondrial dysfunction, oxidative stress and autophagy in progression of Alzheimer's disease. Journal of the Neurological Sciences. 2021;**421**:117253

[14] Vaz M, Silva V, Monteiro C, Silvestre S. Role of aducanumab in the treatment of Alzheimer's disease: Challenges and opportunities. Clinical Interventions in Aging. 2022;**17**:797-810

[15] Alzheimer's Association. FDA-Approved Treatments for Alzheimer's. 2024. Available from: https://www.alz.org/media/Documents/alzheimers-dementia-fda-approved-treatments-for-alzheimers-ts.pdf

[16] Nowak A, Kojder K, Zielonka-Brzezicka J, Wróbel J, Bosiacki M, Fabiańska M, et al. The use of *Ginkgo biloba* L. as a neuroprotective agent in the Alzheimer's disease. Frontiers in Pharmacology. 2021;**12**:775034

[17] Bayram C, Hacimuftuoglu A. Investigation of antioxidant efficacy of *Glycyrrhiza glabra* L. extract in glutamate toxicity-induced primary neuron culture. Anatolian Journal of Biology. 2022;**3**(1):18-24

[18] Gregory J, Vengalasetti YV, Bredesen DE, Rao RV. Neuroprotective herbs for the management of Alzheimer's disease. Biomolecules. 2021;**11**(4):543

[19] Spagnuolo C, Napolitano M, Tedesco I, Moccia S, Milito A, Luigi Russo G. Neuroprotective role of natural polyphenols. Current Topics in Medicinal Chemistry. 2016;**16**(17):1943-1950

[20] da Costa IM, de Moura Freire MA, de Paiva Cavalcanti JR, de Araújo DP, Norrara B, Moreira Rosa IMM, et al. Supplementation with *Curcuma longa* reverses neurotoxic and behavioral damage in models of Alzheimer's disease: A systematic review. Current Neuropharmacology. 2019;**17**(5):406-421

[21] Liu Q, Wang J, Gu Z, Ouyang T, Gao H, Kan H, et al. Comprehensive exploration of the neuroprotective mechanisms of *Ginkgo biloba* leaves in treating neurological disorders. The American Journal of Chinese Medicine. 2024;**52**(4):1053-1086

[22] Cascella M, Palma G, Barbieri A, Bimonte S, Amruthraj NJ, Muzio MR, et al. Role of Nigella sativa and its constituent thymoquinone on chemotherapy-induced nephrotoxicity: Evidences from experimental animal studies. Nutrients. 2017;**9**(6):625

[23] Eltahir AO, Omoruyi SI, Augustine TN, Luckay RC, Hussein AA. Neuroprotective effects of *Glycyrrhiza glabra* total extract and isolated compounds. Pharmaceuticals. 2024;**17**(7):852

[24] Teleanu DM, Niculescu A-G, Lungu II, Radu CI, Vladâcenco O, Roza E, et al. An overview of oxidative stress, neuroinflammation, and neurodegenerative diseases. International Journal of Molecular Sciences. 2022;**23**(11):5938

[25] Madhavadas S, Subramanian S. Cognition enhancing effect of the aqueous extract of *Cinnamomum zeylanicum* on non-transgenic Alzheimer's disease rat model: Biochemical, histological, and behavioural studies. Nutritional Neuroscience. 2017;**20**(9):526-537

[26] Assi A-A, Farrag MM, Badary DM, Allam EA, Nicola MA. Protective effects of curcumin and *Ginkgo biloba* extract combination on a new model of Alzheimer's disease. Inflammopharmacology. 2023;**31**(3):1449-1464

[27] Arab H, Mahjoub S, Hajian-Tilaki K, Moghadasi M. The effect of green tea consumption on oxidative stress markers and cognitive function in patients with Alzheimer's disease: A prospective

intervention study. Caspian Journal of Internal Medicine. 2016;7(3):188

[28] Halim MA, Rosli IM, Jaafar SSM, Ooi H-M, Leong P-W, Shamsuddin S, et al. *Withania somnifera* showed neuroprotective effect and increase longevity in drosophila Alzheimer's disease model. BioRxiv. 2020:2020.04.27.063107

[29] Cuya T, Baptista L, França TCC. A molecular dynamics study of components of the ginger (*Zingiber officinale*) extract inside human acetylcholinesterase: Implications for alzheimer disease. Journal of Biomolecular Structure and Dynamics. 2018;**36**(14):3843-3855

[30] Qi-Hai G, Qin W, Xie-Nan H, An-Sheng S, Jing N, Jing-Shan S. Protective effect of *Ginkgo biloba* leaf extract on learning and memory deficit induced by aluminum in model rats. Chinese Journal of Integrative Medicine. 2006;**12**:37-41

[31] Pandey SN, Rangra NK, Singh S, Arora S, Gupta V. Evolving role of natural products from traditional medicinal herbs in the treatment of Alzheimer's disease. ACS Chemical Neuroscience. 2021;**12**(15):2718-2728

[32] Sanka N, Santhipriya N, Nadendla RR. An updated review on anti-Alzheimer's herbal drugs. Journal of Drug Delivery and Therapeutics. 2018;**8**(6):360-372

[33] Sabaragamuwa R, Perera CO, Fedrizzi B. *Centella asiatica* (Gotu kola) as a neuroprotectant and its potential role in healthy ageing. Trends in Food Science and Technology. 2018;**79**:88-97

[34] Rho T, Choi MS, Jung M, Kil HW, Hong YD, Yoon KD. Identification of fermented tea (*Camellia sinensis*) polyphenols and their inhibitory activities against amyloid-beta aggregation. Phytochemistry. 2019;**160**:11-18

[35] Fernandes L, Cardim-Pires TR, Foguel D, Palhano FL. Green tea polyphenol epigallocatechin-gallate in amyloid aggregation and neurodegenerative diseases. Frontiers in Neuroscience. 2021;**15**:718188

[36] Luo Y, Smith JV, Paramasivam V, Burdick A, Curry KJ, Buford JP, et al. Inhibition of amyloid-β aggregation and caspase-3 activation by the *Ginkgo biloba* extract EGb761. National Academy of Sciences of the United States of America. 2002;**99**(19):12197-12202

[37] Rao PV, Gan SH. Cinnamon: A multifaceted medicinal plant. Evidence-Based Complementary and Alternative Medicine. 2014;**2014**(1):642942

[38] Sharma H, Sharma N, An SSA. Black pepper (*Piper nigrum*) alleviates oxidative stress, exerts potential anti-glycation and anti-AChE activity: A multitargeting neuroprotective agent against neurodegenerative diseases. Antioxidants. 2023;**12**(5):1089

[39] Chao C-L, Huang H-W, Huang H-C, Chao H-F, Yu S-W, Su M-H, et al. Inhibition of amyloid beta aggregation and deposition of *Cistanche tubulosa* aqueous extract. Molecules. 2019;**24**(4):687

[40] Abass S, Latif M, Shafie N, Ghazali M, Kormin F. Neuroprotective expression of turmeric and curcumin. Food Research. 2020;**4**(6):2366-2381

[41] Lerose V, Ponticelli M, Benedetto N, Carlucci V, Lela L, Tzvetkov NT, et al. *Withania somnifera* (L.) Dunal, a potential source of phytochemicals for

treating neurodegenerative diseases: A systematic review. Plants. 2024;**13**(6):771

[42] Dziwenka M, Coppock RW. *Ginkgo biloba*. In: Nutraceuticals. Amsterdam: Elsevier; 2021. pp. 835-852

[43] Rao RV, Descamps O, John V, Bredesen DE. Ayurvedic medicinal plants for Alzheimer's disease: A review. Alzheimer's Research and Therapy. 2012;**4**(3):22

[44] Ferreira A, Rodrigues M, Fortuna A, Falcão A, Alves G. Huperzine A from *Huperzia serrata*: A review of its sources, chemistry, pharmacology and toxicology. Phytochemistry Reviews. 2016;**15**:51-85

[45] Qu J, Xu N, Zhang J, Geng X, Zhang R. Panax notoginseng saponins and their applications in nervous system disorders: A narrative review. Annals of Translational Medicine. 2020;**8**(22):1525

[46] Singh A, Agarwal S, Singh S. Age related neurodegenerative Alzheimer's disease: Usage of traditional herbs in therapeutics. Neuroscience Letters. 2020;**717**:134679

[47] Sharma N, Tan MA, An SSA. Mechanistic aspects of Apiaceae family spices in ameliorating Alzheimer's disease. Antioxidants. 2021;**10**(10):1571

[48] Liu C-g, Wang J, Li L, Xue L-x, Zhang Y-q, Wang P-c. MicroRNA-135a and-200b, potential biomarkers for Alzheimer's disease, regulate β secretase and amyloid precursor protein. Brain Research. 2014;**1583**:55-64

[49] Sayad-Fathi S, Zaminy A, Babaei P, Yousefbeyk F, Azizi N, Nasiri E. The methanolic extract of *Cinnamomum zeylanicum* bark improves formaldehyde-induced neurotoxicity through reduction of phospho-tau (Thr231), inflammation, and apoptosis. EXCLI Journal. 2020;**19**:671

[50] Zhang X, Wang X, Hu X, Chu X, Li X, Han F. Neuroprotective effects of a *Rhodiola crenulata* extract on amyloid-β peptides (Aβ(1-42)) -induced cognitive deficits in rat models of Alzheimer's disease. Phytomedicine. 2019;**57**:331-338

[51] Ibrahim Fouad G, Zaki Rizk M. Possible neuromodulating role of different grape (*Vitis vinifera* L.) derived polyphenols against Alzheimer's dementia: Treatment and mechanisms. Bulletin of the National Research Centre. 2019;**43**(1):108

[52] Valverde-Salazar V, Ruiz-Gabarre D, García-Escudero V. Alzheimer's disease and green tea: Epigallocatechin-3-gallate as a modulator of inflammation and oxidative stress. Antioxidants. 2023;**12**(7):1460

[53] Zhang R, Zhang L, Li Z, Zhang P, Song H, Yao D-a, et al. Green tea improves cognitive function through reducing AD-pathology and improving anti-oxidative stress capacity in Chinese middle-aged and elderly people. Frontiers in Aging Neuroscience. 2022;**14**:919766

[54] Li F, Kim MR. Effect of aged garlic ethyl acetate extract on oxidative stress and cholinergic function of scopolamine-induced cognitive impairment in mice. Preventive Nutrition and Food Science. 2019;**24**(2):165

[55] Kaur A, Tiwari R, Tiwari G, Ramachandran V. Resveratrol: A vital therapeutic agent with multiple health benefits. Drug Research. 2022;**72**(01):5-17

[56] Veerendra Kumar M, Gupta Y. Effect of *Centella asiatica* on

cognition and oxidative stress in an intracerebroventricular streptozotocin model of Alzheimer's disease in rats. Clinical and Experimental Pharmacology and Physiology. 2003;**30**(5-6):336-342

[57] Akram M, Nawaz A. Effects of medicinal plants on Alzheimer's disease and memory deficits. Neural Regeneration Research. 2017;**12**(4):660-670

[58] Albohy A. 2023. Available from: https://www.sciencedirect.com/science/article/abs/pii/S0378874123004993?via%3Dihub

[59] Kure C, Timmer J, Stough C. The immunomodulatory effects of plant extracts and plant secondary metabolites on chronic neuroinflammation and cognitive aging: A mechanistic and empirical review. Frontiers in Pharmacology. 2017;**8**:117

[60] Zhang X, Li Y, Hu Y. Green synthesis of silver nanoparticles and their preventive effect in deficits in recognition and spatial memory in sporadic Alzheimer's rat model. Colloids and Surfaces A: Physicochemical and Engineering Aspects. 2020;**605**:125288

Chapter 5

Exploring the Antioxidant Activity of Selected Aromatic and Medicinal Plants

Amin Salhi, Chahid Zannagui, Abdellah Elyoussfi, M'hamed Ahari, Fouad Mourabit, Hassan Amhamdi, El Houssien Akichouh and Soufian El Barkany

Abstract

This study explores the in vitro antioxidant activity of three plants: *Pistacia lentiscus*, *Mentha pulegium*, and *Tetraclinis articulata*. Initially, we quantified the total polyphenol, flavonoid, and flavonol content in each extract. Subsequently, the antioxidant potential was assessed using DPPH radical scavenging, ferric reducing antioxidant power (FRAP), and β-carotene bleaching assays. Our findings revealed that the crude extracts exhibited significant anti-radical and antioxidant activities, correlating with their polyphenol and flavonoid contents. A linear relationship was established, with flavonoid-rich fractions demonstrating the highest activity. However, the intensity of antioxidant activity was solely dependent not only on the flavonoid content but also on their specific nature. Notably, the strong inhibition of lipid oxidation by the dichloromethane and ethyl acetate fractions, despite their low polyphenol concentration, suggested the presence of other bioactive substances. These include waxes, fatty acids, sterols, triterpenes, carotenoids, highly methoxylated flavonoid aglycones, and coumarins, which may act independently or synergistically. This study offers valuable insights into the complex antioxidative properties and potential health benefits of these plant extracts.

Keywords: plant extracts, polyphenols, solvent polarity, DPPH assay, FRAP assay

1. Introduction

Free radicals induce oxidative stress, leading to substantial damage to cellular proteins, membrane lipids, and nucleic acids. This harmful process has been associated with aging and numerous diseases, including cancer, atherosclerosis, and Alzheimer's disease [1, 2].

Due to this, free radicals and related species have attracted significant attention recently. Phenolic antioxidants, both natural and synthetic, have emerged as powerful compounds used extensively in commercial and biological contexts to prevent oxidation. The well-known antioxidant properties of phenolic compounds include their potent chain-breaking activities and their ability to neutralize radicals, which helps protect cells from the adverse effects of reactive oxygen species [3].

In recent years, the structure-activity relationships that determine the antioxidant capacity of these compounds have been extensively studied and clarified. Through experimental studies and quantum chemical analyses, researchers have rationalized these relationships [4–6]. It is well established that the radical scavenging effectiveness of phenolic compounds is significantly influenced by both the number and the spatial arrangement of their phenolic hydroxyl groups.

2. Methodology

2.1 Collection of plant material

The selected species were collected from Al-Hoceima National Park (The Rif) (**Table 1**). Their identification was carried out at the Faculty of Sciences at Mohamed First University.

Freshly harvested plant material was dried in the shade for 2 to 3 weeks before being ground into a fine powder. The resulting powders were stored in glass vials, labeled with the name of the species and the specific part of the plant, and stored in the freezer for preservation.

2.2 Colorimetric analyses by UV-visible spectrophotometry

2.2.1 Total polyphenol content determination

The total polyphenol content was determined using the Folin-Ciocalteu method described by Wong et al. [7], which detects a color change upon oxidation of polyphenols, with maximum absorption at 760 nm. After mixing 200 μL of diluted extract with 1 mL of Folin-Ciocalteu reagent and a 4-minute incubation, 800 μL of 7.5% sodium carbonate solution was added. Following a 2-hour incubation, absorbance was measured, and polyphenol concentration was calculated using a gallic acid standard curve, expressed as micrograms of gallic acid equivalents (GAE) per milligram of extract.

2.2.2 Determination of total flavonoid content

To quantify flavonoids in plant extracts, the method by Djeridane et al. [8] using aluminum chloride ($AlCl_3$) was adapted. After appropriate dilutions, 1 mL of each extract solution and standard (dissolved in ethanol) was mixed with 1 mL of 2% $AlCl_3$ solution in ethanol. Following incubation in darkness at room temperature for

Station	Collection period	Parts studied	Longitude	Latitude
Al-Hoceima National Park	May–July	Leaves	4° 00' 00" W	5° 20' 00" N

Table 1.
Geographical and bioclimatic parameters of the study.

30 minutes and absorbance reading at 430 nm, flavonoid content was determined using a linear calibration curve with quercetin as the standard. The results are expressed as milligrams of quercetin equivalents per gram of dry plant weight (mg QE/g DW).

2.2.3 Determination of flavonol content

The method by Kosalec et al. [9], with slight modifications, was used to assess flavonol content in various extracts. A mixture of distilled water, $AlCl_3$, CH_3COOK, and the extract was incubated, and absorbance at 415 nm was measured after 30 minutes. Results, expressed as milligrams of quercetin equivalents per gram of dry plant weight (mg EQ/g DW), were obtained from a standard curve prepared using a quercetin standard under the same conditions.

2.3 In vitro antioxidant evaluation

The complexity of phytochemicals in plant extracts requires diverse methods for antioxidant activity assessment. Three methods were used: DPPH radical scavenging, β-carotene bleaching, and FRAP assays. These methods rely on color changes, with absorbance readings at specific wavelengths.

2.3.1 DPPH stable radical test

Antioxidants' ability to reduce the DPPH free radical is tracked using UV-visible spectrophotometry, measuring absorbance decrease at 517 nm upon extract addition. Initially purple, DPPH turns colorless as unpaired electrons pair up, indicative of extract efficacy in neutralizing radicals irrespective of enzymatic activities (**Figure 1**). The stable radical substrate transforms to yellow DPPH-H upon antioxidant interaction, losing characteristic absorbance at 517 nm. Reactions occur at room temperature in an ethanol environment, aiding antioxidant solubility. This widely adopted, rapid, and cost-effective test holds paramount importance in antioxidant assessment and research.

In our study, we utilized the method by Moure et al. [10] to evaluate the activity. A DPPH solution was prepared by dissolving 4.0 mg of DPPH in 100 mL of ethanol. Various concentrations of sample and control solutions were added to 1 mL of the DPPH solution, followed by a 30-minute incubation period in darkness at room temperature. Absorbance readings were taken at 517 nm against blanks, and results were presented as the mean of three measurements ± standard deviation. Ascorbic acid

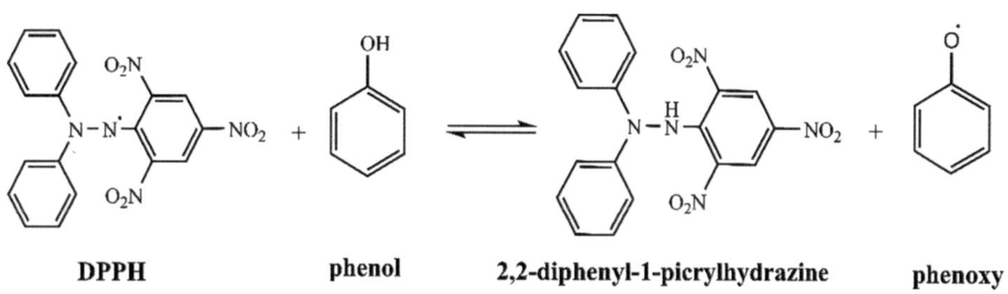

Figure 1.
Reduction of the radical by an antioxidant.

(vitamin C) and BHA (Butyl-hydroxyanisole, E320) were used as standard antioxidants for comparative analysis, with results expressed as percentage inhibition:

$$RSA\% = \left[Abs_{\text{control}} - Abs_{\text{sample}} \, / \, Abs_{\text{control}} \right] \times 100 \quad (1)$$

Additionally, studying the variation of radical scavenging activity with extract concentration allowed determination of the concentration corresponding to 50% inhibition (IC_{50}), where a lower IC_{50} value indicates stronger antioxidant activity against free radicals.

2.3.2 Ferric ion reducing power (frap)

The FRAP assay, based on Oyaizu's method [11], evaluates the reducing activity of antioxidants. This method measures the reduction of Fe^{3+} to Fe^{2+}, indicative of electron donation, a characteristic of polyphenol antioxidants.

To assess the antioxidant activity, samples at varying concentrations were mixed with phosphate buffer and potassium ferricyanide solution. Following an incubation period and subsequent termination of the reaction, the mixture underwent centrifugation, and the resulting supernatant was then combined with ferric chloride solution. Absorbance readings were taken at 700 nm against a blank. As a positive control, ascorbic acid solution was utilized.

This assay serves as a valuable tool for evaluating the reducing power of the tested extracts. Higher absorbance values indicate increased antioxidant activity, providing a quantitative measure of their effectiveness in reducing ferric ions.

2.3.3 β-carotene bleaching test

The β-carotene bleaching test evaluates antioxidant capacity by measuring the inhibition of oxidative degradation of β-carotene (bleaching) by linoleic acid oxidation products, as described by Tepe et al. [12].

A method by Kartal et al. [13] with minor adjustments was used. An emulsion of β-carotene/linoleic acid was prepared, followed by the addition of sample or standard solutions. The mixture was incubated in darkness at 50°C. Emulsion bleaching kinetics were monitored at 470 nm for 120 minutes. Antioxidant activity was determined using the formula:

$$\left(A_{St} \, / \, A_{S0} \right) \times 100\% \quad (2)$$

where A_{s0} is the initial absorbance and A_{St} is the absorbance after 120 minutes.

3. Results and discussion

3.1 Extraction yields of crude extracts

Extracts from the aerial parts of the plants were prepared using solvents of increasing polarity: hexane, dichloromethane, ethyl acetate, ethanol, methanol, and water. This process yielded six distinct crude extracts: hexane (EH), dichloromethane (ED), ethyl acetate (EA), ethanol (EE), methanol (EM), and aqueous (EAq) extracts.

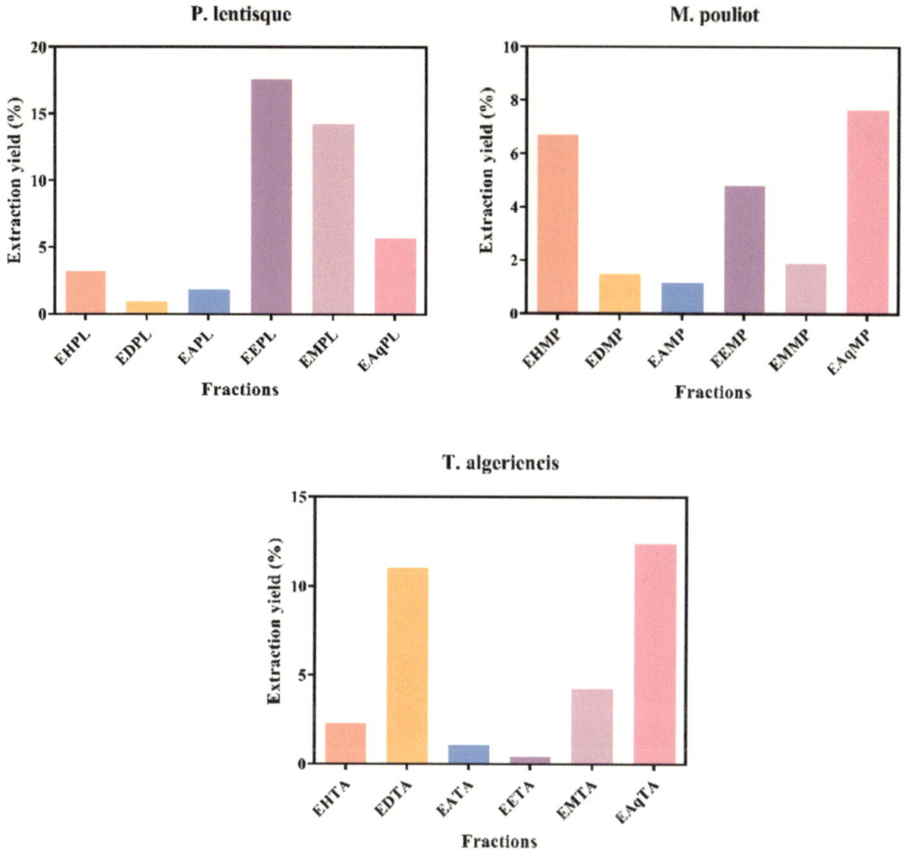

Figure 2.
Average extraction yields (%).

Extraction yields, expressed as a percentage of extract mass relative to the fresh plant mass, are shown in **Figure 2**. The highest yield was from ethanol leaf extract (EEPL) at 17.6%, followed by aqueous extract (EAqTA) at 12.4% and aqueous extract (EAqMP) at 7.6%.

It is important to highlight that the extraction method, including the choice of solvents and the conditions under which the extraction is performed (hot or cold), as well as the specific plant part used, significantly impacts the total phenol and flavonoid content. Consequently, these factors also influence the biological activities mediated by these metabolites [14].

3.2 Determination of phenolic compound content

The various crude extracts obtained through solid-liquid extraction (SLE) were quantitatively analyzed for their polyphenol, flavonoid, and flavonol content using a UV-visible spectrophotometer. The results are expressed in terms of gallic acid equivalents (mg GAE/g), catechin equivalents (mg CE/g), and quercetin equivalents (mg QE/g), respectively (**Table 2**).

The results indicate significant variations in the total polyphenol content among the extracts from different plants. Ethanol extracts exhibited the highest polyphenol levels, with values of 438.20 ± 3.32 mg GAE/g for *M. pouliot* and 70.40 ± 7.07 mg GAE/g for *P.*

Plante	Extrait	Polyphenols	Flavonoids	Flavonols
P. lentisque	EDPL	10.06 ± 0.06	5.81 ± 0.79	2.97 ± 0.10
	EAPL	24.43 ± 2.72	12.63 ± 0.18	7.09 ± 0.29
	EEPL	70.40 ± 7.07	32.06 ± 1.68	14.36 ± 1.68
	EMPL	36.94 ± 1.35	15.12 ± 0.88	8.12 ± 0.88
	EAqPL	62.90 ± 4.80	22.09 ± 0.76	11.61 ± 0.06
M. pouliot	EDPR	41.06 ± 2.04	14.21 ± 0.37	7.94 ± 2.92
	EAMP	51.65 ± 0.70	21.73 ± 0.46	13.62 ± 1.94
	EEMP	438.20 ± 3.32	138.80 ± 16.70	67.97 ± 0.04
	EMMP	270.38 ± 13.59	66.61 ± 17.45	24.87 ± 1.06
	EAqMP	188.70 ± 2.72	40.37 ± 1.06	18.72 ± 0.16
T. algeriensis	EDTA	10.12 ± 0.40	4.87 ± 0.18	2.88 ± 0.03
	EATA	24.13 ± 4.21	8.81 ± 1.32	5.38 ± 0.08
	EETA	147.80 ± 11.60	26.00 ± 1.77	16.96 ± 5.06
	EMTA	169.42 ± 8.16	34.0 ± 2.12	22.96 ± 5.06
	EAqTA	117.50 ± 16.30	17.31 ± 0.08	12.11 ± 0.09

Table 2.
Total polyphenol (mg GAE/g), flavonoid (mg CE/g), and flavonol (mg QE/g) contents of the different extracts obtained by SLE.

lentiscus. Methanol extracts showed the highest polyphenol content for *Thymus algeriensis* at 169.42 ± 8.16 mg GAE/g. In contrast, extracts obtained using solvents of lower polarity, such as dichloromethane and ethyl acetate, had the lowest polyphenol levels.

Furthermore, the data in **Table 2** reveal considerable variation in total flavonoid content across different plants. *M. pouliot* leaves had the highest flavonoid content (EE MP = 138.80 ± 16.70 mg CE/g), followed by *P. lentiscus* (EEPL = 32.06 ± 1.68 mg CE/g) and *T. algeriensis* leaves (EMTA = 34.0 ± 2.12 mg CE/g). Ethanol and methanol were the most effective solvents for extracting flavonoids from the aerial parts of the plants, while dichloromethane and ethyl acetate were less effective.

The findings clearly show that these compounds are present in all the extracts from the various plants studied, with concentrations varying widely. Ethanol extracts of *M. pouliot* had the highest flavonol content at 67.97 ± 0.04 mg QE/g, compared to 16.96 ± 5.06 mg QE/g and 14.36 ± 1.68 mg QE/g for EMTA and EEPL, respectively.

3.3 Study of antioxidant activity of crude extracts

3.3.1 DPPH radical scavenging activity

The free radical scavenging activity was evaluated using the DPPH assay, which measures the ability of the extracts to neutralize the stable $DPPH^{\bullet}$ radical in solution through the donation of a hydrogen atom or electron.

The antiradical activity profiles (**Figure 3a, b**, and **c**) show that the tested extracts exhibit a dose-dependent response. The stabilization phase indicates almost complete reduction of the $DPPH^{\bullet}$ radical to its non-radical form, DPPH-H.

In this study, comparisons were made among the three species to determine the ability of their extracts to eliminate the DPPH• free radical. **Table 3** presents the IC_{50} values of the DPPH test for the extracts of the three plants. The IC_{50} values ranged from 5.34 ± 0.2 to >200 μg/mL. Generally, the results showed that extracts derived from highly polar solvents led to an increase in free radical scavenging activity. Interestingly, the free radical scavenging activities of polar extracts were comparable to the standards (BHA and ascorbic acid).

The variation in IC_{50} values among the extracts of different species could be attributed to differences in their polyphenolic compositions [15]. Therefore, extracts with higher antioxidant activities likely possess higher amounts of polyphenols (**Table 2**). This observation was statistically proven by calculating the Pearson correlation coefficient r (**Table 4**).

The DPPH assay identified the ethanol extract of *P. lentiscus* [5.34 ± 0.2 μg/mL] (the lowest IC_{50} value) as having statistically the highest free radical scavenging activity, followed by the ethanol extract of M. pouliot [11.82 ± 0.4 μg/mL] and the methanol extract of T. algeriensis [14.80 ± 0.4 μg/mL]. Meanwhile, the dichloromethane extract of T. algeriensis, EDTA, showed the lowest activity (> 200 μg/mL).

Previous studies have demonstrated that extracts from the examined plants have a strong capacity to act as antioxidant agents. Specifically, both EEMP and EMMP extracts showed strong antiradical activity compared to the results reported by Mata et al.; Stagos et al.; Teixeira et al. [16–18]. On the other hand, Kamkar et al. corroborated the findings by showing powerful antiradical activity presented by both aqueous and methanol extracts of *M. pulegium* [IC_{50} = 5.5 ± 0.3 μg/mL and IC_{50} = 6.1 ± 0.1 μg/mL] [19]. Regarding the species *T. algeriensis*, the study conducted by Fatma et al. indicated that the inhibition rate of methanol extract (MOK) reached 84 ± 0.034%, which is very close to our results [20].

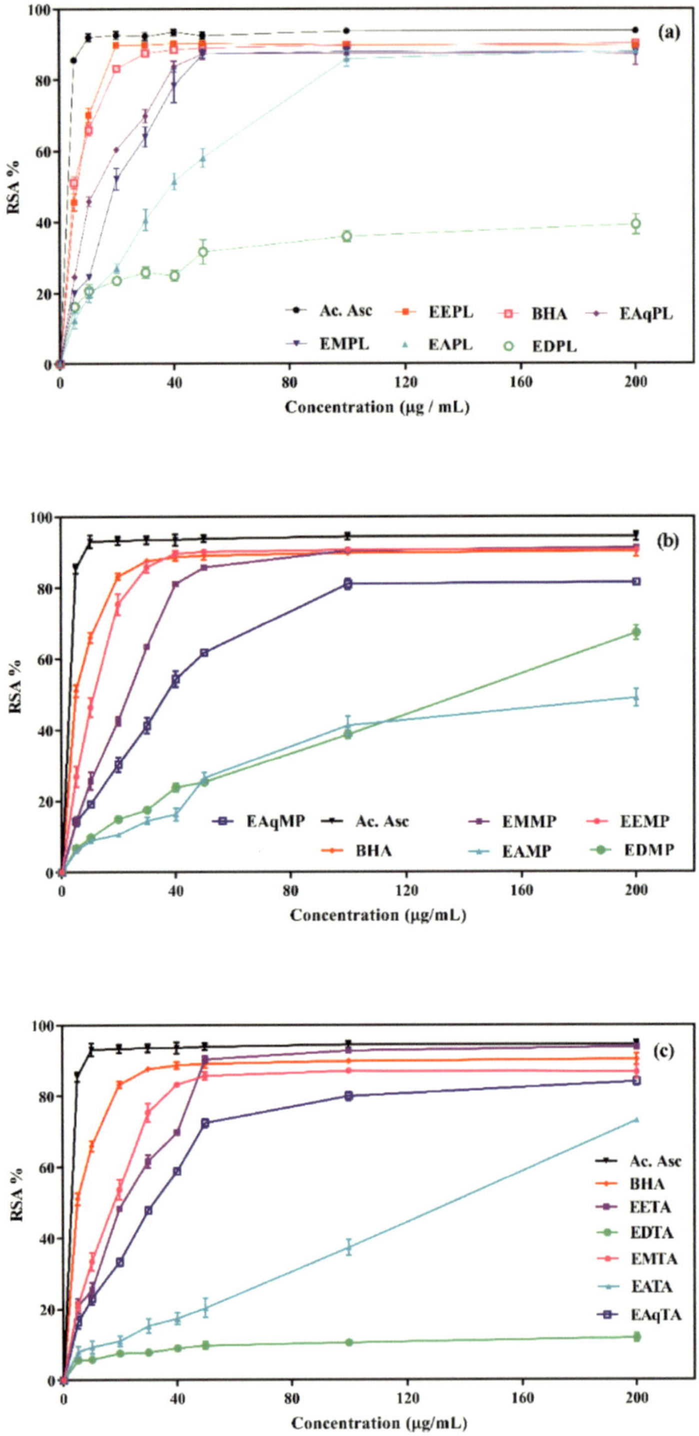

Figure 3.
Profiles of anti-radical activity (DPPH• test) of extracts.

Samples	DPPH		FRAP	βCB
	IC_{50} (µg/mL)	% RSA	Abs	%
EEPL	05.34 ± 0.2	89.5 ± 0.7	1.07 ± 0.02	84.43 ± 1.68
EMPL	17.80 ± 0.8	87.7 ± 0.1	1.20 ± 0.02	79.66 ± 2.00
EAqPL	12.87 ± 0.5	87.3 ± 3.1	1.17 ± 0.03	81.12 ± 4.53
EAPL	39.01 ± 1.0	88.1 ± 0.4	0.26 ± 0.03	87.39 ± 2.00
EDPL	249.8 ± 2.9	39.2 ± 2.8	0.12 ± 0.02	90.32 ± 2.98
EEMP	11.82 ± 0.4	90.7 ± 0.2	0.43 ± 0.03	65.80 ± 4.74
EMMP	23.41 ± 0.2	91.2 ± 0.0	0.34 ± 0.00	68.25 ± 0.00
EAqMP	36.62 ± 0.9	81.5 ± 0.9	0.73 ± 0.03	60.58 ± 8.90
EAMP	211.5 ± 3.1	48.9 ± 2.5	0.14 ± 0.01	82.04 ± 8.75
EDMP	139.18 ± 0.7	67.1 ± 2.1	0.10 ± 0.00	77.16 ± 5.73
EETA	20.40 ± 0.2	93.7 ± 0.1	0.98 ± 0.04	77.60 ± 3.47
EMTA	14.80 ± 0.4	86.7 ± 1.9	0.80 ± 0.01	72.69 ± 10.1
EAqTA	32.40 ± 0.3	79.8 ± 1.2	0.53 ± 0.04	70.39 ± 8.52
EATA	134.66 ± 0.6	73.0 ± 0.0	0.09 ± 0.01	82.49 ± 2.22
EDTA	> 200	11.8 ± 1.2	0.04 ± 0.00	83.50 ± 0.00
BHA	5.55 ± 0.3	90.2 ± 1.6	NT	94.73 ± 3.34
Ac. Asc	2.82 ± 0.1	94.4 ± 1.1	1.29 ± 0.03	81.44 ± 2.50

Table 3.
Various antioxidant activity methods.

		Correlation coefficient (r)					
		RSA	FRAP	βCB	TPC	TF	FV
	RSA	1	—	—	0.861	0.765	0.686
MP	RP	0.645	1	—	0.510	0.361	0.323
	βCB	−0.707	−0.930	1	−0.684	−0.532	−0.436
	RSA	1	—	—	0.779	0.751	0.749
TA	RP	0.764	1	—	0.957	0.915	0.910
	βCB	−0.632	−0.662	1	−0.818	−0.702	−0.736
	RSA	1	—	—	0.933	0.875	0.928
PL	RP	0.940	1	—	0.823	0.722	0.775
	βCB	−0.891	−0.966	1	−0.696	−0.574	−0.659

Table 4.
Pearson correlation coefficient analysis.

3.3.2 Ferric reducing power assay (FRAP)

The FRAP assay, often utilized to assess the capacity of natural antioxidants to donate electrons or hydrogen, is a significant mechanism of action for phenolic antioxidants [21].

The reducing power of various extracts (15.6–100 μg/mL) from the three plants is presented in **Figure 4**. It can be observed that the highest reducing power is achieved by the EMPL extract (1.20 ± 0.02) from P. lentisque, the EETA extract (0.98 ± 0.04)

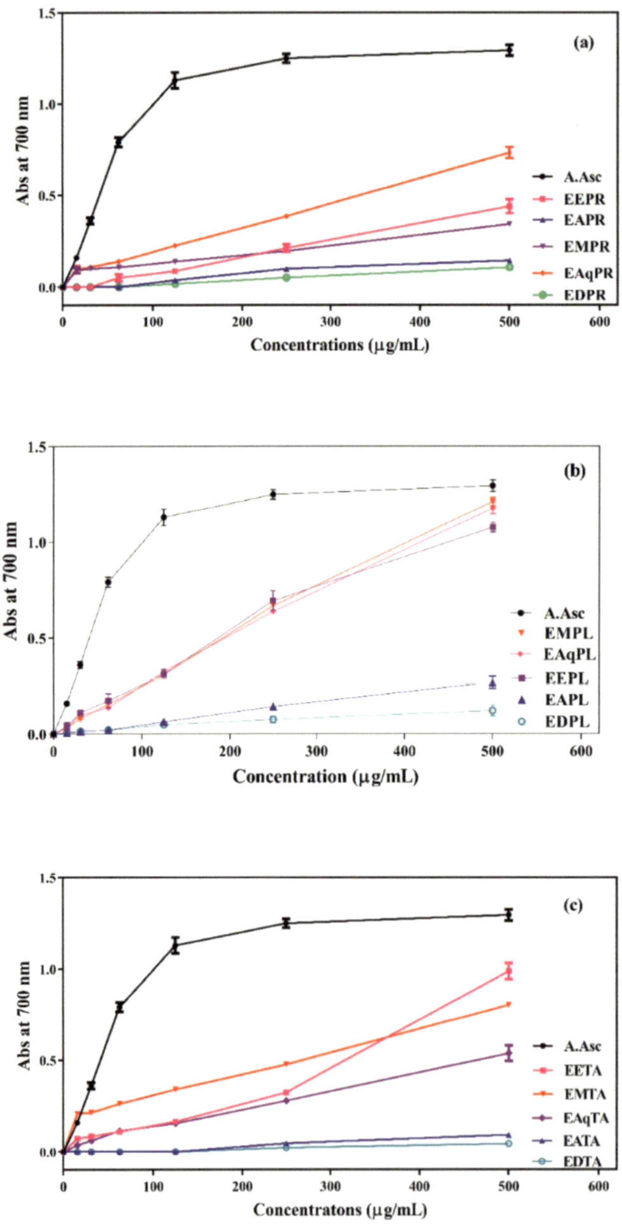

Figure 4.
Profiles of ferric reducing power of crude extracts.

from *T. algeriensis*, and the EAqMP extract (0.73 ± 0.03) from *M. pulegium*, which is comparable to that of the standard ascorbic acid (1.29 ± 0.03).

Additionally, the FRAP assay results were consistent with those of the DPPH free radical assay for the three plants examined. Examination of the reducing power results of the extracts from each species revealed the effect of the extraction solvent. Indeed, extracts with higher polarity for all species exhibited very strong reducing power. In contrast, the ferric ion reducing activity of extracts with lower polarity was lower, except for the two extracts EAPL and EAMP, which were 0.26 ± 0.03 and 0.14 ± 0.01, respectively.

A strong correlation was found between the reducing power and the total phenolic content present in the various extracts, indicating that phenolic compounds play a significant role in the beneficial effects of these medicinal plants.

3.3.3 Inhibition of β-carotene bleaching

In this study, the ability of the extracts to inhibit lipid peroxidation was evaluated using the β-carotene bleaching technique. Any chemical substance that delays or inhibits the bleaching of β-carotene can be considered an antioxidant [22].

To assess the effectiveness of our extracts in slowing down the oxidation rate of lipids, we monitored the reaction of linoleic acid oxidation by measuring the decrease in absorbance over time. The results show that both BHA and the tested extracts from different species effectively inhibit the coupled oxidation of linoleic acid and β-carotene (**Figure 5**).

An exception was noted for the dichloromethane and ethyl acetate fractions of each tested species; these two fractions are very low in phenolic compounds but exhibited remarkably strong inhibitory power compared to the other extracts.

These two extracts are quite complex; they may contain a variety of substances (waxes, fatty acids, sterols, triterpenes, carotenoids, highly methoxylated flavonoid aglycones, and coumarins) that can act independently or synergistically. Mariod and colleagues in 2009 found maximum inhibition with the hexane fraction of *Nigella sativa L* seeds [23]. They indicated that, in addition to the probable contribution of antioxidants to the activity of the two extracts, another parameter seems to intervene the polarity of the solvents.

Frankel and Meyer proposed that within lipid emulsion systems in water, apolar antioxidants demonstrate superior antioxidant properties compared to polar ones [24]. They found that apolar antioxidants concentrate at the lipid-water interface, inhibiting lipid radical formation and β-carotene oxidation. In contrast, polar antioxidants, dispersed in the aqueous phase, are less effective due to their dilution.

3.4 Pearson correlation analysis

Undergoing Pearson correlation analysis, we delved into establishing the linear relationships among all antioxidant activities and between antioxidant activities and phenolic compound contents. What emerged prominently were the highest positive correlation coefficients displayed by DPPH and FRAP across the trio of species under scrutiny: *P. lentiscus* (r = 0.940), *T. algeriensis* (0.764), and *M. pulegium* (0.645) (**Table 4**). This intriguing revelation hints at the consistent polarity alignment between both DPPH and FRAP antioxidant activities and the solvent. To elaborate, it appears that the greater the solvent's polarity, the more potent the antioxidant capacity within the plant extracts. This hypothesis gains traction as we observe the polar nature of the reaction environments governing both processes. Moreover, our

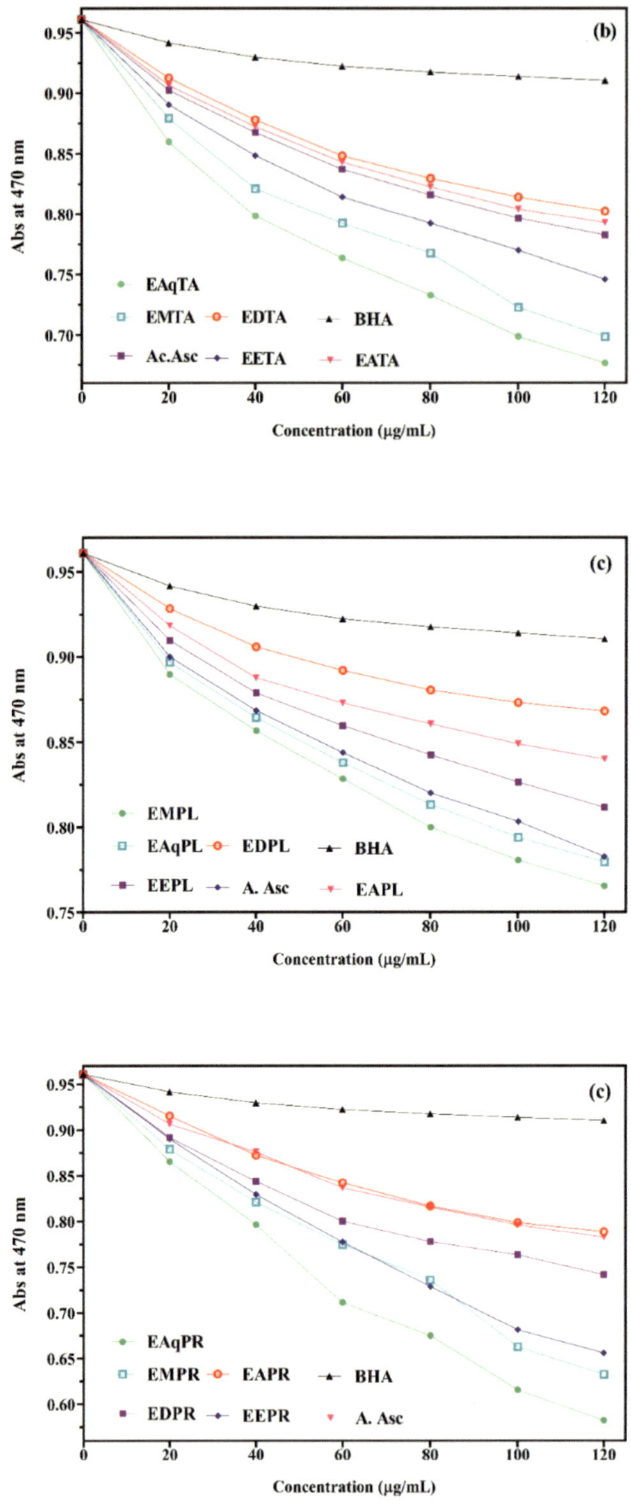

Figure 5.
Profiles of inhibitory activity of extracts.

exploration uncovers the richness of polar compounds in extracts like ethanol, methanol, and aqueous solutions, manifesting as either hydrogen atom donors or singlet electron transfer agents, thus augmenting the antioxidant potency.

However, the β-carotene bleaching test exhibited notably strong negative correlations with both DPPH and FRAP ($r = -0.891$, $r = -0.966$, respectively). These findings are likely supported by the solvent polarity and the hydrophobic characteristics of the reaction environment.

4. Conclusion

The in vitro antioxidant activity of the extracts was assessed using various methods, including DPPH radical scavenging, ferric ion reducing power, and β-carotene bleaching inhibition. We found that the different crude extracts tested exhibited interesting anti-radical and antioxidant activities, which were dependent on total polyphenol and flavonoid contents. A linear relationship was established, with fractions richest in flavonoids showing the highest activity. However, the intensity of antioxidant activity is not solely dependent on the overall flavonoid content but also on their nature. Thus, the strong inhibition of lipid oxidation by the dichloromethane and ethyl acetate fractions of the different plants, despite their low polyphenol concentration, may be attributed to other substances (waxes, fatty acids, sterols, triterpenes, carotenoids, highly methoxylated flavonoid aglycones, and coumarins) that can act independently or synergistically.

Conflict of interest

The authors declare no conflict of interest.

Author details

Amin Salhi[1*], Chahid Zannagui[1], Abdellah Elyoussfi[1], M'hamed Ahari[1], Fouad Mourabit[1], Hassan Amhamdi[1], El Houssien Akichouh[1] and Soufian El Barkany[2]

1 Applied Chemistry Team, FSTH, Abdelmalek Essaâdi University, Tetouan, Morocco

2 Faculty Multidisciplinary Nador, Department of Chemistry, Laboratory of Molecular Chemistry, Materials and Environment (LMCME), Mohamed 1st University, Nador, Morocco

*Address all correspondence to: a.msalhi@uae.ac.ma; amiinsalhii@gmail.com

References

[1] Farbstein D, Kozak-Blickstein A, Levy AP. Antioxidant vitamins and their use in preventing cardiovascular disease. Molecules. 2010;**15**(11):8098-8110. DOI: 10.3390/molecules15118098

[2] Pietta PG. Flavonoids as antioxidants. Journal of Natural Products. 2000;**63**(7):1035-1042. DOI: 10.1021/np9904509

[3] Ndhlala AR, Moyo M, Van Staden J. Natural antioxidants: Fascinating or mythical biomolecules? Molecules. 2010;**15**(10):6905-6930. DOI: 10.3390/molecules15106905

[4] Queiroz AN, Gomes BAQ, Moraes WM, Borges RS. A theoretical antioxidant pharmacophore for resveratrol. European Journal of Medicinal Chemistry. 2009;**44**(4):1644-1649. DOI: 10.1016/j.ejmech.2008.09.023

[5] Mikulski D, Górniak R, Molski M. A theoretical study of the structure–radical scavenging activity of trans-resveratrol analogues and cis-resveratrol in gas phase and water environment. European Journal of Medicinal Chemistry. 2010;**45**(3):1015-1027. DOI: 10.1016/j.ejmech.2009.11.044

[6] Leopoldini M, Russo N, Toscano M. The molecular basis of working mechanism of natural polyphenolic antioxidants. Food Chemistry. 2011;**125**(2):288-306. DOI: 10.1016/j.foodchem.2010.08.012

[7] Wong CC, Li HB, Cheng KW, Chen F. A systematic survey of antioxidant activity of 30 Chinese medicinal plants using the ferric reducing antioxidant power assay. Food Chemistry. 2006;**97**(4):705-711. DOI: 10.1016/j.foodchem.2005.05.049

[8] Djeridane A, Yousfi M, Nadjemi B, Boutassouna D, Stocker P, Vidal N. Antioxidant activity of some Algerian medicinal plants extracts containing phenolic compounds. Food Chemistry. 2006;**97**(4):654-660. DOI: 10.1016/j.foodchem.2005.04.028

[9] Kosalec I, Bakmaz M, Pepeljnjak S, Vladimir-Knezevic S. Quantitative analysis of the flavonoids in raw propolis from northern Croatia. Acta Pharmaceutica. 2004;**54**(1):65-72. DOI: urn.nsk.hr/urn:nbn:hr:163:570058

[10] Moure A, Franco D, Sineiro J, Domínguez H, Núñez MJ, Lema JM. Evaluation of extracts from Gevuina avellana hulls as antioxidants. Journal of Agricultural and Food Chemistry. 2000;**48**(9):3890-3897. DOI: 10.1021/jf000048w

[11] Oyaizu M. Studies on products of browning reaction antioxidative activities of products of browning reaction prepared from glucosamine. The Japanese Journal of Nutrition and Dietetics. 1986;**44**(6):307-315. DOI: 0.5264/eiyogakuzashi.44.307

[12] Tepe B, Daferera D, Sokmen A, Sokmen M, Polissiou M. Antimicrobial and antioxidant activities of the essential oil and various extracts of Salvia tomentosa miller (Lamiaceae). Food Chemistry. 2005;**90**(3):333-340. DOI: 10.1016/j.foodchem.2003.09.013

[13] Kartal B, Rattray J, Van Niftrik LA, Van de Vossenberg J, Schmid MC, Webb RI, et al. Candidatus “Anammoxoglobus propionicus” a new propionate oxidizing species of anaerobic ammonium oxidizing bacteria. Systematic and Applied Microbiology. 2007;**30**(1):39-49. DOI: 10.1016/j.syapm.2006.03.004

[14] Yıldırım A, Mavi A, Kara AA. Determination of antioxidant and antimicrobial activities of *Rumex crispus L*. extracts. Journal of Agricultural and Food Chemistry. 2001;**49**(8):4083-4089. DOI: 10.1021/jf0103572

[15] Kaur C, Kapoor HC. Anti-oxidant activity and total phenolic content of some Asian vegetables. International Journal of Food Science and Technology. 2002;**37**(2):153-161. DOI: 10.1046/j.1365-2621.2002.00552.x

[16] Mata AT, Proença C, Ferreira AR, Serralheiro MLM, Nogueira JMF, Araújo MEM. Antioxidant and antiacetylcholinesterase activities of five plants used as Portuguese food spices. Food Chemistry. 2007;**103**(3):778-786. DOI: 10.1016/j.foodchem.2006.09.017

[17] Stagos D, Portesis N, Spanou C, Mossialos D, Aligiannis N, Chaita E, et al. Correlation of total polyphenolic content with antioxidant and antibacterial activity of 24 extracts from Greek domestic Lamiaceae species. Food and Chemical Toxicology. 2012;**50**(11):4115-4124. DOI: 10.1016/j.fct.2012.08.033

[18] Teixeira B, Marques A, Ramos C, Batista I, Serrano C, Matos O, et al. European pennyroyal (*Mentha pulegium*) from Portugal: Chemical composition of essential oil and antioxidant and antimicrobial properties of extracts and essential oil. Industrial Crops and Products. 2012;**36**(1):81-87. DOI: 10.1016/j.indcrop.2011.08.011

[19] Kamkar A, Javan AJ, Asadi F, Kamalinejad M. The antioxidative effect of Iranian Mentha pulegium extracts and essential oil in sunflower oil. Food and Chemical Toxicology. 2010;**48**(7):1796-1800. DOI: 10.1016/j.fct.2010.04.003

[20] Fatma G, Mouna BF, Mondher M, Ahmed L. In-vitro assessment of antioxidant and antimicrobial activities of methanol extracts and essential oil of *Thymus hirtus sp*. algeriensis. Lipids in Health and Disease. 2014;**13**:1-12. DOI: 10.1186/1476-511X-13-114

[21] Romani A, Pinelli P, Galardi C, Mulinacci N, Tattini M. Identification and quantification of galloyl derivatives, flavonoid glycosides and anthocyanins in leaves of *Pistacia lentiscus L*. Phytochemical Analysis: An International Journal of Plant Chemical and Biochemical Techniques. 2002;**13**(2):79-86. DOI: 10.1002/pca.627

[22] Shimada K, Fujikawa K, Yahara K, Nakamura T. Antioxidative properties of xanthan on the autoxidation of soybean oil in cyclodextrin emulsion. Journal of Agricultural and Food Chemistry. 1992;**40**(6):945-948. DOI: 10.1021/jf00018a005

[23] Mariod AA, Ibrahim RM, Ismail M, Ismail N. Antioxidant activity and phenolic content of phenolic rich fractions obtained from black cumin (*Nigella sativa*) seedcake. Food Chemistry. 2009;**116**(1):306-312. DOI: 10.1016/j.foodchem.2009.02.051

[24] Frankel EN, Meyer AS. The problems of using one-dimensional methods to evaluate multifunctional food and biological antioxidants. Journal of the Science of Food and Agriculture. 2000;**80**(13):1925-1941. DOI: 10.1002/1097-0010(200010)80:13<1925::AID-JSFA714>3.0.CO;2-4

Chapter 6

Medicinal Plants for Controlling of Gastrointestinal Nematodes in Scavenging Chickens: A Systematic Review

Nkanyiso Majola, Mbusiseni Mkwanazi, Sithembile Z. Ndlela and Michael Chimonyo

Abstract

The review investigates medicinal plants published in peer-reviewed journals from 2000 to 2021. The objective of the review is to explore the use of IK to control gastrointestinal nematodes. Chickens contribute extensively to the livelihood of many communities by ensuring food security, women empowerment, and income provision. Scavenging chickens are, however, highly exposed to gastrointestinal nematodes (GIN). In total, 15 ethno-veterinary plant species belonging to 16 families were identified to control GIN. These included *Agave sisalana*, *Aloe forex*, *Gunnera perpensa L.*, and *Aloe marlothii*. The value of these EVM lies in various chemical substances that possess properties such as alkaloids, saponins, and other phenolic compounds that fight diseases and parasites. Farmers collected plants from the bush, around the kraal, and along the homestead fence for easy access. Various administration methods and dosages were used. The use of plants to control nematodes in is attributed to the availability and ease of application. Medicinal plants, either as an alternative to anthelmintics or as a complement to conventional knowledge, need to be documented and promoted. It is necessary to evaluate the appropriate dosages of medicinal plants. Policies that govern the use and threats of medicinal plants need to be developed to conserve valuable remedies.

Keywords: ethnoveterinary remedies, conservation, indigenous knowledge, nematode infestation, natural products

1. Introduction

The demand for organic poultry products from free-range and deep-litter production systems is increasing [1]. Scavenging chickens significantly contribute to households with limited resources, particularly landless women, allowing them to receive healthcare and education. They contribute to sustainable development goals and food security by maintaining biodiverse genomes [2]. Chickens promote gender equality, particularly amongst disadvantaged groups and less helped areas of rural Africa [3]. They are not labour-intensive, can be reared as sideline enterprises, and demand less space than larger animals such as cattle. Keeping chickens is advantageous to women as they manage poultry production and marketing without seeking permission from their husbands. The meat from scavenging chickens is highly preferred, thus suggesting that these genetic resources are promising options to enhance food security.

In large-scale production systems, the rearing of chickens is characterized by low productivity and high mortality [4]. Other challenges that resource-limited farmers face seriously include feed shortages [3]. Chickens are, thus, forced to roam around, scavenging around homesteads in contaminated areas with infective nematode eggs. Gastrointestinal nematodes are far from the most important parasites of chickens and remain the major factor hindering the successful production of village chickens [5]. Nematode infestations lead to decreased productivity and increased morbidity and mortality in chickens. The widespread occurrence of nematode infestations is linked to low management levels and poor hygiene [6, 7]. In intensive production systems, nematodes are usually controlled using anthelmintic; however, they are often out of reach for most farmers with limited resources as they are costly and, occasionally, inconsistently inaccessible. Using anthelmintic drugs has, however, been reported to lead to the development of nematode resistance against anthelmintic if overdosed and due to infrequent applications [3]. Consequently, this has increased the search for alternative control practices, such as using indigenous knowledge (IK). Indigenous knowledge is a set of perceptions, experiences, information, and behavior that guide community members in efficiently utilizing their natural resources [8].

The use of indigenous knowledge has been part of the day-to-day practices of resource-limited farmers for centuries [9]. Although for some years, IK has been neglected and secluded in development, the Department of Science and Technology has developed an IK policy with the main goal of strengthening the contribution of IK to social and economic development [10]. The use of IK and its contribution to veterinary care cannot be underemphasized. According to Luseba and Tshisikhawe, [11] an estimated population of 80% depends on IK in Africa, though IK is not recognized and documented. Ethno-veterinary remedies are effective and locally available to resource-limited farmers. Indigenous knowledge is sustainable and practically sound due to its casc of production and processing [10].

Developing indigenous knowledge systems (IKS) creates opportunities for conventional knowledge to complement and integrate with IK. Both systems have the potential to integrate into educational and lifelong learning frameworks, contributing to sustainable development and enhancing the veterinary care of chickens. Also, sharing IKS is important to ensure that it is used and preserved for the future. The paper explores existing information on the potential utilization of IK to control gastrointestinal nematodes in chickens. The review discusses the role of chickens in empowering women, enhancing food security, promoting organic meat production, and the significance of IK in managing nematode infestations in chickens and the common nematodes that infect them. The review also identifies potential areas that require more research concerning the exploitation of IK.

2. Materials and methods

The study focuses on using IK to control gastrointestinal nematodes in chickens. In this study, indigenous knowledge is the understanding and practices that local people use for survival. It has evolved through extensive trial and error and has been proven to handle changes in their environments [12] effectively. PRISMA guidelines (**Figure 1**)

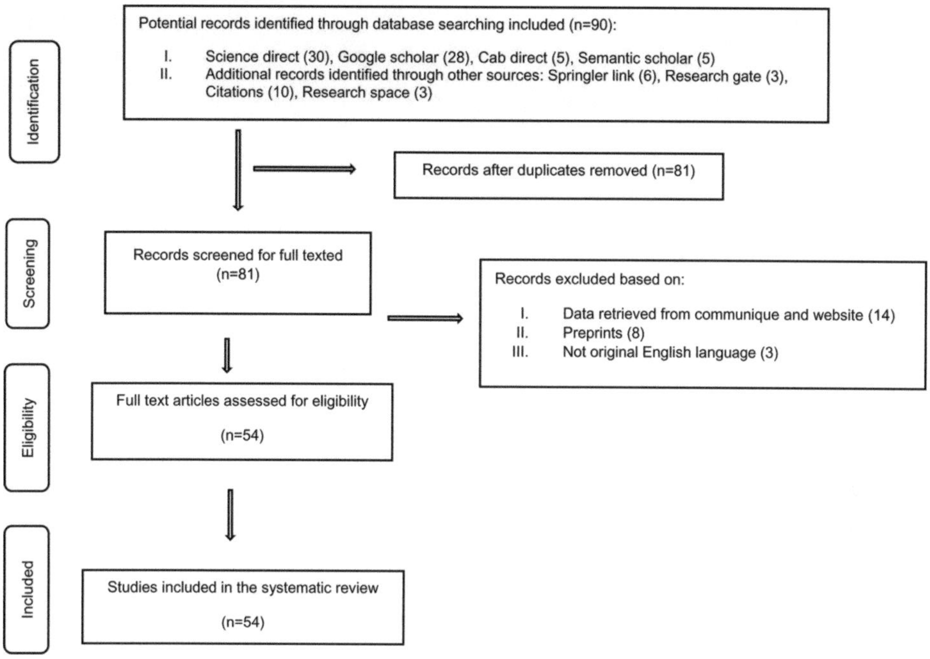

Figure 1.
Diagram illustrating the process for screening literature.

were followed in the systematic review. Science Direct, Google Scholar, and Semantic Scholar were scientific databases used to search for the information. Additional searches were done through the reference lists of key articles to ensure a wide range of articles from different sources. Other sources, such as Springer links and Researchgate, were used in cases where articles were not obtainable from scientific databases. Research space was used in cases where the data found was obtained from a thesis. Keywords used during the article search included nematodes in chickens, medicinal plants, ethno-veterinary plants, indigenous knowledge, traditional animal healthcare, the role of chickens in resource-limited areas, and chicken production. During the search stage, preprints were not considered.

After completing the search, the authors (NGM, SZN, MVM, and MC) eliminated all duplicate articles. Before the qualitative synthesis, information such as article titles, authors, journals, publication type, English articles, indigenous knowledge of nematodes, and the functions and roles of chickens were gathered. Complete article texts were reviewed and dismissed based on the following exclusion criteria: studies providing data irrelevant to the research question, communique, and Website content from organizations such as FAO were rejected, and articles not in the original English language were rejected. Literature was synthesized into a quality metric utilizing four criteria: aim, methodology, results, and application. This review categorized the studies based on quality criteria, dividing them into categories: high referred to >75% of all sub-criteria satisfied, moderate 50–75% satisfied, and weak <50% of criteria fulfilled. The literature was used regardless of the research method employed (qualitative or quantitative). Research published in a language other than English presented abstract only or not peer-reviewed was left out. All pertinent articles were thoroughly reviewed and summarized utilizing a uniform data extraction table within a Word document (**Table 1**). The included articles were examined to find additional records.

Lead author, year	Location	Type of publication	Method used	Number of participants/ sample size (N)	Rank
Abdelqader et al. [1]	Germany	Research paper	*In vivo* and *in vitro* trial	225	H
Ajani et al. [13]	Nigeria	Review	–	–	W
Alam et al. [6]	Bangladesh	Research paper	*In vivo* and *in vitro* trial	–	W
Belete et al. [14]	Ethiopia	Review	–	–	M
Bettridge et al. [15]	Ethiopia	Research paper	Experimental	1056	H
Butboochoo and Wongsawad [7]	Thailand	Research paper	Experimental	120	H
Chander et al. [16]	India	Review	–	–	H
Dasgupta and Roy [17]	India	Research paper	*In vitro* trial	–	H
Giday et al. [18]	Ethiopia	Research paper	Semi-structured interviews	17	M
Gwala [19]	South Africa	MSc-Thesis	–	–	M
Idika et al. [20]	Nigeria	Research paper	Experimental	125	M
Jain et al. [21]	India	Review	–	–	W
Kabeer [22]	–	Review	–	–	W
Karumari et al. [23]	India	Research paper	Experimental	–	M
Khan et al. [24]	Pakistan	Research paper	Experimental	–	M
Katoch et al. [25]	India	Research paper	Experimental	125	H
Kumm [26]	Sweden	Short communication	Experimental	–	H
Kusina et al. [27]	Zimbabwe	Research paper	Semi-structured interviews	416	H
Lalchhandama et al. [5]	India	Research paper	Experimental	–	H
Matos Lopes et al. [28]	Brazil	Research paper	Experimental	–	H
Luseba and Tshisikhawe [11]	South Africa	Research paper	Focus group discussions	37	H
Malatji et al. [4]	South Africa	Research paper	Questionnaire	87	H
Mapiye et al. [29]	Zimbabwe	Review	–	–	H
Mapiye and Sibanda [30]	Zimbabwe	Research paper	Questionnaire	72	W
Melesse [31]	Germany	Review	–	–	M
Mitileni et al. [32]	South Africa	Review	–	–	M
Mathialagan [33]	India	Research paper	Questionnaire	200	W

Lead author, year	Location	Type of publication	Method used	Number of participants/ sample size (N)	Rank
Mkwanazi et al. [12]	South Africa	Research paper	Questionnaire	300	H
Mwale et al. [34]	Zimbabwe	Research paper	Questionnaire	150	M
Mwale and Masika [3]	South Africa	Research paper	Experimental	–	H
Mwale and Masika [3]	South Africa	Research paper	Experimental	14	M
McGlaw and Ellof [9]	South Africa	Review	–	–	H
Muchadeyi et al. [35]	Zimbabwe	Research paper	Questionnaire	100	M
Naphande and Chaudhari [36]	India	Research paper	Experimental	–	W
Ncobela and Chimonyo [37]	South Africa	Research paper	Questionnaire	239	H
Ndlela et al. [38]	South Africa	Research paper	Questionnaire	294	H
Puttalakshmamma et al. [39]	India	Research paper	Experimental	100	M
Prakash et al. [40]	India	Review	–	–	W
Raza et al. [41]	Pakistan	Review	–	–	W
Siamba et al. [42]	Kenya	Research paper	Experimental	–	W
Subash et al. [43]	India	Research paper	Experimental	–	M
Swatson et al. [44]	South Africa	Research paper	Experimental	–	M
Symeonidou et al. [45]	Greece	Review	–	–	W
Sujith et al. [46]	India	Research paper	Experimental	–	M
Sugumar et al. [47]	India	Research paper	Experimental	–	M
Tesfaheywe et al. [48]	Ethiopia	Research paper	Semi-structured interviews	–	M
Tewari et al. [49]	India	Research paper	Semi-structured interviews	210	W
Uhuo et al. [50]	Nigeria	Research paper	Experimental	–	W
Vilakazi et al. [8]	South Africa	Research paper	Semi-structured interviews	400	H
Wuthijaree et al. [51]	Italy	Research paper	Experimental	–	H
Wong et al. [2]	Australia	Review	–	–	H
Zaman et al. [52]	Pakistan	Review	–	–	H

Table 1.
Study characteristics of the final qualified papers.

3. Results

Our search strategies identified a total of 90 articles. Following removing duplicates, an initial review of titles and abstracts was conducted to ascertain relevance, resulting in the identification of 56 articles that met the inclusion criteria for full-text screening. The review process is outlined in **Figure 1**, respectively. The data were taken from the articles provided and then examined:

1. Research attributes, study sites, and sample volume

2. Experimental conditions, such as the method used to collect data.

Out of 56 eligible articles, almost half of the studies were carried out in India (14), South Africa (12), Zimbabwe (6), Ethiopia (4), Nigeria (3), Pakistan (=3), Germany (2), and one article in Bangladesh, Thailand, Brazil, Italy, Greece, Sweden, Kenya, and Australia (**Table 1**).

4. Importance of chickens in rural economies

Women are generally owners and managers of chickens in resource-limited areas. Males largely own cattle and goats. Chickens contribute to livelihoods through women empowerment, ensuring seasonal food security, and providing cash and organic meat.

4.1 Women and youth empowerment

Women empowerment is fundamental to achieving gender equality. The empowerment of women is determined by the increase in economic benefits and role within the household economy [22]. It is also pertinent for increased productivity and improved health and nutrition. Scavenging chickens empower women socially, economically, physiologically, and technically [33]. Scavenging chickens are a valuable tool to empower women and improve their social status. Therefore, public institutions such as government and non-governmental agencies should promote farming by scavenging poultry. Farming chickens increases independent decision-making and enhances the involvement of women in their family affairs. It also promotes the socio-economic development of the rural sector. Participating in poultry-rearing projects positions rural women to develop good business skills. Such projects empower women by developing their economic benefits.

These chickens are raised with minimal financial inputs, feed supplements, land, and housing. Youth unemployment is one of the major challenges in the developing world. For example, in South Africa alone, the youth unemployment rate is estimated to be 66.5% in the current year, making it the leading country with the highest youth unemployment. The youth lack interest in agriculture due to inadequate finance, start-up capital, and their negative perception of agriculture in general [13]. Thus, youth prefer to seek employment opportunities in other sectors to economically empower themselves. Youth can have a safe social environment where they feel valued and supported and can share their ideas in decision-making. Furthermore, youth are interested in engaging and participating in socio-political processes to affect change while contributing to the empowerment of the community. Poultry production presents such opportunities.

4.2 Enhancing food and nutrition security using scavenging chickens

Food security is achieved when all people consistently have both the physical and economical means to access sufficient, safe, and nutritious food to fulfil their dietary requirements and preferences, enabling them to lead active and healthy lives at all times [32]. This definition is based on two interconnected pillars: availability and access to food. Wong et al. [2] characterized food availability as adequate quality foods that are culturally and socially acceptable within a specific community or society. Even if food is accessible, resource-limited households' insufficient purchasing ability and power make them suffer from food insecurity. While many countries are food secure nationally, most resource-limited households grapple with food insecurity. One potential approach to attaining household food security is to enhance the efficiency of scavenging chickens. This is ascribed to their products, such as meat and eggs, consumed at the household level without formal marketing channels. Providing meat and eggs from village chickens is the primary source of proteins to resource-poor households.

Eggs provide important nutrients, such as essential amino acids for human nutrition, and contribute 3–4% of the energy and protein an adult person requires daily [31]. A single egg provides 150.5 kilocalories of energy. It contains 12.4 grams of protein and 0.72 grams of carbohydrates. Regarding vitamins, an egg provides 158 micrograms of Vitamin A, 0.46 milligrams of Vitamin B2, and 1.05 milligrams of Vitamin E [19, 37]. Even though their consumption pattern cannot be quantified because they are consumed when there is a need. Scavenging chickens provide meat, which forms a source of protein in human diets. Consumers favour village chicken meat due to its superior taste and freshness, so much so that people in urban areas are willing to pay more for these birds at local markets (**Table 2**). In resource-limited communal production systems, chickens are kept by four out of five households [37]. Efforts are required to improve the livelihoods of communities by enhancing the availability and access to proper nutrition. Scavenging chickens provide cheap, readily harvestable protein-enriched white meat and eggs with highly digestible protein [30]. Chickens contribute by increasing the availability and accessibility of food supply and nutrients, leading to zero hunger, good health, and well-being [19].

4.3 Provision of household income and organic meat

Scavenging chickens are important to rural households in providing income, though their contribution to the household economy is relatively scant [30] and undocumented. Thus, their economic importance and contribution to food security are unappreciated nationally in most developing countries. Poultry contributes significantly to meeting welfare needs and raising the living standards of resource-limited communities. Chickens serve as reserves or assets, being sold to meet household needs, including school fees and medical costs [37]. Therefore, ensuring the effective advancement of chicken production systems is crucial, especially in this era of the rising human population, serving as a gateway to sustainable household income generation.

Organic meat is produced using ecological resources, such as natural by-products [26]. For example, feed produced without chemical pesticides, artificial fertilizers, and genetically modified organisms can be deemed organic [16]. Chickens raised organically exhibit natural behaviours, such as enjoying outdoor access year-round and using simple structures. Promoting the production of organic meat is vital because it plays an important role in ensuring an enduring supply of food. Producing organic meat from scavenging chickens has the capability to ensure nutritional security for resource-limited households by converting unusable into usable products. Indigenous knowledge could influence the success of producing organic poultry meat. Indigenous knowledge and practices used in producing scavenging chicken products are wholesome, tasty, and safe meat and eggs that can markedly increase nutrition security for women, children, and the elderly.

5. Indigenous knowledge in controlling nematodes in scavenging chickens

Although using IK to control parasites and improve immunity and productivity is humongous, its utilization is slowly diminishing [38]. Farmers utilize IK to identify chickens affected by nematode infestation, including observing their behavior. In chickens infested with nematodes, farmers observed impaired growth, decreased output, diarrhoea, and reduced production in the flock [1]. Farmers monitor various signs of the bird's recovery, including alertness, movement, feeding behavior, and the appearance of the green coloring in faeces, to confirm its full recovery.

Chickens recover at different times; some recover within 24 hours, some within days, while others recover within weeks [34]. The type of remedy, processing, and duration of application can influence the anthelmintic properties used so that some plant extracts act more swiftly than others. This might signify that different medicinal plants may have varying healing properties, thus accounting for the variability in the recovery time. Therefore, determining the active compounds of these plants would be of utmost interest. Resource-limited farmers use ethnoveterinary remedies over anthelmintic drugs because these remedies are locally available, effective, and convenient. The practice of using ethnoveterinary remedies to control nematodes dates back centuries. There are various kinds of medicinal plants that can manage chicken nematodes. *Aloe* is the most commonly utilized plant species [24], containing components such as *Aloe* leaf gel and exudates [32]. Other common plant species that farmers use are shown in **Table 2**.

	% consumption by households		
Village chicken portions	**Male**	**Female**	**Children**
Head	2.8	9.9	73.1
Feet	0.4	16.5	72.7
Neck	21.4	40.0	36.7
Thighs	43.8	53.7	5.7
Drumstick	47.9	47.1	4.9
Wings	47.5	45.0	14.0
Breasts	18.6	31.8	50.0
Back	29.3	38.4	28.9
Intestines and abdominal organs	16.1	11.1	57.4
Eggs	10.3	17.3	69.0

Source: Gwala [19].

Table 2.
Consumption of village chicken products in households.

6. Nematode species infesting chickens

Farmers with limited resources identify and categorize nematodes based on their colour schemes, form, dimensions, and preference sites. Farmers use IK to name nematode species using their various colour schemes and sizes. However, when it comes to nematode control, farmers understand that plant extracts have a wide spectrum, so no plant is specific for a particular nematode. Of the three helminth classes, nematodes are more important than cestodes and trematodes [24]. Nematodes are notably recognized amongst helminths for the extent of harm they inflict on chickens, especially during severe infestations [48]. Nematodes cause significant chronic illnesses and economic losses to farmers [1]. The three nematode species are *Ascaridia galli*, *Heterakis gallinarum*, and *Capillaria* [50]. *Ascaridia galli* is the most common nematode infecting chickens in terms of the number and percentage of infections it causes.

Idika et al. [20] highlighted that *A. galli* is the most common nematode and ranks most frequently found helminth species in the local chickens, at a rate of 22%, followed by *H. gallinarum* a prevalence of 12%, ranking fourth in the overall prevalence. The second most prevalent nematode was *Heterakis gallinarum*, comprising 28% of the total [50], with little pathogenicity. Katoch et al. [25] also identified *Ascaridia galli* as the most common helminth spp. (30%), followed by *Heterakis gallinarum* (24%), *Raillietina cesticillus* (19%) and *Raillietina echinobothrida* (14%) [25]. It is important to highlight that nematode infection rates depend on rainfall patterns, locality, soil type, and feed given to chickens. The widespread availability of intermediate hosts, such as beetles and houseflies, contributes significantly to the high incidence of *Heterakis gallinarum* amongst local scavenging chickens.

Ascaridia galli infests chickens of all age groups, although the most significant damage is usually observed in younger birds aged less than 12 weeks [14]. Furthermore, *Ascari gali* serves as a potential carrier for Salmonella infections. Chickens heavily infested with *Ascari gali* spp. experience decreased feed efficiency, resulting in weight loss. In severe cases, reduced egg production may occur [36]. During a heavy infestation, adult *Ascaridia galli* worms cause intestinal blockage, move up the oviduct, and may be found in eggs. Naphande and Chaudhari [36] reported that *Ascaridia galli* might secrete toxins that could harm the enzyme systems in the chicken's intestinal lining. The life cycle of *Ascaridia galli* does not involve an intermediate host. It lays eggs in the small intestine and proliferates rapidly.

The presence of *Heterakis gallinarum* enhances the danger of transmitting a pathogenic infection called *Histomonas meleagridis* [14]. After becoming infested with *Heterakis gallinarum*, the chicken experiences a thickening of the caecal wall, leading to cloacal dirtiness [50]. Bettrige et al. [15] reported that *Heterakis gallinarum* infestation suppresses the immune system. *Capillaria* species are highly pathogenic and are common in scavenging chickens [51]. In deep-litter systems, there is a growing build-up of infective eggs from *Capillaria* species. Severe infestations cause the oesophagus to thicken and the crop wall to inflame. In heavy infestations, chickens become emaciated, weak, and anaemic, and they excrete bloody diarrhoea and suffer from haemorrhagic enteritis. *Capillaria* species pose a threat to young birds under three months old because of their underdeveloped immunity, while adult birds can tolerate infestations [11]. Even though research has consistently reported the effects of nematodes on chicken productivity, the definite thresholds of nematode infestations have not been clearly defined. Therefore, additional research is needed. This will help producers comprehend and handle the interaction between nematode and their host, offering strategies for managing nematode infestations. It is necessary to identify management strategies to decrease nematode infestation in chickens. Extension services may assist farmers by offering capacity-building initiatives in management.

7. Efficacy of medicinal plants used to control nematodes in chickens

Ethno-veterinary medicine (EVM) practices are widespread due to numerous socio-economic difficulties, especially the lack of sufficient veterinary services [12]. The worth of these EVM is found in various chemical compounds that can potentially reduce and kill nematode burden. Several medicinal plants possessing anthelmintic properties have been used to reduce nematode burden (**Table 3**). In total, 15 ethno-veterinary plant species belonging to 11 families were identified to control nematodes. The efficacy of EVM has been tested by grinding seeds, leaves, bark, or any other part of the plant that possesses active ingredients [52]. Techniques, such as mass spectrophotometer and liquid chromatography, have been used to identify active plant ingredients. Validation of plants against nematodes based on *in vitro* and *in vivo* studies is not the goal of all ethnoveterinary studies [53]. To promote the use of the ethno-veterinary in sustaining the health of scavenging chickens, participatory studies involving farmers need to be conducted, and appropriate validation studies should be designed to affirm claims made by IK custodians. *Aloe forex*, *Gunnera perpensa* L., and *Agave sisalana Perrine* have successfully controlled nematodes [3] in chickens.

At a dosage of 100 mg/kg of *Aloe ferox*, the egg count was reduced by 81%. A notable reduction was observed in the 50 mg/kg dosage from the 7th to the 14th day (**Table 3**). A comparable pattern was observed on *Gunnera perpensa* L., whereas *Agave* sisalana *Perrine* decreased the egg count by 86% at 50 mg/kg dosage on day 7 and completely eliminated it by day 14. Kaingu et al. [53] tested the efficacy of *Aloe secundiflora* Engl. *in vitro.* The crude extracts were shown to inhibit the development of larval stages of *Ascarida galli*. Other plant species showing anthelmintic properties against nematodes include *Ozoroa reticulata* and *Strychnos spinosa* [34]. Other authors have reported plants that are specific to a particular helminth species, for example, *Vernonia amygdalina* [42], *Murraya koeniggi* [46], and *Azdirachta indica* [41] are known to have properties that destroy *A. galli*. A study examining *in vitro* anthelmintic properties of *Bassia latifolia* found that an aqueous extract from dried seeds caused more mortality in adult *A. galli* than alcoholic extract.

Treatment	**Dose (mg/kg)**	**Mean worm egg count (±SE)**			**Egg count reduction (%)**	
			Day		**Day**	
		0	**7**	**14**	**7**	**14**
Aloe ferox	50	1150.00 ± 934	350.00 ± 235	62.50 ± 453	96	83
	100	1312.50 ± 934	37.50 ± 244	375.00 ± 453	81	99
Gunnera perpensa	50	9400.00 ± 934	350.00 ± 244	137.50 ± 453	91	89
	100	987.50 ± 934	25.00 ± 244	525.00 ± 453	71	92
Agave sisalana	50	262.50 ± 934	12.50 ± 244	62.50 ± 453	86	100
	100	212.50 ± 934	50.00 ± 244	150.00 ± 453	33	67
Source: Mwale and Masika [3].						

Table 3.
Efficacy of indigenous medicinal plants in controlling nematodes of scavenging poultry.

Oil from *Piper betle* L. was administered at a dosage rate of 200 mg/kg body weight for a 24-hour interval and reduced worm burden by 13.9% after the first dose. *Piper betle* L., after a second dose of treatment, reduced the worm burden by 51.4%. Fruits from *Anacardium occidentale* L. were extracted with alcohol and aqueous extract (250 and 500 mg/ml) and showed significant anthelmintic properties at higher concentrations [41]. Both extracts showed anthelmintic activities in a dose-dependent manner, with the shortest time of paralysis. The aqueous extract of *Solanum torvum* fruits proved more effective, as it was lethal to the *Ascaridia galli* at a reduced concentration following 36 hours of exposure, compared to the leaves of *Sageraea grandiflora* [23]. However, during the initial 12–24 hours of exposure, the aqueous leaf extract of *S. grandiflora* proved more effective. The aqueous extract of *Agave sisal* waste demonstrated limited effectiveness against parasitic-stage parasites [54]. However, the extract exhibited moderate efficacy against both the eggs and free-living stages of the parasite without posing any toxicity risk to the goats [49]. Leaf extracts of *Eupatorium triplinerve* showed greater anthelminthic efficacy in both the study's worms compared to the standard albendazole [35].

8. Discussion

Scientific evidence of the contribution of IK to control nematodes in scavenging chickens amongst resource-limited farmers was reviewed [3]. Accessibility to a year-round provision of adequate nutrition remains a major challenge in developing countries. Amongst the most vulnerable groups are widows, women, children under the age of five, and lastly, elderly people. In communal areas, 35% of women earn income from poultry [2]. Chickens are favored among households as the most democratic and popular livestock species, as all members, including children, can own them. In addition, amongst resource-limited farmers, chickens contribute to food variability and diversity [35]. Although chickens are an asset to resource-limited households, several constraints that limit their contribution have been identified. These include housing, predation, low productivity exacerbated by the high prevalence of nematode infestation, and poor veterinary and extension services. As such, IK plays a vital role in improving and eradicating high nematode burdens. For the sustainable intensification of chickens in rural communal areas, there is a need to explore and understand the contribution of IKS to alleviating nematodes in chickens.

The findings from the current review provided insight into how chickens empower women and children and enhance food security by providing organic meat. The observation that chickens are used to empower women could be influenced by the fact that most chickens in the village are owned by females [32]. Women actively engage in various activities, assuming complementary roles and collaborating with their male counterparts, with their contribution surpassing that of men, particularly in chicken production. Women facilitate cleaning, feeding, vaccinating, and selling chickens and eggs [27]. This finding is, however, also contrary to Mapiye et al. [29]. As much as chickens contribute to food security, however, their eating behavior is usually skewed because of culture [19]. The bigger portions of the meat, such as thighs and breasts, are usually given to men rather than women and children. Such patriarchal structures may also contribute to children's malnutrition challenges in Africa and may need to be addressed. The type of production system chickens are kept in is also associated with sub-optimal management, predisposing chickens to high nematode infestation. Such findings agree with Mwale et al. [34] and Swatson et al. [44]. The high nematode burden in chickens is even reported in other parts of the world, such as India and Pakistan [25]. These results are comparable to Puttalakshmamma et al. [39], who reported 77.3 and 71% helminthic infections in local chickens, respectively. Since the advent of anthelmintic resistance and meat safety concerns, searching for alternative approaches to control nematodes has prompted the need to explore IKS (**Table 4**).

The study finds that using IK has proven effective and beneficial due to its active compound against nematodes. There is no risk of drug residues in poultry products

Scientific name	Family	Disease	Method of preparation	References
Aloe maculata *(syn.* Aloe saponaria*)*	Asphodelaceae	Internal worms	Leaf infusions	McGaw and Eloff [9]
Aloe secundiflora	Asphodelaceae	Parasites and diarrhoea	Infusion administered through drench	Kaingu et al. [53]
Aloe marlothii	Asphodelaceae	Parasites, diarrhoea	Leaves	McGaw and Eloff [9]
Aloe ferox	Asphodelaceae	Parasites and diarrhoea	Infusion made of leaves	Mwale and Masika [3]
Acacia karroo	Fabaceae	Intestinal parasites and diarrhoea	Bark and leaves	McGaw and Eloff [9]
Agave sisalana	Agavoideae	Internal worms	Leaves sliced and grounded	Mwale and Masika [3]
Gunnera perpensa	Gunneraceae	Internal parasites	Leaves sliced, grounded, put in water	Mwale and Masika [3]
Sageraea grandiflora	Fabaceae	Ascarida galli	Leaves	Karumari et al. [23]
Centella asiatica	Apiaceae	Internal worms	Cut the whole plant, boil, cool it, and give it to chickens to drink	Mwale and Masika [3]
Xysmalobium undulatum L. R. (Br.)	Apocynaceae	Internal parasites	Cut the whole plant, boil, cool it, and give it to chickens to drink	Mwale and Masika [3]
Millettia grandis (E.Mey.) Skeels	Fabaceae	Internal worms	Soak the leaves in cold water, then give birds to drink	Mwale and Masika [3]
Vernonia colorata (Willd.) Drake subsp. colorata	Asteraceae	Internal Worms	Take the roots and soak them until the color changes to dark brown (like coke), and give the animal 1 L	Luseba and Tshisikhawe [11]
Acacia oxyphylla	Leguminosae	Internal worms	Cut the bark and add to the water; allow it to release the darkish fluid and give chickens to drink	Symeonidou et al. [45]
Alpinia galanga	Zingiberaceae	Pheritima posthuma	Dried rhizome	Subash et al. [43]
Eupatorium triplinerve	Asteraceae	Internal worms	Cut the leaves and soak in the water	Symeonidou et al. [45]

Table 4.
Indigenous plants used for nematode control in scavenging chickens.

compared to synthetic anthelmintics [52]. Using locally available and cheap IK is the most sustainable method for limited households to control nematodes [35]. Using IK covers people's knowledge, methods, skills, and beliefs about the care of chickens and, through trial and error, uses this knowledge to control GIT parasites. Often at times farmers also include the use of Western medicine in combination with IK [3]. Plants from the genus *Aloe* have a long history of use in Africa to eradicate nematodes; however, no medication has been produced. This vividly reveals the need to decolonize veterinary structures as these organizations only accept Western medicine and disparage IKS. Research has consistently been conducted on the efficacy of ethno-veterinary plants against nematodes. However, there is still a lack of valid knowledge about compound activity and toxicology against nematodes and poultry hosts, hence the need for further investigations. *Aloe* species have been reported to possess numerous anthelmintic properties, such as antibacterial, antifungal, and antivenin [29]. These properties are thought to be responsible for paralysing nematodes and preventing their multiplication, respectively.

Acacia spp. has been reported to possess anthelmintic activity against *Ascarida galli*, though no scientific evidence is available for *Acacia karoo*. The degree of anthelmintic activity reported in *Sesbania grandiflora* leaves and *Solanum torvum* fruits aqueous extract could be due to the variations in phytochemicals, such as alkaloids, saponins, and tannins. The study also revealed that different plant parts are exploited during remedy preparation, and different methods are used to prepare plants. The primary plant parts used are roots, leaves, bark, fruits, as well as young shoots and flowers [41]. The efficacy of *Piper betle* L. could be attributed to the active ingredients present in plants, such as alkaloids, flavonoids, polyphenols, and terpenes. These phytochemicals may damage the nematode mobility and cuticle, thus causing paralysis or mortality of the parasites [45]. *Aloe secundiflora* L. is mainly utilized for its exudates and leaf gel, sourced from inner epidermal layers [53]. The secretions from *Aloe secundiflora* L. contain well-known phenolic compounds, including phenyl pyrones, athrones, chromones, tannins, polysaccharides, phenolic compounds, and terpenoids, while the gel mainly consists of polysaccharides [45]. Compounds such as monoterpenes, which are part of essential oils, tend to disrupt the tubulin polymerization in the intestinal cells of the nematode, leading to their degeneration and death [21]. Substances such as tannins possess the ability to bind free protein in the digestive tract, limiting the availability of nutrients and thereby causing larval starvation [21]. In addition, tannins may cause a decrease in gastrointestinal metabolism by inhibiting oxidative phosphorylation, leading to larval death. The leaves of the *Azadirachta indica L*. plant hold significant medicinal value. This plant's chemical constituents include numerous biologically active substances, such as alkaloids, carotenoids, flavonoids, steroids, triterpenoids, ketones, and phenolic compounds [41].

The presence of secondary metabolites might decrease egg hatching, larvae development rate, and egg production by adult parasites. The use of the *Agave sisalana* plant is based on the richness of phytoconstituents responsible for potent medical activities, such as the presence of tannins, flavonoids, coumarins, steroids, and triterpenes [49]. Other authors have reported using *Agave sisalana* with other plants, particularly *M. pyriflora* roots and Aloe sp. leaves, to treat fowl pox in chickens [18]. *Eupatorium triplinerve* is widely used in folk medicine due to its analgesic, anticoagulant, antianorexic, antiparasitic, anthelmintic, sedative, antifungal, and antibacterial properties. The major chemical groups of *E. triplinerve* are saponins, reducing sugars, alkaloids, steroids, triterpenoids, phenols, tannins, and flavonoids [28]. *Eupatorium triplinerve* revealed the presence of Coumarins and phenolic compounds as chemical constituents. Phenolic compounds have anthelmintic and antiparasitic properties (Ascaris) [47]. Likewise, anthelmintics such as oxyclozanide, niclosamide, and bithionol are classified as synthetic phenols and have been proven to disrupt energy production in helminths. In the study by Subash et al. [43], it was found that the phenolic contents in extracts of *Eupatorium triplinerve* exhibited effects comparable to and even surpassed those found in *Alpinia galanga*. The same authors concluded that the anthelmintic activity of *Alpinia galanga* on *Ascaridia galli* has a specific activity, while *Eupatorium triplinerve* has a broad spectrum of anthelmintic activity when used on *Ascaris lumbricoides*.

The aerial parts and roots of *Centella asiatica* are used for medicinal purposes, and its chemical constituents have broad therapeutic benefits, including antimicrobial, antioxidant, anti-inflammatory, anticancer, neuroprotective, and wound healing properties [40]. Asiatic acid, asiaticoside, and madecassoside are the primary constituents contributing to their pharmacological value and are abundant in flavonoids and terpenoids. Centelloid was coined to reflect diverse secondary metabolites produced by plants, primarily pent acyclic, triterpenoid, and saponins. Analysis from the gas chromatography-mass spectrometry revealed that the essential oil of *C. asiatica* contained significant levels of P-cymene-(44%) and various other volatile compounds [40]. *Acacia spp*. are effectual anthelmintic, anti-bacterial, and antifungal agents. The most active components of this genus are condensed tannins (CTs), a type of phenolic secondary metabolites that seldom exhibit toxic effects. The genus also contains saponins like *Acaciaside A* and B, which have been proven to have nematocidal and cestocidal properties. *Acacia oxyphylla* is used widely against gastrointestinal worms in traditional rural medicine. *Acacia oxyphylla* is also responsible for altering the surface ultrastructure in cestodes [17]. The observation that farmers used roots, leaves, and barks during remedy preparation could be influenced by the seasonal effects as the growth of different plant forms varies with season. Indigenous knowledge custodians, however, do not recommend using roots as they can potentially destroy the whole plant.

9. Concluding remarks and further research

Using plant extracts to combat nematodes offers significant benefits, such as reducing contamination in meat and eggs. It can replace synthetic drugs, which pose numerous health risks, such as drug resistance in local pathogen populations and residues in poultry meat. Scavenging chickens play a crucial role in enhancing food security and empowering women while supplying nutritious organic meat. Promoting scavenging chickens could serve as a sustainable way of poverty reduction and improving food security at the household level in many developing countries. Scavenging birds are raised in outdoor production systems which are known to have a high burden of nematode infestations. Although farmers abundantly rely on ethnoveterinary remedies to mitigate nematode challenges, the drawbacks to medicinal plants include inconveniences in using or preparing remedies and the seasonal availability of most medicinal plants. Understanding the remedy preparation methods for treating chickens is crucial to reducing worm counts effectively.

Indigenous knowledge helps control nematodes and enhance both chicken immunity and production. This includes the widespread use of plants, such as *Aloe marlothii A. berger* and *Aloe maculata All.* However, their potential efficacy needs to be validated. It is necessary to evaluate suitable dosages for potential medicinal plants. Policies regulating the utilization and protection of medicinal plants need to be implemented to ensure the preservation and future availability of ethnoveterinary remedies. Farmers' classification of diseases and treatments needs to be comprehended. Efforts are required to evaluate the potential nutritional advantages of these medicinal plants, as certain nutrients can enhance birds' immunity, thereby promoting recovery. Therefore, investigating the potential impact of these ethno-veterinary plants on the carcass attributes and meat quality of scavenging birds is essential. This could include potentially utilizing these ethno-veterinary plants as natural growth promoters. For example, plants such as *Lippia Javanica* leaves have been used as growth promoters in chickens. Other types of *Acacia* plants have been noted to improve the quality of meat. To ensure the safety of organic meat and egg production, biological activity or toxic effects of ethnoveterinary medicine need to be assessed.

There is also a need for the government and other research institutions to invest in studying how indigenous plant products can be commercially developed. They should also offer support to emerging businesses that sell these plants in formal markets. Other opportunities that need to be explored, such as promoting the development of processing skills of medicinal plants, are important because they will assist in plant conservation considering the global issues of climate change and plant species migrating to other areas. There is also a need to explore the development of business skills from IK; for example, in South Africa, the indigenous plant trade has been reported to be worth about 62 million annually. Indigenous plants are processed to make products sold in the informal markets, and such opportunities could be useful in eradicating household hunger. In addition, plants such as *Acacia* leaves and *marula* trees have been tested on meat and carcass quality, growth performance, and antioxidants of various species due to their nutritional contents, such as high protein content. This demonstrates that these plants provide anthelmintic properties and are highly esteemed as feed alternatives. Hence, investing in using plants for medicinal purposes could also lead to discovering plants useful to nutritionists as feed shortages are becoming erratic.

Acknowledgements

The authors would like to acknowledge the University of KwaZulu-Natal Competitive Research Grant (funding code: P530) for funding the project. We also acknowledge the staff at Ukulinga Research Farm, UKZN, and Pietermaritzburg for caring for the birds.

Author's contributions

MC conceived the research idea. NGM reviewed papers and drafted the manuscript, and MVM, SZN, and MC edited the manuscript. MC and MVM did the critical revision of the manuscript.

Disclosure of potential conflict

The authors declare no competing interests.

Author details

Nkanyiso Majola[1], Mbusiseni Mkwanazi[2], Sithembile Z. Ndlela[1] and Michael Chimonyo[2]*

1 Animal and Poultry Science, School of Agricultural, Earth and Environmental Sciences, University of KwaZulu-Natal, Pietermaritzburg, South Africa

2 Faculty of Science, Engineering and Agriculture, University of Venda, Thohoyandou, Limpopo Province, South Africa

*Address all correspondence to: michael.chimonyo@univen.ac.za

References

[1] Abdelqader A, Qarallah B, Al-Ramamneh D, Daş G. Anthelmintic effects of citrus peels ethanolic extracts against *Ascaridia galli*. Veterinary Parasitology. 2012;**188**(1):78-84

[2] Wong JT, de Bruyn J, Bagnol B, Grieve H, Li M, Pym R, et al. Small-scale poultry and food security in resource-poor settings: A review. Global Food Security. 2017;**15**:43-52

[3] Mwale M, Masika PJ. Ethno-veterinary control of parasites, management and role of village chickens in rural households of Centane district in the Eastern Cape, South Africa. Tropical Animal Health and Production. 2009;**41**(8):1685-1693

[4] Malatji DP, Tsotetsi AM, van Marle-Köster E, Muchadeyi FC. A description of village chicken production systems and prevalence of gastrointestinal parasites: Case studies in Limpopo and KwaZulu-Natal Provinces of South Africa. Onderstepoort Journal of Veterinary Research. 2016;**83**(1):1-8

[5] Lalchhandama K, Roy B, Dutta BK. Anthelmintic activity of Acacia oxyphylla stem bark against *Ascaridia galli*. Pharmaceutical Biology. 2009;**47**(7):578-583

[6] Alam M, Alam K, Begum N, Amin M. Comparative efficacy of different herbal and modern anthelmintics against gastrointestinal nematodiasis in fowl. International Journal of Biological Research. 2014;**2**(2):145-148

[7] Butboonchoo P, Wongsawad C. Occurrence and HAT-RAPD analysis of gastrointestinal helminths in domestic chickens (*Gallus gallus domesticus*) in Phayao province, Northern Thailand. Saudi Journal of Biological Sciences. 2017;**24**(1):30-35

[8] Vilakazi BS, Zengeni R, Mafongoya P. Indigenous strategies used by selected farming communities in KwaZulu Natal, South Africa, to manage soil, water, and climate extremes and to make weather predictions. Land Degradation & Development. 2019;**30**(16):1999-2008

[9] McGaw LJ, Eloff JN. Ethnoveterinary use of southern African plants and scientific evaluation of their medicinal properties. Journal of Ethnophamarcology. 2008;**119**(3):559-574

[10] Mkwanazi MV, Ndlela SZ, Chimonyo M. Utilization of indigenous knowledge to control ticks in goats: A case of KwaZulu-Natal Province, South Africa. Tropical Animal Health and Production. 2020;**52**:1375-1383

[11] Luseba D, Tshisikhawe MP. Medicinal plants used in the treatment of livestock diseases in Vhembe region, Limpopo province, South Africa. Journal of Medicinal Plants Research. 2013;**7**(10):593-601

[12] Mkwanazi MV, Ndlela SZ, Chimonyo M. Indigenous knowledge to mitigate the challenges of ticks in goats: A systematic review. Veterinary and Animal Science. 2021;**13**:100190

[13] Ajani EN, Mgbenka RN, Onah O. Empowerment of youths in rural areas through agricultural development programmes: Implications for poverty reduction in Nigeria. International Journal of Research. 2015:34-38

[14] Belete A, Addis M, Ayele M. Review on major gastrointestinal parasites that

affect chickens. Journal of Biology, Agriculture and Healthcare. 2016;**6**(11)

[15] Bettridge JM, Lynch SE, Brena MC, Melese K, Dessie T, et al. Infection-interactions in Ethiopian village chickens. Preventive Veterinary Medicine. 2014;**117**(2):358-366

[16] Chander M, Bodapati S, Mukherjee R, Kumar S. Organic livestock production: An emerging opportunity with new challenges for producers in tropical countries. Scientific and Technical Review of the O.I.E. 2011;**30**(3):569-583

[17] Dasgupta S, Roy B. Antiparasitic activity of methanolic extract of *Acacia oxyphylla* (Leguminosae) against Raillietina echinobothrida. Journal of Parasitic Diseases. 2010;**34**(1):14-19

[18] Giday M, Asfaw Z, Elmqvist T, Woldu Z. An ethnobotanical study of medicinal plants used by the Zay people in Ethiopia. Journal of Ethnopharmacology. 2003;**85**(1):43-52

[19] Gwala MP. Contribution of village chickens to resource-poor households [Msc. thesis]. South Africa: University of KwaZulu-Natal; 2014

[20] Idika IK, Obi CF, Ezeh IO, Iheagwam CN, Njoku IN, et al. Gastrointestinal helminth parasites of local chickens from selected communities in Nsukka region of Southeastern Nigeria. Journal of Parasitic Diseases. 2016;**40**(4):1376-1380

[21] Jain P, Singh S, Singh SK, Verma SK, Kharya MD, Solanki S. Anthelmintic potential of herbal drugs. International Journal Research Development Pharmacy Life Sciences. 2013;**2**(3):412-427

[22] Kabeer N. Gender equality and women's empowerment: A critical analysis of the third millennium development goal 1. Gender and Development. 2005;**13**(1):13-24

[23] Karumari RJ, Sumathi S, Vijayalakshmi K, Ezhilarasi B. Anthelmintic efficacy of *Sesbania grandiflora* leaves and *Solanum torvum* fruits against the nematode parasite *Ascaridia galli*. American Journal of Ethnomedicine. 2014;**1**(5):326-333

[24] Khan L, Qureshi AW, Shah MN, Feroz K, Mansoor A et al. Prevalence and Identification of Nematodes in Chickens from District Charsadda, KPK, Pakistan. 2016

[25] Katoch R, Yadav A, Godara R, Khajuria JK, Borkataki S, et al. Prevalence and impact of gastrointestinal helminths on body weight gain in backyard chickens in subtropical and humid zone of Jammu, India. Journal of Parasitic Diseases. 2012;**36**(1):49-52

[26] Kumm KI. Sustainability of organic meat production under Swedish conditions. Agriculture, Ecosystems & Environment. 2002;**88**(1):95-101

[27] Kusina J, Kusina NT, Mhlanga J. A survey on village chicken losses: Causes and solutions as perceived by farmers. In: ACIAR Proceedings. 2001;**12**(2):148-155

[28] Matos Lopes TR, de Oliveira FR, Malheiros FF, de Andrade MA, Monteiro MC, Baetas Goncalves AC. Antimicrobial bioassay-guided fractionation of a methanol extract of *Eupatorium triplinerve*. Pharmaceutical Biology. 2015;**53**(6):897-903

[29] Mapiye C, Mwale M, Mupangwa JF, Chimonyo M, Foti R, et al. Research review of village chicken production constraints and opportunities in Zimbabwe. Asian-Australian Journal of Animal Science. 2008;**21**(11):1680-1688

[30] Mapiye C, Sibanda S. Constraints and opportunities of village chicken production systems in the smallholder sector of Rushinga district of Zimbabwe. Livestock Research for Rural Development. 2005;**17**(10):34-45

[31] Melesse A. Significance of scavenging chicken production in the rural community of Africa for enhanced food security. World's Poultry Science Journal. 2014;**70**(3):593-606

[32] Mitileni BJ, Muchadeyi FC, Maiwashe A, Chimonyo M, Dzama K. Conservation and utilisation of indigenous chicken genetic resources in Southern Africa. World's Poultry Science Journal. 2012;**68**(4):727-748

[33] Mathialagan P. Empowering Self-help Group Women Through Backyard Poultry Farming Training. 2014;**14**(2):1-9

[34] Mwale M, Bhebhe E, Chimonyo M, Halimani TE. Use of herbal plants in poultry health management in the Mushagashe small-scale commercial farming area in Zimbabwe. International Journal of Applied Research in Veterinary Medicine. 2005;**3**(2):163-170

[35] Muchadeyi FC, Sibanda S, Kusina NT, Kusina JF, Makuza SM, et al. Village chicken flock dynamics and the contribution of chickens to household livelihoods in a smallholder farming area in Zimbabwe. Tropical Animal Health Production. 2005;**37**(4):333-344

[36] Naphade ST, Chaudhari KV. Studies on the seasonal prevalence of parasitic helminths in Gavran (desi) chickens from Marathwada region of Maharashtra. International Journal of Fauna Biological Studies. 2013;**1**(2):4-7

[37] Ncobela CN, Chimonyo M. Farmer perceptions on the use of non-conventional animal protein sources for scavenging chickens in semi-arid environments. African Journal of Agricultural Research. 2015;**10**(32):3107-3115

[38] Ndlela SZ, Mkwanazi MV, Chimonyo M. Characterisation of the indigenous knowledge used for gastrointestinal nematode control in smallholder farming areas of KwaZulu-Natal Province, South Africa. BMC Veterinary Research. 2022;**18**(1):1-10

[39] Puttalakshmamma GC, Ananda KJ, Prathiush PR, Mamatha GS, Rao S. Prevalence of gastrointestinal parasites of poultry in and around Banglore. Veterinary World. 2008;**1**(7)

[40] Prakash V, Jaiswal NISHITA, Srivastava MRINAL. A review on medicinal properties of *Centella asiatica*. Asian Journal of Pharmaceutical and Clinical Research. 2017;**10**(10):69

[41] Raza A, Muhammad F, Bashir S, Aslam B, Anwar MI, Naseer MU. In-vitro and in-vivo anthelmintic potential of different medicinal plants against Ascaridia galli infection in poultry birds. World's Poultry Science Journal. 2016;**72**(1):115-124

[42] Siamba DN, Okitoi LO, Watai MK, Wachira AM, Lukibisi FB, Mukisira EA. Efficacy of *Tephrosia vogelli* and *Vernonia amygdalina* as anthelmintics against *Ascaridia galli* in indigenous chicken. Livestock Research for Rural Development. 2007;**19**(12):2007

[43] Subash KR, Jagan Rao N, Cheriyan BV, Bhaarati GM, Kumar KS. The anthelmintic activity of *Eupatorium triplinerve* and *Alpinia galanga* in *Pheritima posthuma* and *Ascardia galli*: A comparative study. Journal of Clinical & Diagnostic Research. 2012;**32**(1)

[44] Swatson HK, Tshovhote J, Nesamvumi E, Ranwedzi NE, Fourie C.

Characterization of Indigenous Free-ranging Poultry Production Systems Under Traditional Management Conditions in the Vhembe District of the Limpopo Province, South Africa. 2002

[45] Symeonidou I, Bonos E, Moustakidis K, Florou-Paneri P, Christaki E, Papazahariadou M. Botanicals: A natural approach to control ascaridiosis in poultry. Journal of the Hellenic Veterinary Medical Society. 2018;**69**(1):711-722

[46] Sujith S, Sreedevi R, Deepa CK, Asif MM, Pramod VS, Priya MN, et al. Anthelmintic activity of methanolic extracts of three medicinal plants against *Ascaridia galli*. Life Sciences International Research Journal. 2015;**1**(1):84-86

[47] Sugumar N, Karthikeyan S, Gowdhami T. Chemical composition and antimicrobial activity of essential oil from Eupatorium triplinerve Vahl. aerial parts. International Letters of Natural Sciences. 2015;**4**

[48] Tesfaheywe TZ, Amare E, Hailu Z. Helminthosis of chickens in selected small-scale commercial poultry farms in and around Haramaya Woreda, Southeastern Ethiopia. Journal of Veterinary Advances. 2012;**2**(9):462-468

[49] Tewari D, Tripathi YC, Anjum N. Agave sisalana: A plant with high chemical diversity and medicinal importance. World Journal of Pharmaceutical Research. 2014;**3**(8):238-249

[50] Uhuo AC, Okafor FC, Odikamnoro OO, Onwe CS, Abarike MC, et al. Common gastrointestinal parasites of local chicken (*Gallus domesticus*) slaughtered in some selected eatery centres in Abakaliki, Ebonyi State: Implication for meat quality. International Journal of Development and Sustainability. 2013;**2**(2):1416-1422

[51] Wuthijaree K, Lambertz C, Gauly M. Prevalence of gastrointestinal helminth infections in free-range laying hens under mountain farming production conditions. British Poultry Science. 2017;**58**(6):649-655

[52] Zaman MA, Abbas RZ, Qamar W, Qamar MF, Mehreen U, Shahid Z, et al. Role of secondary metabolites of medicinal plants against *Ascaridia galli*. World's Poultry Science Journal. 2020:1-17

[53] Kaingu F, Kibor A, Waihenya R, Shivairo R, Mungai L. Efficacy of *Aloe secundiflora* crude extracts on *Ascaridia galli* in vitro. Sustainable Agriculture Research. 2013;**2**(2):49

[54] Botura MB, Silva GD, Lima HG, Oliveira JVA, Souza TS, Santos JDGD, et al. In vivo anthelmintic activity of an aqueous extract from sisal waste (*Agave sisalana* Perr.) against gastrointestinal nematodes in goats. Veterinary Parasitology. 2011;**177**(1-2):104-110

Chapter 7

Role of Herbal Medicine, Acupressure and Acupuncture in the Treatment of Irritable Bowel Syndrome

Ankita Wal, Biplab Debnath, Neha Verma, Sumanta Bhattacharya, Rahul Shivajirao Solunke, Mohd Masih Uzzaman Khan and Pranay Wal

Abstract

Irritable bowel syndrome (IBS), is a chronic functional gastrointestinal disease that is characterized by a variety of symptoms that have a major negative impact on patients' quality of life. It affects 9–23% of the total population of the world. At this time, no medication that is capable of addressing all symptoms associated with IBS in an effective manner (antispasmodics, antidiarrheals, sedatives). More than half of patients may seek treatment for their gastrointestinal problems via the use of complementary and alternative medicine (CAM), which includes treatments like herbal medicine, acupuncture, and acupuncture. The objective of this chapter is to evaluate the effectiveness and safety of a herbal preparation, acupuncture, and acupressure treatment in patients diagnosed with IBS. Several sources were used to acquire the material, including review articles published in various publications that had keywords such as herbal drugs, acupuncture, acupressure, IBS and so on. The information was also gathered from the Internet. Herbal therapy and plant products are widely utilized to treat IBS. Acupuncture and acupressure have long been used successfully by patients to treat functional gastrointestinal problems. Multiple clinical studies have shown that their effectiveness and safety are superior to those of placebo and conventional medications. Herbal medications, acupressure, or acupuncture show clinically and statistically significant alleviation of IBS symptoms.

Keywords: acupuncture, herbal medicine, irritable bowel syndrome, acupoint, acupressure

1. Introduction

Irritable bowel syndrome (IBS) is a prevalent gastrointestinal disorder that occur as stomach discomfort, gas, diarrhea, and constipation. IBS involves around 10–15% of the regular populace and it has a negative impact on the sufferer's standard of

IntechOpen

IBS with diarrhea (IBS-D)	IBS with constipation (IBS-C)	IBS with mixed bowel habits or cyclic pattern (IBS-M)
Stools that are loose more than 25% of the time and solid less than 25% of the time	Hard stools more than 25% of the time and watery stool less than 25% of the time	More than 25% of the time, both hard and soft stool
Men have a higher prevalence of this condition.	Men have a higher prevalence of this condition.	

Table 1.
Different kinds of irritable bowel syndrome.

living [1]. In addition, many IBS patients experience extracolonic symptoms such as insomnia, anxiety, sadness, and myofascial pain [2, 3]. Females and young individuals are more likely to be affected [4]. According to stool pattern, IBS is categorized into different subclasses: constipation-predominant IBS (IBS-C), diarrhea-predominant IBS (IBS-D), mixed IBS (IBS-M), and unspecified IBS (IBS-U) (**Table 1**) [5].

Many elements are linked in the etiology, which is unknown. Understanding the pathophysiology of IBS is critical since novel pharmacological treatments are starting to target IBS's well-recognized pathophysiologic mechanisms. Gastrointestinal mobility, visceral sensitivity, post-infectious response, brain-gut connections, alterations in fecal microbiota, bacteria overpopulation, food allergy, and intestinal swelling have all been implicated in the development of IBS (**Figure 1**).

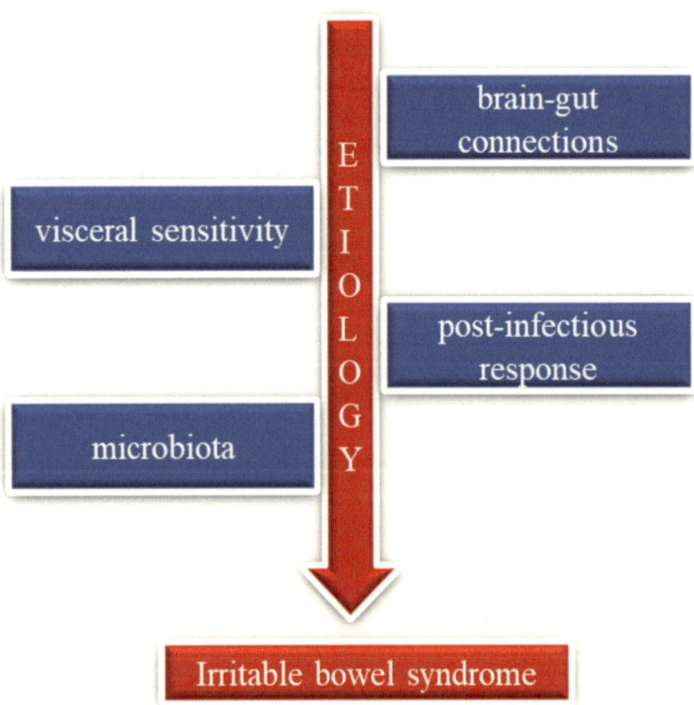

Figure 1.
Etiology of irritable bowel syndrome.

The reported symptoms associated with these mechanisms, include Stomach-ache, gas, diarrhea, and constipation. Not all complaints are related to gastrointestinal; for example, fatigue seems quite prevalent. Medical care of these particular issues has emphasized symptomatic relief [6]. A significant amount of serotonin is found in enterochromaffin cells, which are found in the stomach or intestine, and perform a vital role in the regulation of the peristaltic reflex and sensory relays in the gastrointestinal tract [7]. It is supported by the evidence suggesting the 5-hydroxytryptamine (5HT) system is dysfunctional in people having IBS. Those suffering from constipation-predominant IBS (IBS-C) have a lower plasma serotonin release, whereas those suffering from diarrhea-predominant IBS (IBS-D) have a higher plasma serotonin release [8].

The standard treatment for irritable bowel syndrome (IBS) consists mostly of adopting dietary changes, using medications, and participating in psychotherapy. Medications may include anticholinergics, stool softeners, and laxatives. Examples of these medications are dicyclomine for abdominal cramps, lubiprostone for irritable bowel syndrome type C, and loperamide for irritable bowel syndrome type D [9]. Even while conventional methods of therapy generate good results, there have been reports of negative effects from patients using these medicines. Although it has been shown that loperamide is successful in reducing the frequency of bowel movements, reducing the amount of water in the stool, and slowing the motility of the gut, there have been reports that nausea, cramps, and constipation may be adverse effects of using this medication [10]. Antispasmodics like dicyclomine alleviate the pain and discomfort associated with irritable bowel syndrome (IBS), but they may also cause adverse effects such as sleepiness, dry mouth, impaired vision, or the inability to pee [11]. However, such drugs only give temporary relief from symptoms, and substantial recurrence rates (40 percent on treatment termination after 3 months) have been seen. A high majority of the sufferers (60.1 percent) reportedly discontinued treatment due to dissatisfaction with the lack of symptom relief [12].

Long-term usage may result in serious adverse effects (AEs) such as cardiovascular diseases and ischemic colitis [13], unsatisfactory medication results and adverse events linked with pharmacologic therapy have increased desire for alternative medicines [14]. Acupuncture, acupressure, and herbal medications are regarded as effective complementary treatments for functional gastrointestinal diseases. Various clinical trial.

1.1 Material method

An extensive literature search was done on the various herbs, acupuncture and acupressure using standard databases such as Scopus, PubMed, and Elsevier. Terms like "ginger acupuncture, acupressure, turmeric, and acupoint". Herbs, acupuncture, and acupressure were studied using preclinical and clinical data, as well as hypothesized mechanisms for their effect in the prevention and treatment of irritable bowel syndrome.

1.2 Selection

We included double-blind, randomized controlled studies; randomized placebo controlled multi-centre trials; and a pilot study that compared the effects of herbs, acupuncture, and acupressure therapy (dose and duration of treatment) with placebo in patients with IBS.

2. Herbal drug management

Clinically, herbal medications are used by over 80% of the people in developing nations for primary healthcare. Aside from its popularity in China and India, it is also popular in European countries [15]. They have long been utilized in Asian nations due to their safety, and the Cochrane library determined in 2006 that several herbal medicine may relieve IBS symptoms. Herbal medicine has a range of compounds that can operate on many targets with potentially synergistic action; those that have been used to manage IBS-related symptoms for millennia with good results will be the best choice. There have been various systematic reviews (SRs) on the usefulness of HMs for IBS [16].

Because of the wide range of symptoms that can occur in a single patient, various studies suggest that specific herbs such as peppermint, bitter candytuft, and artichoke leaf may provide some relief for irritable bowel syndrome (IBS), but no single herb should be relied on to provide complete relief. Instead, an herbal blend should be employed. Every herb used to treat irritable bowel syndrome has a specific purpose and is classified as anti-diarrheal, anti-spasmodic, or anti-inflammatory, like peppermint oil and Fumaria officinalis are anti-inflammatory [17, 18] while psyllium act as anti-diarrheal [19].

There have been a number of clinical trials conducted on a variety of herbs, all of which demonstrate good effects in the treatment of irritable bowel syndrome.

2.1 Antispasmodic herbs

Irritable bowel syndrome is characterized mostly by abdominal discomfort, and treatment with antispasmodic herbs is strongly recommended. As a result of the predominance of this symptom, the therapy for IBS often consists of more than one antispasmodic.

Antispasmodics, such as wild yam root, crampbark or blackhaw bark, have a tendency to possess a favorable impact when used in IBS formulations. Despite the fact that these plants have been used for a very long time, very little study has been done on the spasmolytic impact that they have. Viburtinosides derived from a crampbark were shown to have a considerable and quick spasmolytic action on the isolated rabbit jejunum in one animal research [20]. Other plants that are effective in the treatment of spasms include chamomile, glycyrrhiza uralensis, anethum graveolens, atropa belladonna, and acorus calamus.

A physician who had extensive expertise in the therapeutic use of botanicals, Dr. Weiss recommended for the use of Atropa belladonna as an antispasmodic for the gastrointestinal system. He noted that belladonna is the most effective antispasmodic for the gastrointestinal tract [21]. He discovered that it was useful in treating spasms of the stomach, intestine, and bile ducts, and it was equally successful in treating all of these disorders. Dr. Weiss often combined belladonna with chamomile, peppermint, and/or wormwood because he believed that these herbs made the effect of the plant more potent. Because of the herb's potential for toxicity, it should only be used by qualified professionals who have extensive knowledge in the field. On the other hand, when administered by such a practitioner, belladonna often demonstrates a high level of effectiveness for treating more challenging and excruciating instances of IBS.

Fennel mainly contains anethol. It has a molecular similarity to the neurotransmitter dopamine and is found in fennel oil seeds. It has a relaxing action on intestinal smooth muscle, isolated rat uterus, and guinea pig trachea rings. in a pilot study, people who suffer from irritable bowel syndrome experienced relieved stomach discomfort. a mechanism that is most commonly regulated by anethole-dependent relaxation of intestinal smooth muscle [22].

2.2 Antidiarrheal herbs

One of the most concerning elements of irritable bowel syndrome (IBS), from the patient's point of view, is the possibility of having diarrhea, which may lead to fecal incontinence. There are a few different types of herbs that are effective in treating both constipation and diarrhea. Formulations for IBS should always include at least one herb that is shown to be useful in the treatment of diarrhea.

The Indian fumitory is a plant that has a history of usage in traditional medicine for the treatment of both diarrhea and constipation [23]. The results of preliminary pharmacologic and animal research appear to support both of these applications.

Psyllium (Plantago spp.) seed is another effective component that may be included to an IBS treatment regimen. In individuals with irritable bowel syndrome (IBS), psyllium was shown to delay stomach emptying and lower the acceleration of colon transit, as shown in one research [24]. A number of the herbal remedies for diarrhea are astringent, in nature.

Aloe barbadensis Mill., more often known as aloe, is a medicinal plant that is widely known for its numerous therapeutic applications. Aloe is an alternative medicine that is frequently used to alleviate the symptoms of IBS. Although there have been some clinical studies in the past that indicated the positive benefits of aloe in relieving IBS symptoms, AV is most generally used as a powerful laxative and as a drug that improves the motility of the gastrointestinal tract [25].

The majority of them are quite high in tannins, which tie up fluid in the colon and hinder the excretory function of diarrhea, which is meant to be protective [26]. Mild astringents, including bayberry (Morella cerifera) root bark and meadowsweet (Filipendula ulmaria) leaves, may be beneficial in a standardized IBS formulation.

2.3 Bitters

Bitters are a category of herbs that improve the activity and motility of the gastrointestinal system. These herbs have a tendency to enhance gastric productions, have a tonic influence on the gastrointestinal system and give support for the exocrine pancreas. Bitters are used to restore digestive function in irritable bowel syndrome (IBS), which, in turn, tends to balance the intestinal flora and minimize gas and bloating symptoms [21].

Some bitters, such as those made from dandelion (Taraxacum officinalis) leaf, fumitory (Fumaria officinalis) leaf, or any of the herbs in the Artemisia spp. (wormwood and allied species), also contain choleretic, cholagogue, and antibacterial properties. Artichoke leaf and bitter candytuft plant are two examples of bitters that have shown efficacy in the treatment of IBS in early research [27, 28].

2.4 Carminatives herbs

IBS is characterized by flatulence, abdominal discomfort, and other symptoms. The bitters mentioned above will help decrease flatulence significantly by aiding digestion, but herbs with carminative action will help lessen these typical symptoms.

Caraway is a popular herb, and one research found that its volatile oil, when coupled with peppermint oil, was just as efficient in treating dyspepsia as the drug cisapride [29] Because irritable bowel syndrome (IBS) and dyspepsia are both functional disorders of the gastrointestinal system, many therapies that are helpful for people with dyspepsia will also be helpful for sufferers with IBS.

Peppermint is used in Western treatments for irritable bowel syndrome (IBS), and there have been a number of clinical studies that appear to confirm the benefits of peppermint oil in IBS [30]. According to the findings of one research, some peppermint constituents, particularly those that are more polar (or water-soluble), have antiulcerogenic and cholagogue properties. The investigator hypothesizes that these compounds might be responsible for the spasmolytic impact that peppermint has on the intestines and the bowel.

Caraway, dill fruit, anise fruit, peppermint leaf, and chamomile flower are all examples of carminatives, which were used for centuries both in the kitchen and as medicine to aid digestive health.

2.5 Anti-inflammatory herbs

Herbs that help decrease inflammation are known as anti-inflammatory herbs. Such as curcuma, ginger, green tea etc.

Curcumin, the most significant secondary metabolite of C. longa, is responsible for the plant's anti-inflammatory properties [31]. Curcumin has anti-inflammatory action in vitro, and it lowers mucosal damage in an animal model of colitis. Mechanisms include the regulation of I-kappa B kinase activity, which is caused by the suppression of nuclear factor B (NF-kB) and pro-inflammatory cytokines (Tumor necrosis factor alpha, interleukin 1 beta, and interleukin 6) [22]. Turmeric (Curcuma longa) has long been used in Indian, Chinese, and Western herbal therapy to treat stomach discomfort and bloating. Hence it is beneficial in irritable bowel syndrome (IBS) treatment [32].

Ginger is one of the most widely used natural remedies for IBS. The US Food and Drug Administration considers ginger to be a safe food; it mostly contains 1–3 percent oil. Ginger has been shown in studies to influence pain and bowel movements, suggesting that it may help decrease discomfort and stool changes in IBS-D. The quantity of prostaglandin E2 (PGE2) produced is closely linked to the severity of IBS-D with stomach discomfort. The conversion of arachidonic acid to prostanoids, mediated by cyclooxygenase-1 and-2 (COX-1, COX-2) is an important step in the generation of PGE2. Previous research has demonstrated that 6-gingerol may suppress PGE2 generation and inflammation [33].

2.6 Antimicrobial herbs

According to research, infection is most likely a problem in at least some of the individuals who have irritable bowel syndrome (IBS). up to one third of sufferers who have bacterial enteritis may end up with "postinfectious" IBS. According to recent research, the majority of individuals with symptomatic Giardia lamblia have IBS and are not improved by antiparasitic medication [34].

Goldenseal, also known as Hydrastis canadensis is a powerful antimicrobial for the intestines and a very suitable option for treatment of intestinal infection.

DOI: http://dx.doi.org/10.5772/intechopen.108757

3. Acupressure and acupuncture

Acupressure is a kind of acupuncture. Both acupuncture and acupressure are based on the principle of stimulating acupoints along the body's meridians in order to achieve therapeutic effects. By applying pressure to certain acupoints with the palms of one's hand or the tips of one's thumbs, acupressure may be utilized to influence the flow of energy inside the body [35, 36].

3.1 Acupuncture

Acupuncture is one of the complementary and alternative treatments that has gained the most popularity throughout the ages. Acupuncture is a kind of therapy that was developed in China more than three thousand years ago and is now widely used throughout the majority of the globe. From 1970s, the therapy has been gaining acceptance in Western world. Acupuncture involves placing tiny, solid needles (typically 32 to 36 gauge) into specific bodily regions. Various literature mention 365 points that are positioned in a methodical manner on meridians or "channels of energy flow" that are mapped onto the body's surface. According to the principles of traditional Chinese medicine (TCM), a disturbance in the relationship between yin and yang is the root of all disease. Yin represents the feminine aspect of life: nourishing, lower, cold, incomplete, inward, sensitive, protecting, gentle, giving. Yang is the masculine polarity: hard, dominating, energetic, higher, hot, excessive, outer, and creative. The movement of these opposing forces, known as Qi, is regarded as a crucial component in TCM therapy. It is best conceived of as energy manifesting itself, a vitalistic force that runs incessantly through the body's meridians, or energy channels. Disease, pain, and susceptibility to sickness are caused by disturbances in the movement of Qi among the meridians, organs, and five elements. TCM practitioners and medical acupuncturists use needles put at important locations along these meridians to balance elements like as heat, cold, wetness, and dryness in both the outer and inner domains [37].

Over the course of the last several decades, Western cultures have shown a growing openness to the practice of acupuncture. Although it may seem to be a mystery, the acupuncture philosophy does display specific gut physiologic reactions in terms of neuro-, humoral-, opioid-, and serotonergic pathways. Therefore, normalized motility, suppressed acid output, an antinociceptive impact through activation of autonomic pathways, decreased rectal hypersensitivity, and changed 5-hydroxytryptamine functions are described. In clinical practice, it is said to be beneficial for cases of nausea, vomiting, inadequate stomach emptying, some FGIDs, peptic ulcer, Crohn's disease, and postoperative ileus [15].

Acupuncture has a long history of successful treatment for functional gastrointestinal conditions including irritable bowel syndrome (IBS). Irritable bowel syndrome still lacks an effective medication therapy for many people in many regions of the world, but alternative medicine provides therapeutic choices for all suffering individuals [38]. Acupuncture seems to be effective in treating IBS because of its influence on rectal sensation. In IBS sufferers, the combination of acupuncture and massage was more effective than either treatment method when used alone [39]. It has been hypothesized that certain acupoints might alleviate problems of irritable bowel syndrome (IBS), including D-IBS, C-IBS, constipation, as well as abdominal discomfort [40].

3.2 Working

Irritable bowel syndrome (IBS) is characterized by the presence of chronic visceral hypersensitivity, often known as CVH. It is possible that the antihyperalgesic action of acupuncture is mediated by the opioidergic, adrenergic, and serotonergic pathways that are present in both the central nervous system and the peripheral nervous system. Electro-acupuncture at the acupoint ST-36 in both of the rats' hind limbs for a period of thirty minutes substantially reduced the hypersensitive reactions to colonic distention in rats who were subjected to heterotypic intermittent stress (HIS). In contrast, the analgesic effects were inhibited when the patients were pre-treated with naloxone, which is an opioid receptor antagonist. This finding led researchers to conclude that the opioid pathway was involved in the modulation of visceral hypersensitivity by acupuncture. It is well established that an increase in visceral sensitivity in the enteric nervous system may be attributed to hyperactivity in serotonin (5-HT). This is supported by the fact that an antagonist for the 5-HT3 receptor is beneficial in treating irritable bowel syndrome. EA administered at ST-36 reduced visceral sensitivity and had an analgesic effect in rats with chronic visceral hypersensitivity by acting on the serotonergic system [41].

3.3 Acupuncture point used in irritable bowel syndrome

The Zusanli point of the lower limb (stomach-36; ST-36) and the Neiguan point (pericardium-6; PC-6) at the wrist are the most widely utilized acupuncture sites in treating Gastrointestinal problems (**Figure 2**).

ST-36 is placed in a depression between the muscles of the cranial tibia and the long digital extensor on the proximal one-fifth of the craniolateral surface of the back leg, distal to the head of the tibia. PC-6 is found in the groove between the flexor carpi radialis and the superficial digital flexor muscles [40].

Acupuncture at the ST-36 point activates the parasympathetic system and accelerates the rate of intestinal transit [42]. Patients who suffer from IBS who have constipation as their primary symptom may benefit from acupuncture treatment at the

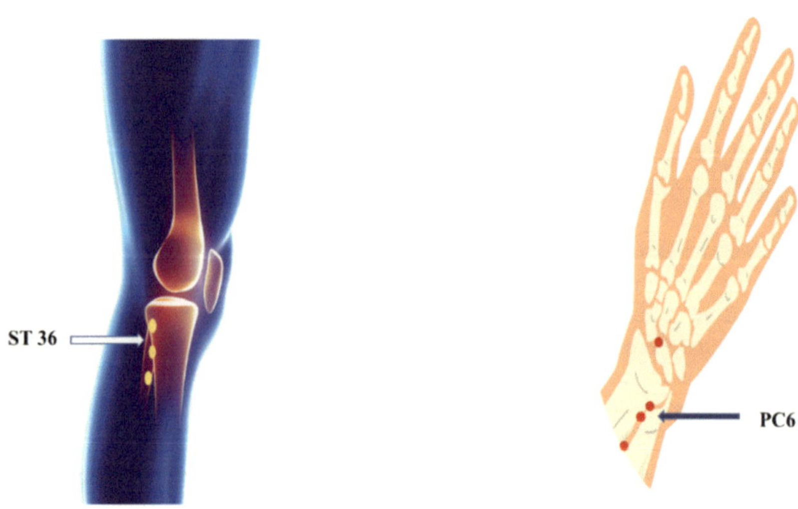

Figure 2.
The sites of the acupuncture points ST36 and PC-6 on the human body.

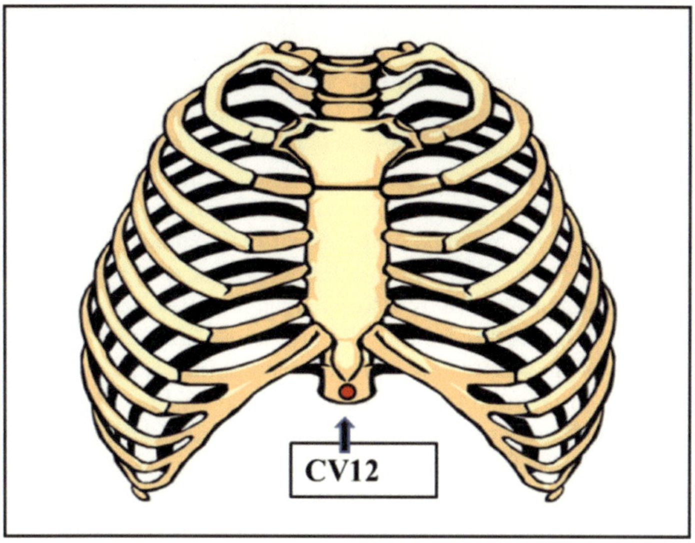

Figure 3.
Acupuncture at the CV-12 location.

ST-36 point, which has a stimulatory impact on intestinal motility. Patients who suffer from stomach discomfort have been treated by acupuncture at the CV-12 location [43, 44]. There is a possibility that activating the sympathetic efferent pathway with acupuncture at CV-12 slows down the rate of colonic transit (**Figure 3**) [45].

3.4 Safety and harmful effects

Acupuncture is an invasive procedure, thus there are certain risk associated with it. These risks include organ puncture, such as pneumothorax, damage to neurological and vascular systems, infection, metal allergy, local discomfort and the creation of a hematoma [46, 47]. The most frequent possible risk is a minor but alarming syncope or presyncope, sometimes known as a "needle shock response," in which the patient feels dizzy and faint. This response may be stopped by withdrawing the needles and providing smelling salts. It is more common on the first visit, although it may be reduced by keeping a careful eye on the sufferer and delivering the therapy in a recumbent rather than sitting posture. Hematoma development is possible, although bleeding is uncommon with acupuncture [37].

3.5 Contraindications

Most sufferers are unable to tolerate acupuncture because they are afraid of needles or are unable to stay in a comfortable posture throughout treatment. Patients who are septic or exceedingly debilitated, as well as those who are not stable due to delusions and hallucinations, are also inappropriate. Electroacupuncture should never be performed on the brain and the heart. These areas are especially vulnerable to injury. Acupuncture therapy should not be given to patients who have serious bleeding problems such as hemophilia or other similar conditions [48]. Acupuncture is not harmful in pregnancy; however, an acupuncturist must be adequately educated and avoid administering sites that might induce uterine contractility.

3.6 Acupressure

Acupressure is a technique across the globe. It is a manual, needle-free, non-invasive, cost-effective, and non-pharmacological healing strategy used to improve the well-being of patients. Muscular tension is relieved in acupressure by putting pressure with the hand at certain acupoints or with the thumbs on specific points, or by putting pressure to acupoints to equalize the flow of physiological energy [36]. Acupressure is similar to reflexology, however with reflexology, the therapeutic response was achieved by working on a predefined reflux zone [49]. Acupressure requires the application of physical pressure to trigger points/acupoints/specific pressure points located along meridians. Meridians are the pathways inside the human body that serve to sustain Qi and consequently the stability of health. Each meridian is linked to different organs and tissues in the human body [50]. It involves applying pressure to certain acupoints in order to activate them. Stimulating these points may rectify an imbalance in the flow of Qi via channels, which in turn treats the disease [36]. In order to attain therapeutic advantages, re-equilibration of Qi, which improves the physiological functioning of bodily systems or Zang-fu in the process, is necessary [51]. Zang-fu is a combined word for the human internal organs; the heart, liver, spleen, lungs, and kidneys are the five Zang organs, while the gallbladder, stomach, small intestine, large intestine, urinary bladder, and sanjiao are the six fu organs [52]. It is essentially a non-pharmacological treatment on the body to cure a variety of illnesses by applying pressure to certain acupoints [53]. Acupuncture refers to the practice of massaging acupoints with the fingers, thumbs, elbows, or any other suitable tools in order to provide effective therapy that lasts from some couple of minutes to hours after a one session. It is a hand-mediated energy healing therapy that is believed to be a useful strategy for the management of a wide variety of ailments. Additionally, it is believed to provide excellent bodily comforts, gratification, and economy [36, 54].

3.7 Acupoints

Pressure points are dispersed across the entire of the human body [55]. The acupoint is the point on the body that lies just under the surface of the skin, and activating the acupoint is the first step in acupressure [56]. Specific acupoint stimulation is known to induce functional responses that may be utilized to cure disorders [57]. Each acupoint has a unique sensation depending on the portion of the body that is experiencing pain or a particular issue. Simply applying pressure to various locations results in a variety of outcomes [36].

Within human bodies, there are a total of 14 meridians that are responsible for the movement of bioenergy (Chetana). Twelve of these fourteen meridians are situated in pairs, one on each side of the body (right and left), with the other two meridians being situated singly. The 12 paired meridians are made up of six 'Yin' meridians, which correspond to the power of negative energy, and six 'Yang' meridians, which correspond to the force of positive energy. These meridians, each of which is connected to one of the body's primary organs, are responsible for regulating the flow of bioenergy. These meridians, which link to the body's major organs, keep the flow of bio-energy going. Each meridian has been named for the organ to which it is linked. One end of the meridian is located in the palm of our hands, legs, or face, while the other end is located in one of our major organs. When pressure is applied to a certain spot on the hand or the leg to which the corresponding organ is linked, the effect is felt in the distant organ. Acupressure employs light to forceful figure pressure. When the acupressure points are stimulated, they help to alleviate muscle tension, boost circulation of blood, and enhance the body's life force energy, all of which contribute to the body's ability to heal itself [58].

3.8 Acupressure point in irritable bowel syndrome

Various acupressure point used in the management of irritable bowel syndrome such as CV6, ST25, SP4, UB25, ST37, and LI14 [59].

3.9 SP4

This point may be found on the medial portion of the inside of the foot, just above the depression on the bottom of the foot. When pressure is applied to this spot, it may help relieve symptoms of irritable bowel syndrome, including stomach discomfort, loss of appetite, diarrhea, and bloody stool (**Figure 4**) [60].

3.10 UB25

Urinary Bladder 25 is positioned in the back, 1.5 cun lateral to the bottom margin of the 4th lumbar vertebra. This pressure point is very beneficial in the treatment of irritable bowel syndrome, as well as abdominal distension, constipation, hemorrhoids, diarrhea, lumbar discomfort, and Urticaria (**Figure 5**) [61].

3.11 L.I.14

Large Intestine 14 or the Upper Arm is a powerful acupuncture point for IBS that may assist with acid regurgitation, IBS complaints, depression, and hiccups (**Figure 6**) [62].

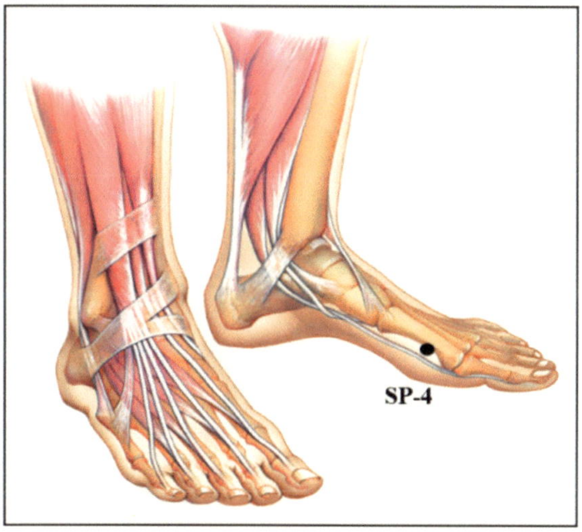

Figure 4.
SP4 site of acupressure.

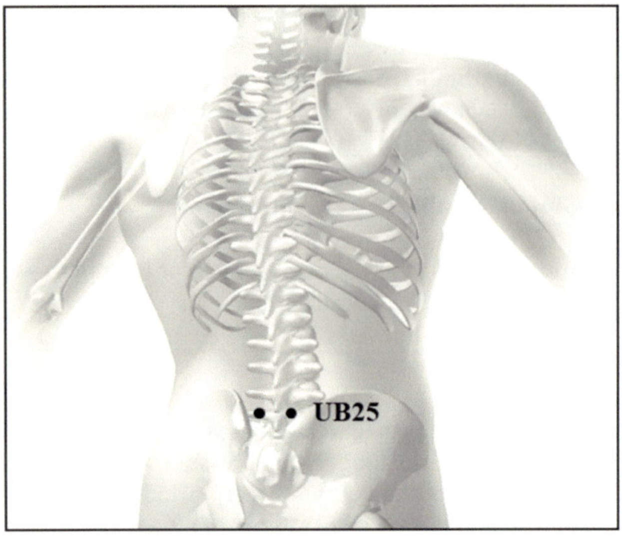

Figure 5.
UB25 location of acupressure.

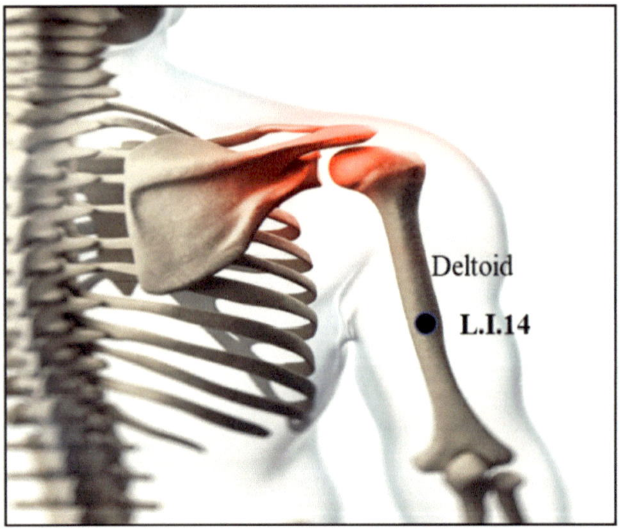

Figure 6.
Acupressure location of L.I.14.

3.12 CV6

CV6, also known as the Sea of Energy, is considered to be one of the most effective acupressure spots for the treatment of irritable bowel syndrome. It is a longevity point that may be helpful in boosting the general health of the body. This point is situated near the center of the lower abdomen, two finger widths below the belly button. Stimulating this spot gently with a soft circular motion stimulates and strengthens the large intestine, which aids in the relief of constipation, IBS, abdominal cramps, and stomach discomfort (**Figure** 7) [63].

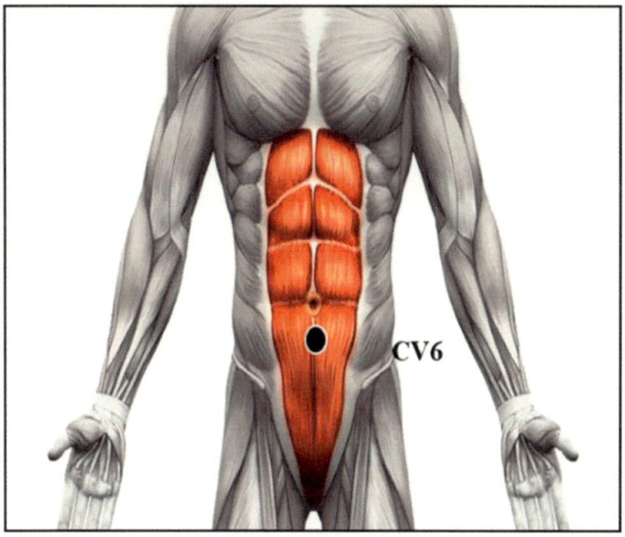

Figure 7.
CV6 site of acupressure.

4. A SUMMARY of many studies on acupuncture, acupressure, and herbal medications

Various clinical trials proven that Acupuncture, acupressure, and herbal medications are safe and effective in the management of irritable bowel syndrome (**Table 2**).

5. Summary

Irritable bowel syndrome (IBS) is a functional gastrointestinal disorder that affects a large percentage of people. The current diagnostic criteria for IBS include the presence of a characteristic symptom profile (abdominal pain or discomfort, bloating or distension, and alterations in defecatory function). Although the pathophysiology of IBS is not fully understood, it is hypothesized that nutrition, gene mutations, psychosocial factors, and immune-mediated mechanisms all have a role. The pathogenesis of IBS is thought to be influenced by visceral hypersensitivity and dysregulation of central pain perception in the brain-gut axis. There is currently no known cure for IBS, and treatment options might vary. Avoiding certain foods, using bulk laxatives and stool softeners for constipation, antimotility drugs for diarrhea, and antispasmodics, antimuscarinics, and antidepressants for pain and spasm are all components of conventional symptom management. As a result, more than 80% of people in developing countries rely on herbal medicine and other alternative therapies for their primary medical needs. This is because there have been so few reports of adverse effects from patients receiving conventional treatment, so they are turning to alternative treatments such as herbal drugs, acupuncture, and acupressure. The Cochrane Library published a study in 2006 that claimed herbal therapy may be able to reduce IBS symptoms. Herbal medicine is made up of a wide number of unique compounds, each of which is capable of operating on a diverse range of targets and, in some instances, performing more successfully when coupled with other compounds.

AUTHOR	CONDITION	DESIGN	INTERVENTION	OUTCOME	MECHANISM	REFERENCE
Zheng H et al.	Irritable Bowel Syndrome	Randomized Controlled trials	Analysis comprised 41 RCTs with 3340 participants.8 RCTs compared acupuncture to sham acupuncture; among which 3 trials verified acupuncture's biological benefit, mainly in treating stomach pain, discomfort and stool frequency.	Acupuncture had no benefits over sham controls in treating IBS while the advantage over western medicine was significant.	Acupuncture	[60]
Pei L et al.		Randomized Controlled trials	In this study participants in each group were randomly randomized to receive acupuncture (18 session) or PEG 4000 (20 g/d for IBS-C)/ pinaverium bromide (150 mg/d for IBS-D) in a 2:1 ratio over a 6-week period.	For the treatment of IBS acupuncture may be more successful than PEG 4000 or pinaverium bromide with result lasting up to 12 weeks	Acupuncture	[12]
Miri B M et al.	Irritable Bowel Syndrome	Randomized Double blinded Controlled trials	In this study, 15 and 65 -year – olds with Rome -III -diagnosed IBS were selected. Control patient were given three tablets of 10 mg hyoscine butyl bromide daily. The participants in the intervention group were daily treated with two 25 mg herbal medicine (Soft gel) capsule containing sunflower oil (28%) as an excipient and pure essentials oils of Zataria multiflora Boiss (28.8%), Anethum graveolens (21.6%) and Trachyspermum ammi (21.6%) for two weeks).	The result of this study showed that the herbal medication was much more effective than hyoscine in relieving the symptoms of IBS	Herbal medicine (Antiseptic, carminative and antispasmodic)	[61]

DOI: http://dx.doi.org/10.5772/intechopen.108757

AUTHOR	CONDITION	DESIGN	INTERVENTION	OUTCOME	MECHANISM	REFERENCE
Madisch A et al.	Irritable Bowel Syndrome	Double blind, Randomized placebo Controlled multi-centre trials	In this study two hundred and eight IBS suffers were randomly allocated to one of four treatments: commercially available herbal products STW 5(n = 51), research herbal preparations STW 5-II (n = 52), bitter candytuft mono – extract (n = 53) or placebo (n = 52).	The result indicates that STW 5, a commercially available herbal product, and STW 5-II, a research formulation, are both beneficial in treating irritable bowel syndrome symptoms.	Clarifications is required regarding the exact workings of the action mechanism.	[62]
Van Tilburg MA et al.	Irritable Bowel Syndrome	Double blind Randomized Controlled trials	Forty -five patients suffering from irritable bowel syndrome (IBS) were divided into three groups given a placebo, on gram of the ginger, or two grams of ginger each day for a period of 28 days.	This study found that ginger was well tolerated but did not perform better than placebo	Ginger (antiemetic, analgesic, sedative, anti-bacterial)	[63]
Liu JH et al.	Irritable Bowel Syndrome	Randomized, Double blind, placebo Controlled trial	In a clinical trial involving 110 people who suffer from irritable bowel syndrome. The peppermint oil was administered three to four times per day, 15 to 30 minutes before meals, for a period of one month	Patients in the active treatment group felt much less pain and discomfort than those in the placebo group. Therefore, peppermint oil was useful in this experiment, and it was well tolerated by the participants.	Peppermint oil (antispasmodic, anti-inflammatory effect)	[17]
Bijerk DW et al.	Irritable Bowel Syndrome	Randomized placebo Controlled trial	In a study conducted by Bijkerk et al. (2009), the dietary intake of soluble fiber (psyllium, 10 grams, n = 85), or insoluble fiber (bran, 10 grams, n = 97), was analyzed in 275 individuals diagnosed with irritable bowel syndrome (IBS)	They demonstrated that patients in the psyllium group experienced a reduction in the intensity of their symptoms that was 90 points more than what was seen in the bran group three months following therapy. They suggested that people in primary care who suffer from IBS might benefit from using psyllium.	Psyllium (the fiber contents increase the weight and size by soften it, A bulky stool is easier to pass and it reduce the chance of constipation)	[18]

AUTHOR	CONDITION	DESIGN	INTERVENTION	OUTCOME	MECHANISM	REFERENCE
Bundy R et al.	Irritable Bowel Syndrome	Partial blinded, Randomized, two dose, pilot study	An eight-week, partly blinded, randomized, two-dose pilot investigation evaluating turmeric extract's effects on individuals with irritable bowel syndrome, two hundred and seven (207) suitable volunteers were randomized.	Approximately two thirds of all patients reported a reduction in the severity of their symptoms after receiving turmeric extract	Turmeric (anti-inflammatory effect, supress proinflammatory molecules in the gut)	[32]
Rahimi R et al.	Irritable Bowel Syndrome	Randomized, double-blind, placebo-controlled trial	The randomized, double-blind, placebo-controlled trial was conducted in IBS patients over a period of 18 weeks using the whole plant of Fumaria officinalis.	The fumitory group experienced a greater reduction in the discomfort associated with IBS compared to the placebo group. Distension caused by IBS was enhanced in the fumitory group whereas it was reduced in the placebo group.	F. officinalis (Anti-spasmodic, anti-inflammatory)	[19]

Table 2.
Summary of different clinical trials on acupuncture, acupressure, and herbal medications.

Herbal medicine may be broken down into three categories: It is believed that they are excellent complementary treatments for disorders that affect the functional gastrointestinal tract. Herbal medicine has a wide variety of compounds, each of which might act on a different target, potentially in a synergistic effect.

Acupuncture and acupressure are the most famous alternative medicine techniques that have been used for digestive system disorders. It may impact the visceral system by activating the somatic system in accordance with the visceral hyperalgesia theory of the central nervous system. When pressure is applied to this region, it may help ease symptoms of irritable bowel syndrome such as pain in the stomach, lack of appetite, diarrhea, bloody stool, abdominal distension, constipation, and bloating.

The herb has numerous uses in Ayurvedic medicine. It is used to treat liver ailments, stomach diseases, and digestive issues, as well as to stimulate the digestive system. Every herb that is used in the treatment of irritable bowel syndrome serves a different purpose. For example, curcuma longa and Zingiber officinale work as anti-inflammatory, while Aloe barbadensis has both laxative effects and anti-inflammatory properties. Whereas peppermint oil decreases gastric motility by directly acting on gut calcium channels to relax gastrointestinal smooth muscle.

Artichoke works as a bitter, and so on. Several clinical trials have shown that these herbs are beneficial in treating irritable bowel syndrome, with minimal adverse effects, and are more cost-effective than traditional medications, which only provide short-term relief.

In patients with irritable bowel syndrome, the practice of acupressure and acupuncture has been shown to have numerous additional beneficial effects on stomach distress and bowel movement. Regularity of bowel movements and hypersensitivity. Irritable bowel syndrome can be managed by applying pressure to certain acupoints throughout the body. These acupoints include SP4 for stomach discomfort, bloody stool, and abdominal distension; UB25 as well as CV6 for abdominal distension and constipation; CV12 alleviates gastrointestinal distress and slows down the rate of colonic transit. Whereas ST 36 accelerates the rate of intestinal transit in IBS-C patients.

6. Conclusion

Since the beginning of the 21st century, herbal medication, acupuncture, and acupressure have captivated both medical professionals and patients around the world. This is due to a number of factors, including the simplicity of their use, their efficacy, and their cost-effectiveness, as well as the fact that conventional medications can cause a greater number of unwanted side effects, such as impaired vision and dry mouth. Alternative and complementary medicine (CAM) therapies are the true culture-based treatments that are used in countries all over the globe. Herbal medications, acupuncture, and acupressure are nonpharmacological interventions that are used in the treatment and management of irritable bowel syndrome. These treatments provide patients with a multitude of benefits and functions that are beneficial for this condition.

Author details

Ankita Wal[1*], Biplab Debnath[2], Neha Verma[1], Sumanta Bhattacharya[3], Rahul Shivajirao Solunke[4], Mohd Masih Uzzaman Khan[5] and Pranay Wal[1]

1 Pranveer Singh Institute of Technology, UP, India

2 Bharat Technology, Uluberia, West Bengal, India

3 Research Scholar Department of Textile Technology, MAKAUT, West Bengal, India

4 Department of Pharmaceutics, Maharashtra College of Pharmacy, Latur, India

5 Department of Pharmaceutical Chemistry and Pharmacognosy, Unaizah College of Pharmacy, Unaizah, Saudi Arabia

*Address all correspondence to: walankita@gmail.com

References

[1] Hungin AP, Whorwell PJ, Tack J, Mearin F. The prevalence, patterns and impact of irritable bowel syndrome: An international survey of 40 000 subjects. Alimentary Pharmacology & Therapeutics. 2003;**17**(5):643-650

[2] Lu CL, Chen CY, Lang HC, Luo JC, Wang SS, Chang FY, et al. Current patterns of irritable bowel syndrome in Taiwan: The Rome II questionnaire on a Chinese population. Alimentary Pharmacology & Therapeutics. 2003;**18**(11-12):1159-1169

[3] Talley NJ. Functional gastrointestinal disorders as a public health problem. Neurogastroenterology & Motility. 2008;**20**:121-129

[4] Lovell RM, Ford AC. Effect of gender on prevalence of irritable bowel syndrome in the community: Systematic review and meta-analysis. Official Journal of the American College of Gastroenterology|ACG. 2012;**107**(7):991-1000

[5] Kibune-Nagasako C, García-Montes C, Silva-Lorena SL, Aparecida-Mesquita M. Irritable bowel syndrome subtypes: Clinical and psychological features, body mass index and comorbidities. Revista Española de Enfermedades Digestivas. 2016;**108**(2):59-64

[6] Occhipinti K, Smith JW. Irritable bowel syndrome: A review and update. Clinics in Colon and Rectal Surgery. 2012;**25**(01):046-052

[7] Talley NJ. Serotoninergic neuroenteric modulators. The Lancet. 2001;**358**(9298):2061-2068

[8] Dunlop SP, Coleman NS, Blackshaw E, Perkins AC, Singh G, Marsden CA, et al. Abnormalities of 5-hydroxytryptamine metabolism in irritable bowel syndrome. Clinical Gastroenterology and Hepatology. 2005;**3**:349-357. DOI: 10.1016/S1542-3565(04)00726-8

[9] Jailwala J, Imperiale TF, Kroenke K. Pharmacologic treatment of the irritable bowel syndrome: A systematic review of randomized, controlled trials. Annals of Internal Medicine. 2000;**133**(2):136-147

[10] Trinkley KE, Nahata MC. Medication management of irritable bowel syndrome. Digestion. 2014;**89**(4):253-267

[11] Brandt LJ, Chey WD, Foxx-Orenstein AE, Schiller LR, Schoenfeld PS, Spiegel BM, et al. American College of Gastroenterology task force on irritable bowel syndrome. An evidence-based position statement on the management of irritable bowel syndrome. The American Journal of Gastroenterology. 2009;**104**:S1-S35

[12] Pei L, Geng H, Guo J, Yang G, Wang L, Shen R, et al. Effect of acupuncture in patients with irritable bowel syndrome: A randomized controlled trial. Mayo Clinic Proceedings. 2020;**95**(8):1671-1683

[13] Nam Y, Min YS, Sohn UD. Recent advances in pharmacological research on the management of irritable bowel syndrome. Archives of Pharmacal Research. 2018;**41**(10):955-966

[14] Tillisch K. Complementary and alternative medicine for functional gastrointestinal disorders. Gut. 2006;**55**(5):593-596

[15] Chang FY, Lu CL. Treatment of irritable bowel syndrome using complementary and alternative

medicine. Journal of the Chinese Medical Association. 2009;**72**(6):294-300

[16] Jun H, Ko SJ, Kim K, Kim J, Jung HS, Park JW. Herbal medicine for irritable bowel syndrome: An overview of systematic reviews protocol. Medicine. 2021;**100**(24):e26364

[17] Liu JH, Chen GH, Yeh HZ, Huang CK, Poon SK. Enteric-coated peppermint-oil capsules in the treatment of irritable bowel syndrome: A prospective, randomized trial. Journal of Gastroenterology. 1997;**32**(6):765-768

[18] Bijerk DW, Muris W. Knottnerus & Hoes (2009): Soluble or insoluble fibre in irritable bowel syndrome in primary care? Randomised placebocontrolled trial. BMJ. 2009;**339**:b3154

[19] Rahimi R, Abdollahi M. Herbal medicines for the management of irritable bowel syndrome: A comprehensive review. World Journal of Gastroenterology: WJG. 2012;**18**(7):589

[20] Cometa MF, Mazzanti G, Tomassini L. Sedative and spasmolytic effects of Viburnum tinus L. and its major pure compounds. Phytotherapy Research: An International Journal Devoted to Pharmacological and Toxicological Evaluation of Natural Product Derivatives. 1998;**12**(S1):S89-S91

[21] Abascal K, Yarnell E. Combining herbs in a formula for irritable bowel syndrome. Alternative & Complementary Therapies. 2005;**11**(1):17-23

[22] Portincasa P, Bonfrate L, Scribano ML, Kohn A, Caporaso N, Festi D, et al. Curcumin and fennel essential oil improve symptoms and quality of life in patients with irritable bowel syndrome. Journal of Gastrointestinal & Liver Diseases. 2016;**25**(2):151-157

[23] Gilani AH, Bashir S, Janbaz KH, Khan A. Pharmacological basis for the use of Fumaria indica in constipation and diarrhea. Journal of Ethnopharmacology. 2005;**96**(3):585-589

[24] Washington N, Harris M, Mussellwhite A, Spiller RC. Moderation of lactulose-induced diarrhea by psyllium: Effects on motility and fermentation. The American Journal of Clinical Nutrition. 1998;**67**(2):317-321

[25] Ahluwalia B, Magnusson MK, Böhn L, Störsrud S, Larsson F, Öhman L, et al. Aloe barbadensis mill. Extract improves symptoms in IBS patients with diarrhoea: Post hoc analysis of two randomized double-blind controlled studies. Therapeutic Advances in Gastroenterology. 2021;**14**:17562848211048133

[26] Yarnell E. Book Review: Second Edition of "Natural Approach to Gastroenterology". Vol. 206. Healing Mountain Publishing; 2011. pp. 341-357

[27] Bundy R, Walker AF, Middleton RW, Marakis G, Booth JC. Artichoke leaf extract reduces symptoms of irritable bowel syndrome and improves quality of life in otherwise healthy volunteers suffering from concomitant dyspepsia: A subset analysis. Journal of Alternative & Complementary Medicine. 2004;**10**(4):667-669

[28] Reichling J, Saller R. Iberis Amara L. (bitter candytuft)--profile of a medicinal plant. Forschende Komplementarmedizin und Klassische Naturheilkunde= Research in Complementary and Natural Classical Medicine. 2002;**9**:21-33

[29] Madisch A, Heydenreich CJ, Wieland V, Hufnagel R, Hotz J. Treatment

of functional dyspepsia with a fixed peppermint oil and caraway oil combination preparation as compared to cisapride. Arzneimittel-Forschung. 1999;**49**(11):925-932

[30] Pittler MH, Ernst E. Peppermint oil for irritable bowel syndrome: A critical review and metaanalysis. The American Journal of Gastroenterology. 1998;**93**(7):1131-1135

[31] Jurenka JS. Anti-inflammatory properties of curcumin, a major constituent of Curcuma longa: A review of preclinical and clinical research. Alternative Medicine Review. 2009;**14**(2):141-153

[32] Bundy R, Walker AF, Middleton RW, Booth J. Turmeric extract may improve irritable bowel syndrome symptomology in otherwise healthy adults: A pilot study. Journal of Alternative & Complementary Medicine. 2004;**10**(6):1015-1018

[33] Zhang C, Huang Y, Li P, Chen X, Liu F, Hou Q. Ginger relieves intestinal hypersensitivity of diarrhea predominant irritable bowel syndrome by inhibiting proinflammatory reaction. BMC Complementary Medicine and Therapies. 2020;**20**(1):1

[34] D'Anchino M, Orlando D, De Feudis L. Giardia lamblia infections become clinically evident by eliciting symptoms of irritable bowel syndrome. Journal of Infection. 2002;**45**(3):169-172

[35] Tournaire M, Theau-Yonneau A. Complementary and alternative approaches to pain relief during labor. Evidence-Based Complementary and Alternative Medicine. 2007;**4**(4):409-417

[36] Mehta P, Dhapte V, Kadam S, Dhapte V. Contemporary acupressure therapy: Adroit cure for painless recovery of therapeutic ailments. Journal of Traditional and Complementary Medicine. 2017;**7**(2):251-263

[37] Sierpina VS, Frenkel MA. Acupuncture: a clinical review. Southern Medical Journal. 2005;**98**(3):330-337

[38] Chao GQ, Zhang S. Effectiveness of acupuncture to treat irritable bowel syndrome: A meta-analysis. World Journal of Gastroenterology: WJG. 2014;**20**(7):1871

[39] Huang ZD, Liang LA, Zhang WX. Acupuncture combined with massage for treatment of irritable bowel syndrome. Zhongguo Zhen jiu= Chinese Acupuncture & Moxibustion. 2006;**26**(10):717-718

[40] Takahashi T. Acupuncture for functional gastrointestinal disorders. Journal of Gastroenterology. 2006;**41**(5):408-417

[41] Li H, He T, Xu Q, Li Z, Liu Y, Li F, et al. Acupuncture and regulation of gastrointestinal function. World Journal of Gastroenterology: WJG. 2015;**21**(27):8304

[42] Iwa M, Matsushima M, Nakade Y, Pappas TN, Fujimiya M, Takahashi T. Electroacupuncture at ST-36 accelerates colonic motility and transit in freely moving conscious rats. Physiology. 2006;**290**(2):G285-G292

[43] Diehl DL. Acupuncture for gastrointestinal and hepatobiliary disorders. The Journal of Alternative and Complementary Medicine. 1999;**5**(1):27-45

[44] Yuehua G. Treatment of acute abdomen by electro-acupuncture-a report of 245 cases. Journal of Traditional Chinese Medicine. 1992;**12**(2):110-113

[45] Tada H, Fujita M, Harris M, Tatewaki M, Nakagawa K, Yamamura T, et al. Neural mechanism of acupuncture-induced gastric relaxations in rats. Digestive Diseases and Sciences. 2003;**48**(1):59-68

[46] Peuker ET, White A, Ernst E, Pera F, Filler TJ. Traumatic complications of acupuncture: Therapists need to know human anatomy. Archives of Family Medicine. 1999;**8**(6):553

[47] Ernst E, White A. Life threatening adverse reactions after acupuncture?A systematic review. Pain. 1997;**71**(2):123-126

[48] Wilson K. The desktop guide to complementary and alternative medicine: An evidence-based approach. BMJ Evidence-Based Medicine. 2002;**7**(3):72

[49] Zhu D, Gao Y, Chang J, Kong J. Placebo acupuncture devices: Considerations for acupuncture research. Evidence-Based Complementary and Alternative Medicine. 2013;**2013**

[50] Narongpunt V, Datcu S, Ibos L, Adnet F, Fontas B, Candau Y, et al. Monitoring acupressure stimulation effects by infrared thermography. Quantitative InfraRed Thermography Journal. 2004;**1**(2):185-204

[51] Lu AP, Jia HW, Xiao C, Lu QP. Theory of traditional Chinese medicine and therapeutic method of diseases. World Journal of Gastroenterology: WJG. 2004;**10**(13):1854

[52] Mehta P, Dhapte V. Cupping therapy: A prudent remedy for a plethora of medical ailments. Journal of Traditional and Complementary Medicine. 2015;**5**(3):127-134

[53] Weaver MT. Acupressure: An overview of theory and application. The Nurse Practitioner. 1985;**10**(8):38-39

[54] Luo D, Wang X, He J. A comparison between acute pressure block of the sciatic nerve and acupressure: Methodology, analgesia, and mechanism involved. Journal of Pain Research. 2013;**6**:589

[55] Cook A, Wilcox G. PRESSURING PAIN alternative therapy for labor pain management. AWHONN Lifelines. 1997;**1**(2):36-41

[56] Kwan RY, Leung MC, Lai CK. Acupressure for agitation in nursing home residents with dementia: Study protocol for a randomized controlled trial. Trials. 2014;**15**(1):1-7

[57] Choi EM, Jiang F, Longhurst JC. Point specificity in acupuncture. Chinese Medicine. 2012;**7**(1):1-5

[58] Mahesh M, Vikrant K, Omkar K. Design and implementation of acupressure therapy using pancake vibrators to trigger palm points. International Journal of Advances in Science Engineering and Technology. 2016;**4**(4):99-102

[59] Devi Gajendran. 8 Effective Acupressure Points for Irritable Bowel Syndrome Treatment. 2015. Available from: https://www.modernreflexology.com/8-effective-acupressure-points-for-irritable-bowel-syndrome-treatment

[60] Zheng H, Chen R, Zhao X, Li G, Liang Y, Zhang H, et al. Comparison between the effects of acupuncture relative to other controls on irritable bowel syndrome: A meta-analysis. Pain Research and Management. 2019;**2019**:2871505

[61] Bordbar G, Miri MB, Omidi M, Shoja S, Akhavan M. Efficacy and safety of a novel herbal medicine in the treatment of irritable bowel syndrome: A randomized double-blinded clinical trial.

Gastroenterology Research and Practice. 2020;**2020**:8213082

[62] Madisch A, Holtmann G, Plein K, Hotz J. Treatment of irritable bowel syndrome with herbal preparations: Results of a double-blind, randomized, placebo-controlled, multi-Centre trial. Alimentary Pharmacology & Therapeutics. 2004;**19**(3):271-279

[63] van Tilburg MA, Palsson OS, Ringel Y, Whitehead WE. Is ginger effective for the treatment of irritable bowel syndrome? A double blind randomized controlled pilot trial. Complementary Therapies in Medicine. 2014;**22**(1):17-20

Section 3

Overall Therapeutic Properties of Herbs

Chapter 8

Phytochemistry, Pharmacological Activities, and Drug Interactions of Pomegranate, *Punica granatum* L. (Punicaceae)

Douglas O. Ochora, Thrineshen Moodley and Rose Hayeshi

Abstract

Pomegranate (*Punica granatum* L.) is a Mediterranean plant that has been used in various countries for the treatment of various diseases in traditional medicine for many generations. These reported medicinal properties of pomegranate are mainly attributed to the presence of various phytochemical compounds in the plant. Scientific literature search was done in PubMed and Google Scholar databases. Full articles published in English for the last 25 years were selected. Pomegranate juice is the widely studied product of a plant. This is because of its wide medicinal and dietary use. Approximately 500 pure compounds have been isolated and characterized from different parts of the plant species. Phytochemically, the juice, seeds, flowers, and peels of *P. granatum* are the most studied parts of the plant. Major phytochemical compounds isolated from the plant include alkaloids, flavonoids, phenolics, tannins, sterols, and terpenes. Most of the compounds isolated from *P. granatum* belong to ellagitannins (punicalagins) and gallotannins. Medicinally, the use of different parts of pomegranate for the treatment of different types of cancer and cardiovascular diseases is the most widely reported in both preclinical and clinical researches. The herb/food-drug interactions of pomegranate juice with approved drugs have shown that pomegranate juice has the potential to inhibit some drugs, especially those metabolized by cytochrome CYP3A and CYP2C9. The current chapter gives a broad overview of the phytochemical, pharmacological, and herb/food-drug interactions of pomegranate.

Keywords: cytochrome, herb/food-drug interactions, *Punica granatum*, pomegranate, phytochemistry

1. Introduction

Punica granatum L., commonly known as the pomegranate, is an ancient plant that is associated with different cultures and religions in the world. Pomegranate is mentioned in the authorized King James Bible version (eight times in the Old Testament), the Koran (three times) [1], and in Buddhist and Chinese arts [2]. The plant is considered native to regions across central Asia, especially Iran and northern India. Its medicinal, nutritional, and ornamental properties have led to its popularity and widespread medicinal use [2, 3].

Since the pomegranate has been known for over 4000 years [4], its medicinal use has been widely studied at both preclinical and clinical levels. Various reviews have been done previously and in recent years on pomegranate; phytochemistry [5], therapeutic/health benefits [6–10], nutritional benefits [11], ethnobotany [8–11], and pharmacokinetics (PK) of different parts of the plant [5]. Related research studies and reviews continue to be published. Therefore, research on pomegranate is still at the exploratory stage and therefore still incomplete [5].

The genus *Punica* has only two species, *P. granatum* (the common pomegranate) and its sister plant, *P. protopunica* Balf. [3]. Most research articles have focused on *P. granatum* and seem to have overlooked *P. protopunica.* Most people are not even aware of the existence of *P. protopunica*. The taxonomy, phytochemical, medicinal, and nutritional values of the forgotten "sister" plant should also be explored [3]. The continued research studies on *P. granatum* depict a potential plethora of medicinal, phytochemical, and nutritional knowledge in the plant species. Consequently, further in-depth study and reporting of research findings on pomegranate is necessary. This will contribute to resolving unclear issues on the plant species and contribute to knowledge in the medical world [5].

The phytochemistry, pharmacokinetics (PK), and pharmacodynamics (PD) of different parts of *P. granatum* (the common pomegranate) have recently been compiled [5]. However, review studies on the effects of *P. granatum* on the metabolism and pharmacokinetics of drugs are limited, and we could only access two that were reported in 2013 and 2023 [12, 13]. This requires an update on previous and current research to guide the current concomitant use of pomegranate with drugs. This happens when people get sick and use *P. granatum* in traditional medicine for the treatment of various diseases [8]. When they are not healed, they seek orthodox treatment in hospitals. Similarly, people also take pomegranate juice during drug medication. This could lead to herb/food-drug interactions [14]. This chapter focuses on the reported effects of pomegranate phytochemicals and pomegranate juice on the PK/PD of approved medicinal drugs since the herb/food-drug interactions are likely to affect the overall pharmacological effects of the co-administered drug.

Based on the wide medicinal use of *P. granatum* in treating various diseases in traditional medicine, coupled with its concurrent use with conventional drugs, a knowledge of the effects of pomegranate on the therapeutic activity of the co-administered drugs remains vital. Moreover, the chapter provides an overall abstract view of previous research on phytochemical, pharmacological, and herb/food-drug interactions of pomegranate that is expected to guide further research on pomegranate and perhaps contribute to a healthy life for its users.

2. Discussion

2.1 Taxonomy

The spelling of the botanical name of pomegranate, *Punica granatum* L. (Punicaceae), was confirmed by checking the *World Flora Online* (WFO) website, https://www.worldfloraonline.org/ (accessed on August 31, 2023). The plant species has 36 heterotypic synonyms, according to the *Plants of the World Online* of the Royal

Botanical Gardens-KEW (accessed on August 31, 2023). The plant is a native of the region covering Iran to the Himalayas of Northern India. This region is considered to be the origin of pomegranate, but the plant has spread to Asia, Europe, America, and Africa (especially North Africa, East Africa, and South Africa) [3, 15]. Pomegranate belongs to a monogeneric family, Punicaceae, which has only two species, *Punica granatum* L. and its sister *P. protopunica* Balf. [3, 16]. *Punica protopunica* is considered the ancestral species of the family. It is less common and occurs only in the northwestern parts of the Indian Ocean, while *P. granatum* is most common and occurs in most parts of the world (Guerrero-Solano et al., 2020). Some of the distinguishing morphological features of the two species include (i) axile placentation in flowers of *P. protopunica,* whereas flowers of *P. granatum* have both axile and parietal, (ii) leaves of *P. protopunica* are dark green while *P. granatum* has shiny green leaves, and (iii) the fruits of *P. protopunica* are less palatable, while those of *P. granatum* are more palatable [3, 16].

Punica granatum grows up to 10 meters high with a pale-brown bark and shiny evergreen leaves. The leaves are oblong with wavy margins, opposite or sub-oppositely arranged, and can grow up to 7 cm long and 2 cm wide (**Figure 1**). Phenological studies of buds and leaves of *P. granatum* revealed that the plant is heterophyllous, having two types of leaves whose shape can be differentiated especially at the apex in dormant stages [17]. The anatomical features of the leaves are similar, but they develop differently to form lanceolate and obcordate final shapes [17]. The flowers are actinomorphic, with a hypanthium that is brightly colored [16]. Pomegranate has three types of flowers: the male flowers, hermaphrodite, and intermediate forms. Heterostyly is the most common form of arrangement of the flowers. The fruit of

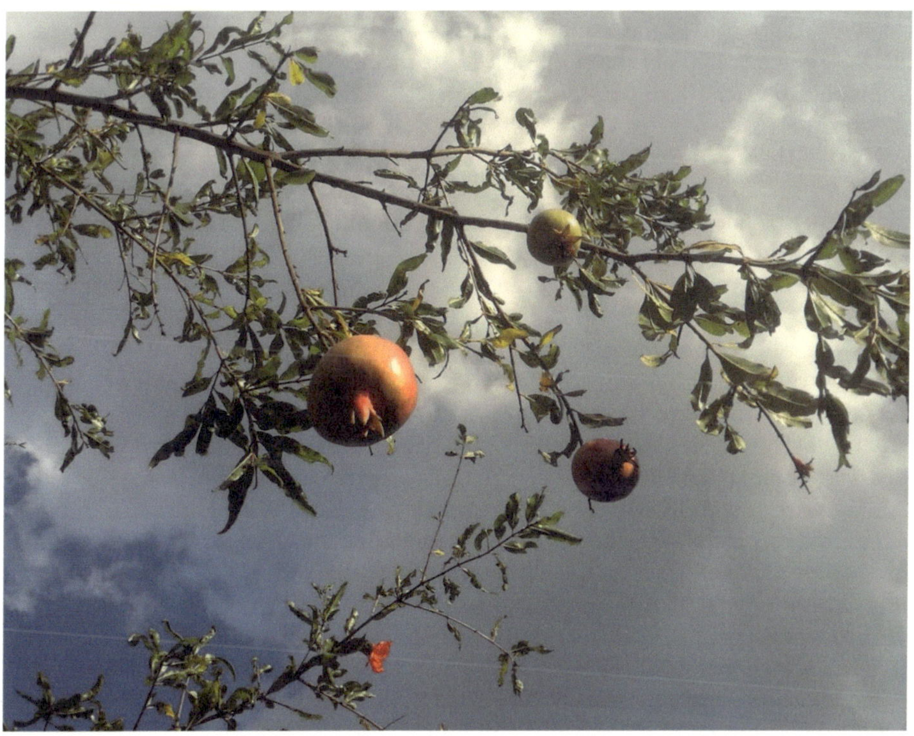

Figure 1.
Punica granatum leaves, fruits, and flower.

pomegranate is globose with a thick tubular calyx. The pericarp is smooth, and the mesocarp is spongy and divided into several parts filled with many seeds [16]. The fruit changes its color from green when young to sun-kissed orange-red (**Figure 1**), which makes it attractive [18].

2.2 Materials and methods

This is a book review chapter on the phytochemistry, pharmacological properties, and herb-drug interactions (HDIs) of *Punica granatum* (pomegranate). Based on the wide medicinal use of pomegranate and published articles and review papers, the current book chapter aimed to compile the phytochemistry, pharmacology, and HDIs of the plant. A review of scientific and relevant literature was therefore selected from PubMed and Google Scholar databases using the following subject headings as keywords: "pomegranate," "*Punica granatum*," "pomegranate phytochemistry," "pomegranate pharmacological properties," "pomegranate herb/food-drug interactions," "pomegranate taxonomy," "pomegranate ethnobotany," "pomegranate anticancer," "pomegranate cardiovascular," "pomegranate antimalarial," and "pomegranate toxicity." Relevant papers were selected based on the following inclusion criteria: full-text original papers written in English, published within the last 25 years for research articles, and last 10 years for review articles. The exclusion criteria included abstracts and articles written in languages other than English. No article was excluded because of affiliation.

2.3 Pomegranate phytochemistry

Plants produce various phytochemical compounds that contribute to the pharmacological activities of medicinal plants. These compounds can act in synergism, especially when the plant is used in its crude form or when isolated compounds are combined. About 500 compounds have been isolated and characterized from different parts of *P. granatum* (leaves, fruit rind, peel, seeds, juice, flowers, and stem bark) [5]. Most of these compounds have been isolated from pomegranate juice. Isolation and characterization of these compounds have been done in various ways. Structure elucidation of 92 compounds such as punicalagin, punicalin, and corilagin was done through nuclear magnetic resonance (NMR) and mass spectroscopy (MS) [5], and recently, other compounds like ellagic acid have been isolated through reverse iontophoresis [19]. In a single study, 88 compounds (flavonoids, coumarins, and phenolic acids) were isolated and identified from pomegranate seeds through ultra-high-performance liquid chromatography (UHPLC) coupled with quadrupole orbitrap high-resolution mass spectrometry (Q Orbitrap HRMS) [20].

Various phytochemical compounds have been isolated from different parts of *P. granatum*: pomegranate juice (180 compounds), seeds (164 compounds), flowers (113 compounds), and peels (108 compounds), based on the basic structures. About 41 compounds have also been isolated from pomegranate leaves and six from the stem bark of the plant species [5]. These compounds include flavonoids, alkaloids, sterols, tannins, ellagitannins, gallotannins, lignans, organic acids, fatty acids, saccharides, anthocyanins, anthocyanidins, proanthocyanidins, coumarins, terpenes, triterpenes, terpenoids, phenolics, phenolic acids, xanthones, xanthonoids, ellagic acid and hydroxycinnamic acid [5, 21, 22], and punicalagin [23]. Based on the review by [5], most compounds belong to ellagitannins and gallotannins.

A total of 88 ellagitannins and 31 gallotannins have been isolated and identified from seeds, juice, flowers, and fruit peels of pomegranates. Most of these compounds have ≥2 constitutional isomers with similar major MS fragments, the same molecular formula, and the same name but different structures [5]. These phytochemicals have shown high health benefits, especially in fruits (pomegranate, strawberry, blackberry, raspberry, and muscadine grapes) and nuts (walnuts) that contain ellagitannins [6].

About 45 anthocyanins have been isolated from *P. granatum*. Considering that these anthocyanins are pigments, they are responsible for the diversified pomegranate flowers and fruit colors [24]. Different substitutions of monosaccharides and disaccharides with aglycone structures corresponding to different chemical structures of anthocyanins have also been isolated from pomegranate. For example, glucose, galactose, xylose, rutinose, and caffeoyl moieties are usually located at different positions of aglycone structure therefore yielding different anthocyanin structures [5].

Pomegranate is also considered a flavonoid-rich plant. Most of these flavonoids have been isolated from pomegranate juice and fruit peel [22]. The study [22] reported that 19 flavonoids have been isolated; however, a later review reported that 171 flavonoid compounds have been isolated from the plant species [5]. Other major compounds like phenolic acids (124 compounds) have also been isolated from pomegranate [5]. These phytochemicals play a major role in the therapeutic effects of *P. granatum* against various human diseases.

2.4 Pharmacological properties of pomegranate

Pomegranate is considered as an ancient medicinal plant in various traditional and complementary systems of treatment for various diseases and disease conditions [4]. To validate this, various research studies have been done at preclinical and clinical levels using various parts (juice, flowers, leaves, fruit rind, bark, peel, seeds, and seed oils) of *P. granatum*. Pomegranate juice is the most widely used pharmacologically.

2.4.1 Ethnobotany of pomegranate

Pomegranate is one of the most ancient plants that have been widely used in traditional medicine, homeopathic medication, and complementary systems of treatment such as Unani Tibb/Islamic, Persian [1, 25], Ayurvedic, Chinese medicine [2], and African traditional medicine [24, 26]. Its current use in traditional medicine for the treatment of several types of cancers, diabetes, hypertension, and stomach ulcers dates back to its native use in Asian cultures [2, 3].

In Ayurvedic (traditional Indian) medication, pomegranate is described as the "dalim fruit" (Sanskrit name), and it is used to cure different parasitic diseases and as a blood tonic. In this respect, people in this Asian culture, regard the plant as "a pharmacy unto itself" [25]. Similarly, in the Chinese ethnomedicine systems (traditional Chinese medicine, Uygur medicine, Mongolian medicine, and Tibetan medicine), most people in these regions use different parts of the plant mostly as a sour flavor to treat diarrhea and stomach upsets [4]. The use of pomegranate for the treatment of various diseases in these and other systems of medication has been studied at preclinical and clinical levels.

2.4.2 Pharmacological properties of pomegranate phytochemicals

Pomegranate has various bioactive substances. These phytochemicals have shown potential preventive and curative pharmacological properties when tested at both preclinical and clinical levels [27]. The preventive activities of pomegranates are displayed by improving the immune response and avoiding infection. The synergistic effect of both preventive and prophylactic activities of pomegranate phytochemicals is greater when these phytochemicals are tested in combination than when they are tested alone [28]. While phytochemicals isolated from pomegranates have been used for the treatment of various ailments, most studies have reported on their use against different types of cancers, treatment of cardiovascular diseases, and some for the treatment of malaria.

2.4.3 Anticancer activities of pomegranate phytochemicals

Cancer is considered one of the leading causes of global mortality. The disease caused 9.6 million deaths, with 18.1 million cases reported in 2018 alone [29, 30]. As part of battling this life-threatening disease, pomegranate has been widely used for the treatment of different types of cancers.

A systematic, comprehensive, and critical review by Wong et al. [27] reported on various research studies on the uses of *P. granatum* for the prevention and treatment of various types of cancer. Furthermore, phytochemicals isolated from different parts of the plant species have shown potential use for the treatment of various types of cancers when tested at both the preclinical (*ex vivo, in vitro*, and *in vivo*) and clinical levels [27]. Polyphenols isolated from natural products have shown anticancer activities. A recent review by Teniente et al. [31] reported on anti-cervical cancer properties of polyphenols from pomegranate peels. Phenolic acids such as punican, punicalagin, ellagic acid, gallic acid, caffeic acid, rutin, and quercetin isolated from pomegranate peels showed *in vitro* activity against cervical cancer [30]. Other phenolics isolated from pomegranate seed oil have also shown *in vitro* antioxidant and anticancer activities against lung and colon cancer [32]. A similar review on the *in vitro* anticancer properties of pomegranate polyphenols has also shown preclinical and clinical therapeutic anticancer activity of various polyphenols against breast cancer [33]. Various studies indicated that these polyphenols have different mechanisms of action such as inhibition and arrest of the cell cycle [34], regulation of cellular redox balance [35], modulation of different signaling pathways [36], and antiproliferative, antiestrogenic, antiangiogenetic, and antimetastatic activities [33, 37].

A recent review on anticancer activities of pomegranate by Rahman et al. [38] reported that extracts and pure compounds isolated from different parts of the plant have preventive and therapeutic activities against different types of cancers such as breast, skin, colon, bladder and lung cancers when tested at preclinical (*in vitro* and *in vivo*) and clinical levels. Similarly, galactomannan isolated from the fruit rind showed *in vitro* and *in vivo* anticancer activities against skin and lung cancers [38, 39]. Other pomegranate phytochemicals such as luteolin, ellagic acid, and punicic acid have shown therapeutic activity against prostate cancer [40]. Furthermore, ellagic acid and urolithins A and B showed *in vitro* inhibition activity against breast cancer. *In vitro* and *in vivo* anticancer prevention activities have also been depicted in pomegranate phytochemicals like tannins and punicalagin against colon cancer [38].

Anthocyanins isolated from natural products are considered as natural antioxidants. Anthocyanins isolated from flowers, leaves, and seeds of pomegranates have shown antioxidant activities [39]. The observed diversity in the chemical structure of pomegranate anthocyanins caused by internal and external factors contributes to the variation of different pomegranate anthocyanins [24]. Additionally, *in vitro* antioxidant activity of phenols, tannins, and flavonoids from pomegranate peels [40] and flowers has also been reported [41]. With the continued reports of increased anticancer multidrug resistance [42], these pomegranate phytochemicals that have shown potential anticancer activities can be used as scaffolds for the discovery of novel anticancer drugs.

2.4.4 Anticancer properties of extracts from pomegranate

Extracts from pomegranate seed oil and fermented fruit have shown *in vitro* therapeutic activity against breast cancer [38]. Peel extracts from pomegranate have shown *in vitro* radical scavenging and Fe^{3+} antioxidant activities [43]. In a recent study, phytocomplexes isolated from pomegranate through hydrodynamic cavitation showed selective *in vitro* antiproliferative activity against human breast cancer cell lines without causing harm to healthy cells [44]. Similarly, fruit extracts of pomegranate have also shown *in vitro* and *in vivo* anticancer activities against skin and prostate cancer [38, 45–47]. The same extract showed *in vivo* antiproliferative activity against lung cancer [38, 48], with similar activity being shown in aqueous peel extracts [49]. Likewise, leaf extracts have also shown *in vitro* signaling pathway inhibition activity against lung cancer [50].

Pomegranate seed, peel extracts, and peel oil have also shown *in vitro* activity against breast cancer [38]. Similar anticancer activity against colon cancer has also been observed in pomegranate juice when tested *in vitro* and *in vivo* [51]. Since cancer is considered the most life-threatening disease globally, pomegranate promises a wide area of further research in the world of oncology. It has potential use as a chemopreventive and/or chemotherapeutic anticancer drug since it has no side effects, especially when used naturally [38].

2.4.5 Anti-cardiovascular activities of pomegranate phytochemicals

Approximately a third of the global deaths in 2019 were caused by cardiovascular (CDV) diseases. This amounted to 9.6 million deaths among men and 8.9 million deaths among women in the same year [52]. Pomegranate phytochemicals have shown potential use to prevent and cure various conditions associated with CDV diseases.

Various pomegranate phytochemicals have shown activity against CDV diseases such as atherosclerosis [53], hypertension, peripheral heart disease, and coronary heart disease [22]. Flavonoids, tannins, ellagitanins, ellagic acid, anthocyanins, punicalagin, punicalin, gallic acid, urolithins, puninic acid, and naringin isolated from *P. granatum* have shown potential vasculoprotective properties [22]. Both preclinical (*in vitro* and *in vivo*) and clinical research studies have shown that the vasculoprotective properties of these phytochemicals are generally through platelet aggregation, reduction of oxidative stress, reduced lipid uptake by macrophages [53, 54], enhanced endothelial cell function [55, 56], alleviation of myocardial ischemia [57], and regulation of blood pressure [22]. Based on the high mortality caused by CDV diseases, these and other pomegranate phytochemicals should be explored further.

2.4.6 Antimalarial activities of pomegranate

Increased resistance of malaria-causing parasites to available antimalarial drugs has made malaria one of the most prevalent parasitic diseases in the world, especially in Sub-Saharan Africa. The disease caused 627,000 deaths globally, in 2021 [58]. Different approaches have been employed to counteract antimalarial drug resistance [59]. Extracts and pure compounds isolated from pomegranate have contributed to the same warfare.

In a book on the use of simple natural remedies, Kurain and Perumal [18] reported that a decoction of the bark of pomegranate is taken for the traditional treatment of malaria [18]. Equally, in the Ayurvedic system of treatment, at a place called Orissa, in the northeastern part of India, the sun-dried rind of immature pomegranate fruits is used as a powdered formulation called OMARIA for treatment and prevention of *Plasmodium falciparum* and *Plasmodium vivax* malaria [60].

The methanolic extracts of the fruit rind of pomegranate have also shown potent *in vitro* antimalarial activity with 50 percent inhibition concentration (IC_{50}) values of 2.8 and 4.5 µg/mL when tested against W2 (chloroquine-resistant) and D10 (chloroquine sensitive) strains of *P. falciparum* [61–63]. These reported antimalarial activities of pomegranate rind are mainly attributed to the ellagic acid and punicalagin phytochemicals of the plant. These compounds are likely to work through the pro-inhibition of mechanisms that are involved in the onset of malaria, especially cerebral malaria [62]. Other compounds like punicalagins have also shown good *in vitro* antiplasmodial activities with IC_{50} values of 7.5 and 8.8 µg/mL, and gallagic acid with IC_{50} values of 7.5 and 8.8 µg/mL when both were tested against D6 and W2 strains of *P. falciparum*, respectively [63]. For *in vivo* antiplasmodial assays, methanolic peel extracts of pomegranate showed a percentage chemosuppression of 50% against *P. chabaudi* using the Swiss albino mouse model [64]. Further antimalarial activities of pomegranate should be explored to validate its use in the treatment of malaria.

Other pharmacological activities of pomegranate extracts and pure compounds such as antibacterial, antifungal, antidiabetic, anti-inflammatory, and antiviral (including COVID-19 virus), and control of disease conditions like Alzheimer's disease, ulcers, and coughs are reported in a review on pharmacological activities of pomegranate [21].

2.5 Herb/food-drug interactions

Herb/food-drug interactions often occur as a result of cytochrome P540 (CYP450) and/or P-glycoprotein (Pgp inhibition). Cytochrome P450 (CYP450) is a heme-containing monooxygenase that primarily defends the body against xenobiotics. CYP450 mediates drug bioactivation to intermediates and is responsible for the metabolism of most of the approved drugs. The CYP450s are mainly hepatic and enteric. This metabolism determines the bioavailability and therefore the therapeutic effect of the orally administered drug [65]. P-glycoprotein is an efflux transporter expressed in a variety of epithelial cells such as those of the large and small intestines. P-glycoprotein in epithelial cells is important in ridding the body of xenobiotics by excretion into, for example, the urine and bile, while endothelial Pgp prevents entry of xenobiotics into organs by excretion into the blood. Herbs and food have been implicated in adverse drug reactions when consumed concomitantly with prescription drugs. Xenobiotics from natural products such as medicinal herbs and food can induce or inhibit CYP450s. Inducers of CYP450s cause increased metabolism of the co-used drugs that can lead to reduced bioavailability of the drug(s), which causes therapeutic failure, and inhibitors lead to increased concentration of the co-used drug(s), thereby enhancing its therapeutic activity or making the drug toxic [65].

People use medicinal plants in traditional medicine for the treatment of various ailments. If the condition persists, patients seek orthodox treatment in hospitals which leads to herb-drug interactions (HDIs) [14, 66]. Food-drug interactions (FDIs) can also occur when food or drinks are taken during medication. The herbs, foods, and drinks taken during drug medication can affect the pharmacokinetics and pharmacodynamics of the drugs by modulating CYP450s [67]. In various parts of the world where pomegranate occurs, especially in Asia, the plant is used both medicinally and dietarily [21]. While most reviews and research studies have reported on the pharmacokinetics of pomegranate juice, extracts, and phytochemicals, few have focused on the effects of pomegranate on drugs. Therefore, herb/food-drug interactions of *Punica granatum* are discussed in this chapter.

2.5.1 Food/juice-drug interactions: effect of pomegranate juice on drugs

Foods or drinks taken during drug medication can lead to food-drug interactions (FDIs). The interaction between grapefruit juice (GFJ) and several drugs is one of the most extensively studied food-drug interactions. The juice was shown to increase the oral bioavailability of the dihydropyridine calcium channel blocker felodipine by inhibiting its metabolism by intestinal CYP3A4 [68]. Similarly, most studies on *P. granatum* drug interactions have focused on pomegranate juice (PJ). The juice has shown inhibition of CYP3A4 [69] and CYP2C9 [70]. Pomegranate juice is taken with drugs since it is thought to possess therapeutic and nutritional benefits [21]. Therefore, an understanding of the effects of PJ on the pharmacokinetics and pharmacodynamics and the overall therapeutic activity of the co-administered drug(s) is necessary.

A recent preclinical and clinical review by Mansoor et al. (2023) showed the effects of PJ on drugs metabolized by CYP3A4 and CYP2C9. The review revealed the preclinical effects PJ on eight drugs: carbamazepine (used for the treatment of seizures), tolbutamide (used to reduce blood sugar), buspirone (used for anxiety disorder), nitrendipine (used for hypertension), metronidazole (antibiotic), sildenafil (male dysfunction), saquinavir (HIV/AIDS), and warfarin (anticoagulant) tested in rats and rabbits [12]. According to the analysis by these authors, these preclinical studies suggested that PJ showed intestinal inhibition of CYP3A4 and CYP2C9 rather than hepatic metabolism.

They also reviewed preclinical studies on drugs not metabolized by CYP3A4 and CYP2C9, namely metformin (antidiabetic) [71], piracetam (nootropic) [72], and theophylline (used for treatment of respiratory diseases such as asthma) [67]. There was no interaction with piracetam and theophylline, but the Cmax of metformin was reduced while there was no change to the area under the curve (AUC). The mechanism of interaction between PJ and metformin was not due to CYP450s. Another recent study showed that PJ and GFJ increased the AUC of brexpiprazole (used for the treatment of schizophrenia and major depressive disorders) in rats [73]. Brexpiprazole is metabolized by CYP3A4 and CYP2D6. The reduction in AUC was suggested to be due to inhibition of intestinal CYP3A4. The effect from the GFJ was more pronounced (approximately twofold) than from the PJ. The review [12] further showed that most clinical studies that were done later showed no effect of PJ on flurbiprofen (an anti-inflammatory) [74], simvastatin [75], dapoxetine [76], midazolam [77], cyclosporine [78], and artemether [23].

This shows that the observed preclinical inhibition of CYP3A4 and CYP2C9 by PJ does not necessarily relate to clinical drug interactions in humans [77]. This could be because most of the clinical studies were done using a single dose of PJ [12] and therefore, further clinical studies with prolonged PJ administration of the co-administered drugs are recommended. Moreover, the observed difference in the preclinical effects of PJ on drugs compared to clinical effects could be due to differences in the drugs used across preclinical (*ex vivo, in vitro, and in vivo*) and clinical studies. Consequently, the clinical studies should be done based on previous similar studies for possible comparison. Interestingly, the study on dapoxetine [76] compared the effects of GFJ and PJ. The GFJ was found to affect the pharmacokinetics of dapoxetine, but the PJ had no effect. This is like the brexpiprazole study in rats, where PJ was found to have a lesser effect on the PK of brexpiprazole compared to GFJ.

Most studies on herb-drug interactions of *P. granatum* focused on PJ. Considering the wide use of the plant species in the treatment of various diseases in traditional medicine and its associated use with drugs, it will be necessary to explore further the effects of the pomegranate extracts on the therapeutic activity of co-administered drugs.

2.6 Toxicity studies of pomegranate extracts

Chloroform, acetone, methanol, and water bark extracts of pomegranate have been reported to be safe in Swiss albino mice as no signs of toxicity were observed when the extracts were orally administered at a dosage of 2000 mg/kg of body [78]. Similar results were obtained when ethanolic leaves and fruit peel extracts of the plant species were orally given to Swiss albino mice at dose levels of 500, 1000, and 2000 mg/kg [79]. This suggests that the reported pharmacological activities of pomegranate are not a result of intrinsic toxicity.

3. Conclusions

Pomegranate is an ancient medicinal plant, and most people continue to use it for the prevention, treatment, and management of various diseases and disease conditions. To guide its traditional use, researchers have focused on the chemopreventive and chemotherapeutic activities of pomegranate. Most of these studies have shown that pomegranate is mostly used to treat different types of cancers and CDV diseases. The continued review reports and studies on the medicinal and phytochemical properties of pomegranate call for further plant research to unearth its medicinal potential.

Conflict of interest

The authors declare no conflict of interest.

Author details

Douglas O. Ochora[1,2*], Thrineshen Moodley[1] and Rose Hayeshi[1]

1 DSI/NWU, Preclinical Drug Development Platform, Faculty of Health Sciences, North-West University, Potchefstroom, South Africa

2 Department of Biological Sciences, School of Pure and Applied Sciences, Kisii University, Kisii, Kenya

*Address all correspondence to: ochoraongeri@gmail.com

References

[1] Farhangii H, Ajilian M, Saeidi M, Khodaei GH. Medicinal fruits in holy Quran. International Journal of Pediatrics. 2014;**2**(3):89-102. DOI: 10.22038/ijp.2014.3461

[2] Chandra R, Dhinesh K, Vilas B, Jadha T, Teixeira D, Silva JA. Origin, history and domestication of pomegranate. Fruit, Vegetable and Cereal Science and Biotechnology. 2010;**2**:1-6

[3] Guerrero-Solano JA, Jaramillo-Morales OA, Jiménez-Cabrera T, Urrutia-Hernández TA, Chehue-Romero A, Olvera-Hernández EG, et al. *Punica protopunica* balf., the forgotten sister of the common pomegranate (*Punica granatum* L.): Features and medicinal properties—A review. Plants. 2020;**9**(9):1-15. DOI: 10.3390/plants9091214

[4] Ge S, Duo L, Wang J, GegenZhula Yang J, Li Z, Tu Y. A unique understanding of traditional medicine of pomegranate, *Punica granatum* L. and its current research status. Journal of Ethnopharmacology. 2021;**271**(27):1-14. DOI: 10.1016/j.jep.2021.113877

[5] Yisimayili Z, Chao Z. A review on phytochemicals, metabolic profiles and pharmacokinetics studies of the different parts (juice, seeds, peel, flowers, leaves and bark) of pomegranate (*Punica granatum* L.). Food Chemistry. 2022;**395**:1-28. DOI: 10.1016/j.foodchem.2022.133600

[6] Espín JC, Larrosa M, García-Conesa MT, Tomás-Barberán F. Biological significance of urolithins, the gut microbial ellagic acid-derived metabolites: The evidence so far. Evidence-Based Complementary and Alternative Medicine. 2013;**2013**:1-15. DOI: 10.1155/2013/270418

[7] Giménez-Bastida JA, Ávila-Gálvez MÁ, Espín JC, González-Sarrías A. Evidence for health properties of pomegranate juices and extracts beyond nutrition: A critical systematic review of human studies. Trends in Food Science and Technology. 2021;**114**:410-423. DOI: 10.1016/j.tifs.2021.06.014

[8] Kumari I, Kaurav H, Chaudhary G. *Punica granatum* L. (Dadim), therapeutic importance of World's most ancient fruit plant. Journal of Drug Delivery and Therapeutics. 2021;**11**(3):113-121. DOI: 10.22270/jddt.v11i3.4832

[9] Valero-Mendoza AG, Meléndez-Rentería NP, Chávez-González ML, Flores-Gallegos AC, Wong-Paz JE, Govea-Salas M, et al. The whole pomegranate (*Punica granatum* L.), biological properties and important findings: A review. Food Chemistry Advances. 2023;**2**:1-12. DOI: 10.1016/j.focha.2022.100153

[10] Vučić V, Grabež M, Trchounian A, Arsić A. Composition and potential health benefits of pomegranate: A review. Current Pharmaceutical Design. 2019;**25**(16):1817-1827. DOI: 10.2174/1381612825666190708183941

[11] Kandylis P, Kokkinomagoulos E. Food applications and potential health benefits of pomegranate and its derivatives. Food. 2020;**9**(2):1-22. DOI: 10.3390/foods9020122

[12] Mansoor K, Bardees R, Alkhawaja B, Mallah E, Abuqatouseh L. Impact of pomegranate juice on the pharmacokinetics of CYP3A4- and CYP2C9-mediated drugs metabolism: A preclinical and clinical review. Molecules. 2023;**28**(5):1-11. DOI: 10.3390/molecules28052117

[13] Srinivas NR. Is pomegranate juice a potential perpetrator of clinical drug-drug interactions? Review of the *in vitro*, preclinical and clinical evidence. European Journal of Drug Metabolism and Pharmacokinetics. 2013;**38**(4):223-229. DOI: 10.1007/s13318-013-0137-x

[14] Erhirhie EO, Ikegbune C, Okeke AI, Onwuzuligbo CC, Madubuogwu NU, Chukwudulue UM, et al. Antimalarial herbal drugs: A review of their interactions with conventional antimalarial drugs. Clinical Phytoscience. 2021;**7**(4):1-10. DOI: 10.1186/s40816-020-00242-4

[15] Hussain SZ, Naseer B, Qadri T, Fatima T, Bhat TA. Fruits Grown in Highland Regions of the Himalayas. 1st ed. Springer; 2021. DOI: 10.1007/978-3-030-75502-7

[16] Rana TS, Narzary D, Ranade SA. Systematics and taxonomic disposition of the genus *Punica* L. pomegranate. Fruit, Vegetable and Cereal Science and Biotechnology. 2010;**4**(2):19-25

[17] Rajaei H, Yazdanpanah P. Buds and leaves in pomegranate (*Punica granatum* L.): Phenology in relation to structure and development. Flora: Morphology, Distribution, Functional Ecology of Plants. 2015;**214**:61-69. DOI: 10.1016/j.flora.2015.05.002

[18] Kurain J, Perumal J. Nature's Remedies Made Simple. 1st ed. Sirivatana Interprint Public Company Limited; 1 Jan 2013. 143 pages. ISBN-10: 6163219767. ISBN-13: 978-6163219763. Available from: https://www.amazon.com/NATURES-REMEDIES-SIMPLE-Kurian-Perumal/dp/6163219767

[19] Moore K, Reeksting SB, Nair V, Pannakal ST, Roy N, Eilstein J, et al. Extraction of phytochemicals from the pomegranate (*Punica granatum* L., Punicaceae) by reverse iontophoresis. RSC Advances. 2023;**13**(17):11261-11268. DOI: 10.1039/d3ra01242e

[20] Li G, Chen M, Chen J, Shang Y, Lian X, Wang P, et al. Chemical composition analysis of pomegranate seeds based on ultra-high-performance liquid chromatography coupled with quadrupole-Orbitrap high-resolution mass spectrometry. Journal of Pharmaceutical and Biomedical Analysis. 2020;**187**:1-9. DOI: 10.1016/j.jpba.2020.113357

[21] Maphetu N, Unuofin JO, Masuku NP, Olisah C, Lebelo SL. Medicinal uses, pharmacological activities, phytochemistry, and the molecular mechanisms of *Punica granatum* L. (pomegranate) plant extracts: A review. Biomedicine and Pharmacotherapy. 2022;**153**:1-23. DOI: 10.1016/j.biopha.2022.113256

[22] Wang D, Özen C, Abu-Reidah IM, Chigurupati S, Patra JK, Horbanczuk JO, et al. Vasculoprotective effects of pomegranate (*Punica granatum* L.). Frontiers in Pharmacology. 2018;**9**:1-15. DOI: 10.3389/fphar.2018.00544

[23] Khuda F, Iqbal Z, Khan A, Zakiullah S, Sahibzada MU, Alam M, et al. Effect of fresh pomegranate juice on the pharmacokinetic profile of artemether: An open-label, randomized, 2- period crossover study in healthy human volunteers. Journal of Pharmaceutical and Biomedical Analysis. 2021;**203**:1-17. DOI: 10.1016/j.jpba.2021.114179

[24] Zhao X, Yuan Z. Anthocyanins from pomegranate (*Punica granatum* L.) and their role in antioxidant capacities *in vitro*. Chemistry and Biodiversity. 2021;**18**(10):e2100399. DOI: 10.1002/cbdv.202100399

[25] Dardona Z. Literature review: *Punica granatum* (pomegranate) with an

emphasis on its anti-parasitic activity. Biological and Pharmaceutical Sciences. 2023;**23**(2):100-114. DOI: 10.30574/gscbps.2023.23.2.0192

[26] Viuda-Martos M, Fernandez-Lopez J, Perez-Alvarez JA. Pomegranate and its many functional components as related to human health: A review. Comprehensive Reviews in Food Science and Food Safety. 2010;**9**:635-654. DOI: 10.1111/j.1541-4337.2010.00131.x

[27] Wong TL, Strandberg KR, Croley CR, Fraser SE, Nagulapalli KC, Fimognari C, et al. Pomegranate bioactive constituents target multiple oncogenic and oncosuppressive signaling for cancer prevention and intervention. Seminars in Cancer Biology. 2021;**73**:265-293. DOI: 10.1016/j.semcancer.2021.01.006

[28] Viladomiu M, Hontecillas R, Lu P, Bassaganya-Riera J. Preventive and prophylactic mechanisms of action of pomegranate bioactive constituents. Evidence-Based Complementary and Alternative Medicine. 2013;**2013**:1-19. DOI: 10.1155/2013/789764

[29] Ochora DO, Kakudidi E, Namukobe J, Heydenreich M, Coghi P, Yang LJ, et al. A new benzophenone, and the antiplasmodial activities of the constituents of *Securidaca longipedunculata* fresen (Polygalaceae). Natural Product Research. 2021;**36**:1-9. DOI: 10.1080/14786419.2021.1925272

[30] WHO. World Health Organization Report on Cancer. WHO; 2020. Available from: https://www.medbox.org/pdf/5e3a6502951fa21f520330b2 [Accessed: September 3, 2023]

[31] Teniente SL, Flores-Gallegos AC, Esparza-González SC, Campos-Múzquiz LG, Nery-Flores SD, Rodríguez-Herrera R. Anticancer effect of pomegranate peel polyphenols against cervical cancer. Antioxidants. 2023;**12**(1):1-15. DOI: 10.3390/antiox12010127

[32] Lydia DE, Khusro A, Immanuel P, Esmail GA, Al-Dhabi NA, Arasu MV. Photo-activated synthesis and characterization of gold nanoparticles from *Punica granatum* L. seed oil: An assessment on antioxidant and anticancer properties for functional yoghurt nutraceuticals. Journal of Photochemistry and Photobiology B: Biology. 2020;**206**:1-6. DOI: 10.1016/j.jphotobiol.2020.111868

[33] Moga A, Dimienescu OG, Balan A, Dima L, Toma SI, Bîgiu NF, et al. Pharmacological and therapeutic properties of *Punica granatum* phytochemicals: Possible roles in breast cancer marius. Molecules. 2021;**26**(4):1-20. DOI: 10.3390/molecules26041054

[34] Hsu TH, Chu CC, Hung MW, Lee HJ, Hsu HJ, Chang TC. Caffeic acid phenethyl ester induces E2F-1-mediated growth inhibition and cell-cycle arrest in human cervical cancer cells. FEBS Journal. 2013;**280**(11):2581-2593. DOI: 10.1111/febs.12242

[35] Park WH. Gallic acid induces HeLa cell death via increasing GSH depletion rather than ROS levels. Oncology Reports. 2017;**37**(2):1277-1283. DOI: 10.3892/or.2016.5335

[36] Li L, Na C, Tian SY, Chen J, Ma R, Gao Y, et al. Ellagic acid induces HeLa cell apoptosis via regulating signal transducer and activator of transcription 3 signaling. Experimental and Therapeutic Medicine. 2018;**16**(1):29-36. DOI: 10.3892/etm.2018.6182

[37] Varghese S, Joseph MM, Aravind SR, Unnikrishnan BS, Sreelekha TT. The

inhibitory effect of anti-tumor polysaccharide from *Punica granatum* on metastasis. International Journal of Biological Macromolecules. 2017;**103**:1000-1010. DOI: 10.1016/j.ijbiomac.2017.05.137

[38] Rahman MM, Islam MR, Akash S, Hossain ME, Tumpa AA, Abrar GM, et al. Pomegranate-specific natural compounds as onco-preventive and onco-therapeutic compounds: Comparison with conventional drugs acting on the same molecular mechanisms. Heliyon. 2023;**9**(7):1-22. DOI: 10.1016/j.heliyon.2023.e18090

[39] Zhang L, Fu Q, Zhang Y. Composition of anthocyanins in pomegranate flowers and their antioxidant activity. Food Chemistry. 2011;**127**(4):1444-1449. DOI: 10.1016/j.foodchem.2011.01.077

[40] Mashkoor MAAL. Total phenol, total flavonoids and antioxidant activity of pomegranate peel. International Journal of ChemTech Research. 2014;**6**(11):4656-4661

[41] Hajimahmoodi M, Moghaddam G, Ranjbar AM, Khazani H, Sadeghi N, Oveisi MR, et al. Total phenolic, flavonoids, tannin content and antioxidant power of some Iranian pomegranate flower cultivars (*Punica granatum* L.). American. Journal of Plant Sciences. 2013;**4**(9):1815-1820. DOI: 10.4236/ajps.2013.49223

[42] Assaraf YG, Brozovic A, Gonçalves AC, Jurkovicova D, Linē A, Machuqueiro M, et al. The multi-factorial nature of clinical multidrug resistance in cancer. Drug Resistance Updates. 2019;**46**:100615-100645. DOI: 10.1016/j.drup.2019.100645

[43] Akuru EA, Chukwuma CI, Oyeagu CE, Erukainure OL, Mashile B, Setlhodi R, et al. Nutritional and phytochemical profile of pomegranate ("wonderful variety") peel and its effects on hepatic oxidative stress and metabolic alterations. Journal of Food Biochemistry. 2022;**46**(4):1-17. DOI: 10.1111/jfbc.13913

[44] Minutolo A, Gismondi A, Chirico R, Marco GD, Petrone V, Fanelli M, et al. Antioxidant phytocomplexes isolated from pomegranate (*Punica granatum* L.). Using hydrodynamic cavitation reveal potential application as adjuvants in cancer therapies. Antioxidants. 2023;**12**(8):1-19. DOI: 10.3390/antiox12081560

[45] Afaq F, Malik A, Syed D, Maes D, Matsui MS, Mukhtar H. Pomegranate fruit extract modulates UV-B–mediated phosphorylation of mitogen-activated protein kinases and activation of nuclear factor kappa B in normal human epidermal keratinocytes. Photochemistry and Photobiology. 2005;**81**(1):38. DOI: 10.1562/2004-08-06-ra-264.1

[46] Malik A, Mukhtar H. Prostate cancer prevention through pomegranate fruit. Cell Cycle. 2006;**5**(4):371-373. DOI: 10.4161/cc.5.4.2486

[47] Zaid MA, Afaq F, Syed DN, Dreher M, Mukhtar H. Inhibition of UVB-mediated oxidative stress and markers of photoaging in immortalized HaCaT keratinocytes by pomegranate polyphenol extract POMx. Photochemistry and Photobiology. 2007;**83**(4):882-888. DOI: 10.1111/j.1751-1097.2007.00157.x

[48] Naghma K, Afaq F, Kweon MH, Kim KM, Mukhtar H. Oral consumption of pomegranate fruit extract inhibits growth and progression of primary lung tumors in mice. Cancer Research. 2007;**67**(7):3475-3482. DOI: 10.1158/0008-5472.CAN-06-3941

[49] Bachoual R, Talmoudi W, Boussetta T, Braut F, El-Benna J. An aqueous pomegranate peel extract inhibits neutrophil myeloperoxidase *in vitro* and attenuates lung inflammation in mice. Food and Chemical Toxicology. 2011;**49**(6):1224-1228. DOI: 10.1016/j.fct.2011.02.024

[50] Yali L, Yang F, Zheng W, Hu M, Wang J, Ma S, et al. *Punica granatum* (pomegranate) leaves extract induces apoptosis through mitochondrial intrinsic pathway and inhibits migration and invasion in non-small cell lung cancer *in vitro*. Biomedicine and Pharmacotherapy. 2016;**80**:227-235. DOI: 10.1016/j.biopha.2016.03.023

[51] Adams LS, Seeram NP, Aggarwal BB, Takada Y, Sand D, Heber D. Pomegranate juice, total pomegranate ellagitannins, and punicalagin suppress inflammatory cell signaling in colon cancer cells. Journal of Agricultural and Food Chemistry. 2006;**54**(3):980-985. DOI: 10.1021/jf052005r

[52] Roth GA, Mensah GA, Fuster V. The global burden of cardiovascular diseases and risks: A compass for global action. Journal of the American College of Cardiology. 2020;**76**(25):2980-2981. DOI: 10.1016/j.jacc.2020.11.021

[53] Mele L, Mena P, Piemontese A, Marino V, López-Gutiérrez N, Bernini F, et al. Antiatherogenic effects of ellagic acid and urolithins *in vitro*. Archives of Biochemistry and Biophysics. 2016;**599**:42-50. DOI: 10.1016/j.abb.2016.02.017

[54] Les F, Carpéné C, Arbonés-Maina JM, Decaunes P, Valero MS, López V. Pomegranate juice and its main polyphenols exhibit direct effects on amine oxidases from human adipose tissue and inhibit lipid metabolism in adipocytes. Journal of Functional Foods. 2017;**33**:323-331. DOI: 10.1016/j.jff.2017.04.006

[55] Han Q, Yan C, Wang L, Li G, Xu Y, Xia X. Urolithin a attenuates ox-LDL-induced endothelial dysfunction partly by modulating microRNA-27 and ERK/PPAR-γ pathway. Molecular Nutrition and Food Research. 2016;**60**(9):1933-1943. DOI: 10.1002/mnfr.201500827

[56] Yilmaz B, Usta C. Ellagic acid-induced endothelium-dependent and endothelium-independent vasorelaxation in rat thoracic aortic rings and the underlying mechanism. Phytotherapy Research. 2013;**27**(2):285-289. DOI: 10.1002/ptr.4716

[57] Tang L, Mo Y, Li Y, Zhong Y, He S, Zhang Y, et al. Urolithin a alleviates myocardial ischemia/reperfusion injury via PI3K/Akt pathway. Biochemical and Biophysical Research Communications. 2017;**486**(3):774-780. DOI: 10.1016/j.bbrc.2017.03.119

[58] World Health Organisation. World Malaria Report. World Health Organisation; 2021. Available from: https://www.who.int/teams/global-malaria-programme/reports/world-malaria-report-2021 [Accessed: September 3, 2023]

[59] Ochora DO, Mogire RM, Masai RJ, Yeda RA, Mwakio EW, Amwoma JG, et al. *Ex vivo* and *in vitro* antiplasmodial activities of approved drugs predicted to have antimalarial activities using chemogenomics and drug repositioning approach. Heliyon. 2023;**9**(8):1-7. DOI: 10.1016/j.heliyon.2023.e18863

[60] Ismail T, Sestili P, Akhtar S. Pomegranate peel and fruit extracts: A review of potential anti-inflammatory and anti-infective effects. Journal of Ethnopharmacology. 2012;**143**(2):397-405. DOI: 10.1016/j.jep.2012.07.004

[61] Dell'Agli M, Galli GV, Corbett Y, Taramelli D, Lucantoni L, Habluetzel A, et al. Antiplasmodial activity of *Punica granatum* L. fruit rind. Journal of

Ethnopharmacology. 2009;**125**(2):279-285. DOI: 10.1016/j.jep.2009.06.025

[62] Dell'Agli M, Galli GV, Bulgari M, Basilico N, Romeo S, Bhattacharya D, et al. Ellagitannins of the fruit rind of pomegranate (*Punica granatum*) antagonize *in vitro* the host inflammatory response mechanisms involved in the onset of malaria. Malaria Journal. 2010;**9**(1):1-9. DOI: 10.1186/1475-2875-9-208

[63] Reddy MK, Gupta SK, Jacob MR, Khan SI, Ferreira D. Antioxidant, antimalarial and antimicrobial activities of tannin-rich fractions, ellagitannins and phenolic acids from *Punica granatum* L. Planta Medica. 2007;**73**(5):461-467. DOI: 10.1055/s-2007-967167

[64] Mubaraki MA, Hafiz TA, Dkhil MA, Al-Quraishy S. Beneficial effect of *Punica granatum* peel extract on murine malaria-induced spleen injury. BMC Complementary and Alternative Medicine. 2016;**16**(1):1-9. DOI: 10.1186/s12906-016-1207-9

[65] Zuo HL, Huang HY, Lin YCD, Cai XX, Kong XJ, Luo DL, et al. Enzyme activity of natural products on cytochrome P450. Molecules. 2022;**27**(2):1-18. DOI: 10.3390/molecules27020515

[66] Ochora DO, Kakudidi EK, Namukobe J, Ipulet P, Wakoli DM, Okore W, et al. Synergism in antiplasmodial activities of Artemether and Lumefantrine in combination with *Securidaca longipedunculata*. Plants. 2022;**11**(47):1-14

[67] Alanbaki A, Alani I, Mallah E, Zakareia Z, Arafat T, Dayyih AW. The effect of pomegranate and licorice on pharmacokinetics of theophylline in rat plasma. Fabad Journal of Pharmaceutical Sciences. 2019;**44**(1):9-15

[68] Bailey DG, Dresser GK, Bend JR. Bergamottin, lime juice, and red wine as inhibitors of cytochrome P450 3A4 activity: Comparison with grapefruit juice. Clinical Pharmacology and Therapeutics. 2003;**73**(6):529-537. DOI: 10.1016/S0009-9236(03)00051-1

[69] Hidaka M, Okumura M, Fujita KI, Ogikubo T, Yamasaki K, Iwakiri T, et al. Effects of pomegranate juice on human cytochrome P450 3A (CYP3A) and carbamazepine pharmacokinetics in rats. Drug Metabolism and Disposition. 2005;**33**(5):644-648. DOI: 10.1124/dmd.104.002824

[70] Nagata M, Hidaka M, Sekiya H, Kawano Y, Yamasaki K, Okumura M, et al. Effects of pomegranate juice on human cytochrome P450 2C9 and tolbutamide pharmacokinetics in rats. Drug Metabolism and Disposition. 2007;**35**(2):302-305. DOI: 10.1124/dmd.106.011718

[71] Awad R, Mallah E, Khawaja BA, Dayyih WA, El-Hajji F, Matalka KZ, et al. Pomegranate and licorice juices modulate metformin pharmacokinetics in rats. Neuro Endocrinology Letters. 2016;**37**(3):202-206

[72] Hamad M, Al-Jariri R, Al-Tamimi L, Abu DA, Abu Dayyih W, Mallah EAT. Validation and determination of Piracetam in rat plasma by using high performance liquid chromatography/Uv/Vis spectrometry (Hplc/Uv/Vis) in presence of pomegranate and liquorice juices for pharmacokinetic study. International Journal of Biology, Pharmacy and Allied Sciences. 2017;**6**(12):2431-2449

[73] Thakkar D, Sahu AK, Rathod R, Sengupta P, Kate AS. Investigation of the impact of grapefruit juice, pomegranate juice and tomato juice on pharmacokinetics of brexpiprazole in rats

using UHPLC–QTOF–MS. Biomedical Chromatography. 2021;**35**(11):e5201. DOI: 10.1002/bmc.5201

[74] Hanley MJ, Masse G, Harmatz JS, Court MH, Greenblatt DJ. Pomegranate juice and pomegranate extract do not impair oral clearance of flurbiprofen in human volunteers: Divergence from *in vitro* results. Clinical Pharmacology and Therapeutics. 2012;**92**(5):651-657. DOI: 10.1038/clpt.2012.170

[75] Park SJ, Yeo CW, Shim EJ, Kim H, Liu KH, Shin JG, et al. Pomegranate juice does not affect the disposition of simvastatin in healthy subjects. European Journal of Drug Metabolism and Pharmacokinetics. 2016;**41**(4):339-344. DOI: 10.1007/s13318-015-0263-8

[76] Abdlekawy KS, Donia AM, Elbarbry F. Effects of grapefruit and pomegranate juices on the pharmacokinetic properties of dapoxetine and midazolam in healthy subjects. European Journal of Drug Metabolism and Pharmacokinetics. 2017;**42**(3):397-405. DOI: 10.1007/s13318-016-0352-3

[77] Anlamlert W, Sermsappasuk P. Pomegranate juice does not affect the bioavailability of cyclosporine in healthy Thai volunteers. Current Clinical Pharmacology. 2020;**15**(2):145-151. DOI: 10.2174/1574884715666200110153125

[78] Laaraj N, Bouhrim M, Kharchoufa L, Tiji S, Bendaha H, Addi M, et al. Phytochemical analysis, α-glucosidase and α-amylase inhibitory activities and acute toxicity studies of extracts from pomegranate (*Punica granatum*) bark, a valuable agro-industrial by-product. Food. 2022;**11**(9):1-19. DOI: 10.3390/foods11091353

[79] Salwe KJ, Sachdev DO, Bahurupi Y, Kumarappan M. Evaluation of antidiabetic, hypolipedimic and antioxidant activity of hydroalcoholic extract of leaves and fruit peel of *Punica granatum* in male Wistar albino rats. Journal of Natural Science, Biology and Medicine. 2015;**6**(1):56-62. DOI: 10.4103/0976-9668.149085

Chapter 9

The Healing Power of Plants for Health

Mehtap Kilic

Abstract

The modern pharmaceutical industry has developed through the use of bioactive molecules isolated from plants, which are traditionally used among the public for disease prevention and treatment. In recent years, with the decline in new drug development efforts, there has been a growing market for existing herbal products such as dietary supplements, standardized plant extracts, and herbal medicines. In therapeutic methods like phytotherapy and aromatherapy, medicinal plants containing therapeutic metabolites are used. However, evolutionary changes in the phytochemical composition of plants have led to an increase in the bioactive compound content in some plants while decreasing it in others. Despite these changes, plants remain an invaluable source of therapeutic compounds due to their extensive biosynthetic capabilities. One major benefit of plants is their intricate composition, comprised of groups of related compounds with diverse activities that synergistically interact to yield a greater overall effect.

Keywords: medicinal plants, phytochemistry, herbal medicine, traditional medicine, phytotherapy

1. Introduction

Herbal medicine remains the predominant choice for approximately 75–80% of the global population, especially in developing nations, as a primary healthcare option [1]. This preference stems from the widespread belief that herbal remedies are not only cost-effective and readily available but also generally free from adverse effects [2]. According to the World Health Organization (WHO), the utilization of herbal treatments surpasses that of conventional medications by two to threefold worldwide [3]. The historical use of plants for medicinal purposes predates recorded human history and serves as the foundation of much of modern medicine. Many mainstream pharmaceuticals have their origins in plants; a century ago, the majority of effective drugs were derived from botanical sources. Examples include aspirin (derived from willow bark), digoxin (from foxglove), quinine (extracted from cinchona bark), and morphine (obtained from the opium poppy) [4].

Throughout the annals of medical history, accounts abound of individuals employing herbs to alleviate the ailments of their communities. However, concurrent with the advent of the Industrial Revolution, allopathic medicine emerged as a dominant force. While herbal medicine remained an effective healing modality, its reception waned [5]. Herbal remedies gradually fell out of favor in conventional medical practice during the mid-twentieth century, not necessarily due to their inefficacy but rather because they lacked the economic viability of newer synthetic drugs [6]. As scientific methodologies advanced in the early nineteenth century, botanical healing practices were increasingly disparaged as pseudoscience. Yet, by the 1960s, concerns regarding the curative effects of conventional medicine and a burgeoning desire for self-reliance spurred a renewed interest in "natural health" and herbal remedies. Globally, herbal medicine received a significant impetus when the World Health Organization advocated for the utilization of traditional plant-based remedies in developing nations to address unmet healthcare needs [7].

Recently, the World Health Organization (WHO) has delineated traditional medicine, which encompasses herbal remedies, as encompassing therapeutic methodologies that have persisted for centuries, predating the emergence and dissemination of modern medical practices and still being utilized today. Traditional medicine represents a synthesis of the cumulative therapeutic wisdom passed down through generations of indigenous medical practitioners. Herbal remedies specifically pertain to traditional medicines primarily relying on medicinal plant preparations for therapeutic purposes. The earliest documented evidence of their utilization can be traced back approximately 5000 years in Indian, Chinese, Egyptian, Greek, Roman, and Syrian texts. Classical Indian texts such as the Rigveda, Atharvaveda, Charak Samhita, and Sushruta Samhita offer insight into the historical use of herbal medicines and traditional remedies, which draw upon the rich traditions of ancient civilizations and scientific heritage [1].

This study discusses the importance of plant chemistry and medicinal plants, focusing on the characteristics of medicinal plants effective in preventing diseases, the pharmacological properties of phytotherapeutic plants, the antimicrobial, antiviral, and anti-inflammatory properties of aromatherapeutic plants, traditional medicinal plants, and how plants historically used in women's health are perceived by the public. Thus, once again, emphasis is placed on the importance of plants and their healing power in human health from the past to the present.

2. Phytochemistry

Historically, natural compounds have served as a boundless reservoir of medicinal remedies [8]. Phytochemistry, the study of this chemical compounds found in plants, is crucial for understanding their potential health benefits. These compounds, which vary widely in structure and function, play a role in defending plants against pests and pathogens. They have been used in traditional medicine for centuries across different cultures. Phytochemistry integrates traditional knowledge with modern scientific approaches, aiming to classify and understand the biosynthetic origins of various phytochemical groups.

Phytochemicals are plant-produced compounds that help plants resist infections and consumption by pests. They come in diverse structures and functions and are classified based on their biosynthetic origin, including amino acids, phenolics, terpenoids, alkaloids, and organosulfur compounds. These compounds have been used in traditional medicines worldwide for centuries and show promise for treating metabolic, immunological, and neurological disorders [9].

3. Medicinal plant

A medicinal plant is defined as a plant that contains substances within one or more of its organs that can be utilized for therapeutic purposes or serve as precursors for synthesizing beneficial drugs. This definition allows for the differentiation between medicinal plants with scientifically established therapeutic properties and constituents, and those plants considered medicinal but have yet to undergo comprehensive scientific scrutiny.

Several plants have been utilized in traditional medicine for extensive periods. While some exhibit apparent efficacy, there might not be adequate scientific evidence, such as double-blind trials, to verify their effectiveness. Nonetheless, such plants should be considered medicinal.

3.1 Medicinal plants and disease prevention

Medicinal plants have the potential to play crucial roles in disease prevention, seamlessly integrating into all established prevention strategies. Nevertheless, deliberate endeavors are necessary to accurately identify, acknowledge, and integrate medicinal plants within the framework and execution of these strategies. These approaches offer intriguing and evolving outlooks within the realm of medicinal plants.

3.2 Medicinal plants used to prevent cancer

In his 2012 review, Yasukawa examined the chemopreventive properties of natural sources, foods, supplements, crude drugs, and Kampo medicines (traditional Japanese herbal prescriptions). He noted that cancer chemoprevention currently stands as one of the most pressing priorities in public health. Cancer chemoprevention involves the utilization of specific natural and synthetic chemical agents to counteract or inhibit carcinogenesis and deter the emergence of invasive cancers. Recent studies have highlighted the significant impact of dietary non-nutrient compounds as chemo-preventive agents, with extensive research conducted on their effects in animal models. Epidemiological studies have established a strong correlation between the majority of human cancers and two primary factors: diet and smoking [10]. Furthermore, certain foods consumed daily by the general population have exhibited anticancer properties, underscoring the pivotal role of environmental factors such as diet in cancer chemoprevention [10]. A comprehensive understanding of the mechanisms underlying carcinogenesis is imperative for effective cancer chemoprevention.

The promotion stage of carcinogenesis, unlike initiation and progression, has been observed in animal studies to span a lengthy period and potentially be reversible, particularly in its early phases. This suggests that targeting tumor promotion could be an effective strategy for cancer control [11]. Yasukawa and colleagues have identified various triterpene alcohols, sterols, and their derivatives from edible plants, fungi, and crude drugs that exhibit inhibitory effects on inflammation induced by 12-Otetradecanoylphorbol-13-acetate (TPA) in mouse ears. Primary cancer prevention seeks to thwart cancer development by inhibiting initiation and/or promotion of carcinogenesis. However, since adults may harbor tumor cells that cannot revert to normalcy, effective cancer prevention strategies involve preventing continuous interaction between these cells and promoters and/or aggressively suppressing tumor promoter effects. Thus, discovering plants containing potent compounds (anti-tumor promoters) that impede, inhibit, or halt tumor promotion an inherently reversible and protracted process is crucial [12]. Below are a few examples of such plants of interest.

3.2.1 Rosmarinus officinalis *L (Labiatae) rosemary*

Colorectal cancer ranks as the second leading cause of cancer-related mortality in Australia. Ngo et al. conducted a comprehensive review spanning studies published from 1996 to March 2010, focusing on the protective effects of rosemary (**Figure 1**) against colorectal cancer and other cancer types [13]. Their analysis of evidence from animal and cell culture studies revealed the anticancer potential of rosemary extract and specific constituents, namely carnosol, carnosic acid, ursolic acid, and rosmarinic acid. López-Jiménez further demonstrated the anti-angiogenic properties of carnosol and carnosic acid, highlighting their potential contribution to the chemopreventive, antitumoral, and antimetastatic effects of rosemary extracts [14]. The study suggested the therapeutic potential of these compounds in treating other angiogenesis-related malignancies.

3.2.2 Vitis vinifera *L. (Vitaceae) grape*

Grape skin and seed extracts (**Figure 2**) demonstrate potent abilities to scavenge free radicals, chelate metals, and prevent lipid oxidation in various food and cell models in vitro. The utilization of grape antioxidants shows promise in combating a wide spectrum of cancer cells through multiple mechanisms. These include targeting the epidermal growth factor receptor (EGFR) and its downstream pathways, suppressing the overexpression of COX-2 and prostaglandin E2 receptors or modulating estrogen receptor pathways. These actions lead to cell cycle arrest and apoptosis [15].

3.2.3 Glycine max *or G. soya (Leguminosae) soya milk*

Genistein, the predominant phytoestrogen found in soybeans, has the potential to interact with estrogen receptors and exhibit anticancer effects. Khan et al. investigated whether the consumption of soy isoflavones might confer protection against

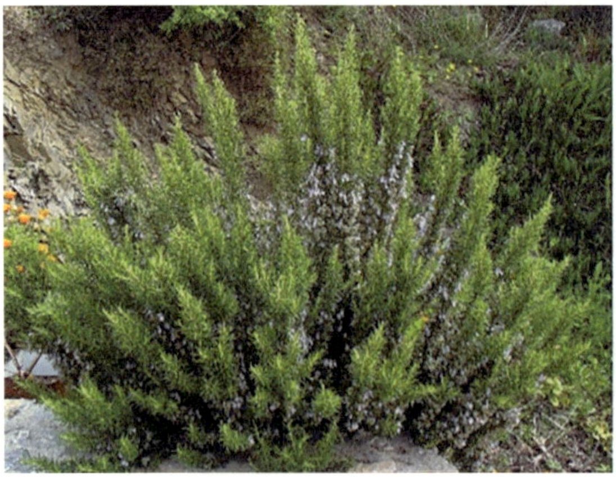

Figure 1.
Rosemary Rosmarinus officinalis *L. (Labiatae) (from: https://www.gardenersworld.com/plants/rosmarinus-officinalis).*

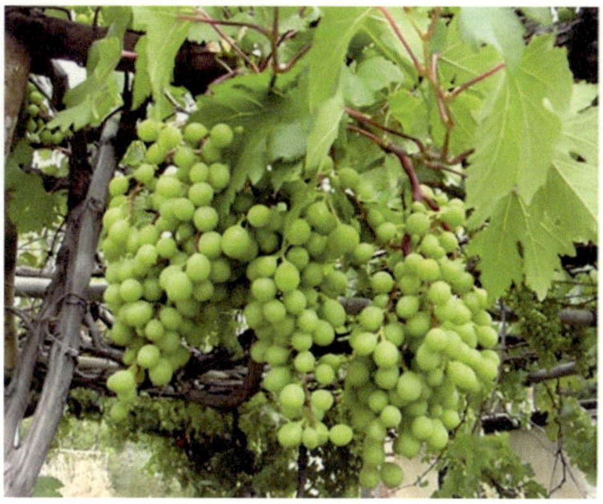

Figure 2.
Grape Vitis vinifera *L. (Vitaceae) (from: https://www.gardenersworld.com/plants/vitis vinifera).*

the development of breast cancer [16]. Their findings revealed a lack of efficacy in breast cancer prevention and a potential adverse effect in premenopausal women. Additionally, Ohta et al. demonstrated that soy milk inhibited mammary carcinogenesis induced by 4-(methylnitrosamino)-1-(3-pyridyl)-1-butanone in rats [17]. Soybeans are rich in isoflavonoids and saponins; isoflavonoids have been reported to possess phytoestrogenic activity (**Figure 3**) [18].

3.2.4 Zingiber officinale *roscoe (Zingiberaceae) ginger*

Dehydrozingerone, a compound found in ginger, shares structural similarities with curcumin, a promising phytochemical known for its potential to inhibit malignant tumors, including colon cancer. Yogosawa et al. investigated the antiproliferative effects of dehydrozingerone on HT-29 human colon cancer cells [19]. They discovered that dehydrozingerone inhibited cell growth at the G2/M phase in a dose-dependent manner, up-regulating p21 expression and inducing intracellular ROS accumulation. These findings suggest that dehydrozingerone analogues could serve as potential chemotherapeutic agents for colon cancer [20]. In another study, Kurapati et al. examined the combined cytotoxic effects of *Curcuma longa* and *Zingiber officinale* (**Figure 4**) on the PC-3 M prostate cancer cell line [21]. While both extracts

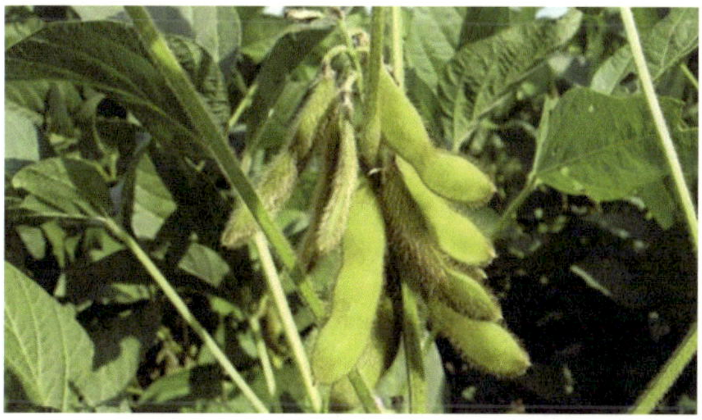

Figure 3.
Soya milk Glycine max *(Leguminosae) (from: https://www.researchgate.net/figure/Soybean-Glycine-max-L-Merr-Fabaceae-family-46_fig4_352376798).*

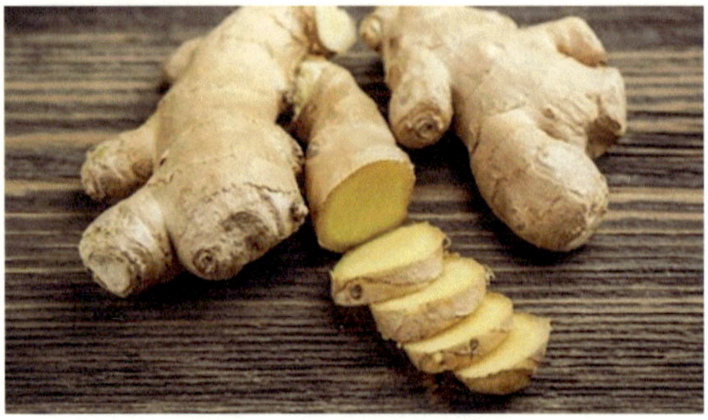

Figure 4.
Ginger Zingiber officinale *(Zingiberaceae) (from: https://www.chandigarhayurvedcentre.com/blog/adrak-zingiber-officinale-ginger//).*

individually inhibited colony formation significantly, their combined effects at equivalent concentrations were even more pronounced, indicating a synergistic mode of action that enhances their beneficial effects.

4. Phytotherapy: an introduction to its history, use, and application

Research on the components of medicinal plants has revealed that their therapeutic potential extends beyond traditional folk medicine usage [22]. While these plants have long been utilized by the public for treating diseases, confirmation of their biological effects has spurred increased therapeutic application. However, it is important to note that despite their benefits, phytotherapeutics derived from medicinal plants may occasionally pose adverse effects.

For centuries, humans have utilized plants as therapeutic remedies. In ancient civilizations, the healing properties of medicinal plants were often imbued with a sense of magic and the supernatural. Some believed these plants influenced the "astral body," leading to both physiological and paranormal phenomena [23]. Even today, medicinal plants continue to hold mystical and religious significance for certain individuals [24].

In 1873, the discovery of the Ebers Papyrus, dating back to 1600 B.C., provided evidence of the ancient Egyptians' use of plants for medicinal purposes [25]. During the Trojan War around 1200 B.C., the plant *Achillea millefolium* was employed to staunch bleeding and promote wound healing among injured soldiers [26]. Additionally, the historical use of poppy dates back to this era [27].

In Greece, around 100 B.C., Pedanius Dioscorides authored a treatise on plants titled "De Materia Medica," which significantly contributed to the field of therapeutic medicine. Conversely, individuals such as Socrates and those who faced execution were put to death using poisons derived from plants [27].

During the Middle Ages, the Swedish doctor Paracelsus was renowned as the pioneer of natural medicine, laying the foundation for many contemporary drugs, including opium. In the eighteenth century, the field of pharmacognosis emerged, combining the Greek terms "pharmakon" (drug) and "gnosis" (knowledge). This multidisciplinary science focuses on identifying and extracting compounds from plants, studying their physical–chemical, biological activity, and pharmaco-toxicological properties [28].

Despite the advancements in the pharmaceutical industry following the Industrial Revolution, phytotherapy remains a valuable therapeutic option [29]. It is imperative for health professionals to undergo training in phytotherapy and its applications to ensure optimal patient care [30].

4.1 Pharmacological characteristics of some of the main medicinal plants

4.1.1 Aesculus hippocastanum

Aesculus hippocastanum (**Figure 5**) comprises a complex combination of compounds including saponins, notably β-escin, tannins, D-catechol, pectin, potassium, volatile oil, calcium, phosphorus, bioflavonoids, and A2 proanthocyanidins [31]. Its mechanism of action facilitates ion transportation through calcium channels while diminishing leukocyte activation [31]. Clinically, it is recommended for conditions such as chronic venous insufficiency, varicose veins, hemorrhoids, decreased inner ear perfusion, and post-operative edema [32]. It enhances the body's antioxidant defense system and exerts anti-inflammatory effects. When combined with anticoagulant medication, it may potentiate its efficacy [31].

At the recommended dosage, adverse effects are rare. Nonetheless, gastrointestinal symptoms, dizziness, headaches, and itching are commonly reported. The standard dosage typically contains 16–20% escin. Oral administration is typically prescribed at 100–150 mg per day, while topical application involves using 2% escin three to four times daily [31].

4.1.2 Cimicifuga racemosa

Cimicifuga racemosa, (**Figure 6**) commonly known as Black Cohosh in North America and Erva-de-São-Cristóvão in Brazil is native to temperate zones. Its extract contains triterpenic glycosides, alkaloids, and aromatic acids, with the extract's

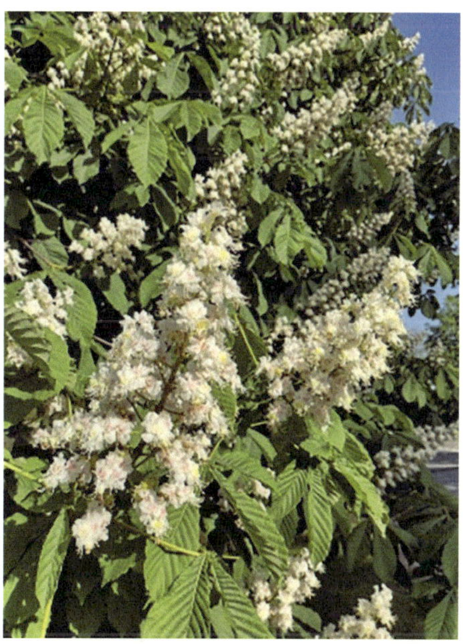

Figure 5.
Horse chestnut Aesculus hippocastanum L. *(Sapindaceae) (from: https: https://www.treesandshrubsonline.org/articles/aesculus/aesculus-hippocastanum).*

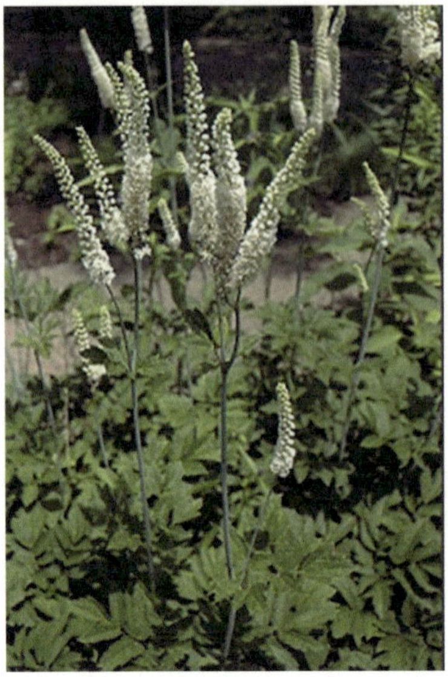

Figure 6.
Black cohosh Cimicifuga racemosa *(Ranunculaceae) (from: https: https://www.plants.longfellowsgreenhouses.com/12100007/Plant/2248).*

activity varying based on its nature [33]. Mechanistically, it reduces serum LH levels through estrogen receptor-negative feedback, acts as a partial agonist at opioid receptors, and exerts hypotensive effects in central vasomotor centers [34]. Recommended for various conditions including menstrual issues, postpartum uterine rhythm normalization, eczema, asthma, migraine, inflammation, and rheumatoid arthritis [33], it can counteract cyclosporine's immunosuppressive effects and is compatible with oral contraceptives and hormones like conjugated estrogen [35]. However, it may lead to side effects such as digestive discomfort, headache, nausea, visual disturbances, tremors, nervousness, abdominal pain, and potential hepatic injury. The recommended daily dosage of the extract is 40 mg, with therapeutic effects typically observed after 2 weeks of treatment [36].

4.1.3 Ginkgo biloba

Ginkgo biloba, (**Figure** 7) utilized globally, contains 24% ginkgo flavone glycosides and 6% terpenoids [37]. It exhibits antioxidant properties [38] and antiapoptotic

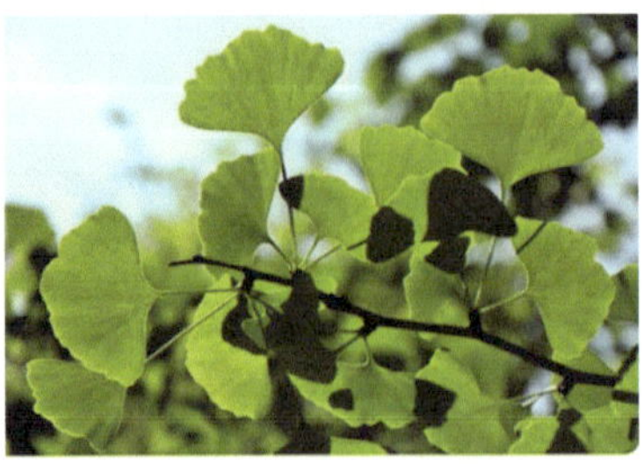

Figure 7.
Ginkgo Ginkgo biloba *(Ginkgoaceae) (from: https://www.vdberk.com/trees/ginkgo-biloba/).*

activity [37], while reducing clastogenic activity and promoting vascular relaxation via nitrous oxide. Additionally, it may enhance acetylcholinesterase effects [39]. Therefore, it is recommended for the clinical treatment of Alzheimer's disease [37], as well as cardiovascular diseases, sexual impotence, hepatic fibrosis, memory enhancement, cerebral vascular insufficiency, PMS, and certain types of cancer [39]. However, caution is advised in patients taking anticoagulants due to potential subdural hematoma formation [40]. Side effects may include nausea, vomiting, salivation, loss of appetite, headaches, dizziness, tinnitus, and hypersensitivity reactions like cutaneous rash.

4.1.4 Hypericum perforatum

This plant is known as "Saint John's Wort" (**Figure 8**). The red substance extracted from the flowers of Hypericum contains hypericins and various compounds such as tannins, resins, pectin, naftodiantrona, and flavonoids, including luteolin, kaempferol, isoquercetine, quercetine, rutine, and myricetin, known for their anti-inflammatory and antiviral properties [41]. Additionally, it contains procianydins, phytosterols, vitamin C, carotene, amino acids, and saponins [41]. Hypericum may inhibit the absorption of serotonin, noradrenaline, and dopamine, potentially contributing to its antidepressant effects, attributed to hypericin, pseudohypericin, or hyperforins [42]. This plant extract is commonly used in Europe for treating mild to moderate depression. Mechanisms of action include interaction with GABA receptors, inhibition of monoamine oxidase enzymes, and catechol-O-methyltransferase [24]. Hypericum may also affect the metabolism of certain medications through cytochrome P450 and CYP1A2, leading to reduced serum concentrations. Side effects include dosage-dependent photosensitivity. Typical dosage ranges from 500 to 1050 mg, taken two or three times daily [42]. Studies also suggest its antiviral activity against various enveloped viruses such as herpes simplex virus type 1, murine cytomegalovirus, and human immunodeficiency virus type 1 [41].

4.1.5 Panax ginseng

Panax ginseng (**Figure 9**), originating from East Asia and Russia, primarily utilizes its root in medicinal applications [43]. It comprises saponins, amino acids, alkaloids, phenols, proteins, polypeptides, and vitamins B1 and B2, contributing to enhanced biochemical resistance and stress management, leading to increased vitality, longevity, and cognitive function [44]. Clinically, it is employed in treating anxiety. *P. ginseng* notably inhibits cytochrome P450 enzymes [45]. Prolonged

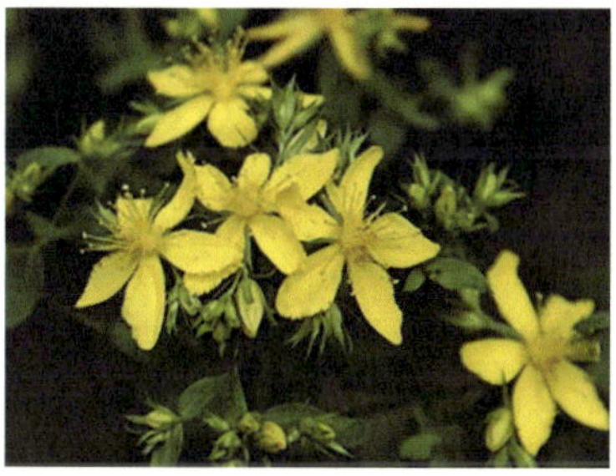

Figure 8.
St John's Wort Hypericum perforatum *(Hypericaceae) (from: https: https://www.wildflowersprovence.fr/plant/hypericum-perforatum/).*

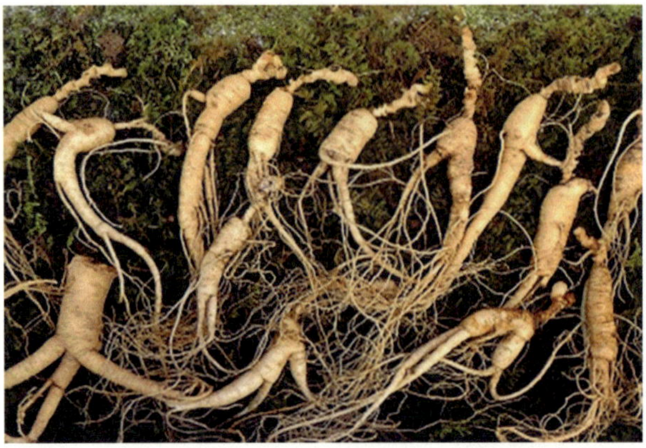

Figure 9.
Ginseng Panax ginseng *(Araliaceae). (from: https: https://www.zellerag.ch/en/phytotherapy/ dictionary-of-medicinal-plants/ginseng/).*

use may result in reversible rash and mild jaundice [46]. The recommended dosage is 50 to 70 mg three times daily to achieve therapeutic effects [46]. Its toxicity is low and dose-dependent, with few reported adverse effects such as hypertension, nausea, diarrhea, headaches, insomnia, and rash. Typical therapeutic dosage involves consuming 1–2 g of raw solid preparations daily for 3 months.

5. Aromatherapy

Aromatherapy involves utilizing highly concentrated essential oils extracted from herbs, flowers, and other plant components to address various ailments [47]. Advocates of aromatherapy often attribute its origins to ancient herbal medicine practices in civilizations such as Egypt and India dating back thousands of years. However, the term itself was coined by the French chemist Gattefossé in a book initially published in 1936 [48]. Nowadays, aromatherapy commonly involves the application of these essential oils through massage onto the skin. The term "aromatherapy" typically denotes the practice of massaging with a variety of aromatic plant extracts, also known as essential oils [49].

The essential oil (EO) industry has experienced significant growth and success in the past decade [50]. Many individuals incorporate products containing essential oils into their daily routines, such as food flavorings, soaps, lotions, shampoos, hair-styling products, colognes, and laundry detergents [51]. Some people perceive essential oils as safer alternatives to conventional pharmacological treatments due to their natural origins. However, despite their widespread use, only limited research has been conducted on essential oils. Consequently, the potential beneficial or adverse effects of these oils remain unclear, underscoring the importance of further investigation to determine their true impact on human health.

EO exposure can occur through various methods, including inhalation, ingestion, massage, and topical application to the skin [52]. These oils are renowned for their diverse health effects, such as antibacterial, antibiotic, and antiviral properties [53]. Additionally, they are valued for their stress-relieving properties and have been utilized in treatments for conditions like sleep disorders, Alzheimer's disease, cardiovascular issues, cancer, and pregnancy-related labor pain [54]. Moreover, essential oils are recognized for their insect-repellent capabilities and antioxidant/anti-inflammatory activity [55]. While most essential oils are generally considered safe, it is crucial to note that adverse effects can occur [55]. Although the majority of these effects are mild, there have been reported instances of serious toxic reactions, including complications such as abortions and pregnancy abnormalities, neurotoxicity, bronchial hyperactivity, hepatotoxicity, prepubertal gynecomastia, and premature thelarche [56].

5.1 Antimicrobial, antiviral, anti-inflamatuar, and antibiotic effects

Essential oils are widely recognized natural products with diverse medical applications. Given the rise of antimicrobial resistance, there has been considerable interest in exploring essential oils as potential antimicrobial agents [57]. Clinical trials have demonstrated their efficacy as bactericidal, virucidal, and fungicidal agents.

Bacterial infections continue to pose a significant threat to human health, contributing to mortality rates worldwide. In response to the growing problem of antibiotic resistance, researchers are exploring alternative therapies against bacterial strains, including essential oils. These oils exhibit antibacterial activity, which can manifest as either bacteriostatic or bactericidal effects. Due to their lipophilic nature, essential oils readily penetrate bacterial cell membranes, disrupting vital cellular processes such as nutrient processing, synthesis of structural molecules, regulation of growth factors, energy production, and modulation of cell-cell communication through quorum sensing networks [58]. The list of specific bacteria targeted by the essential oils is expanding and includes, but are not limited to, *Listeria monocytogenes*, *Bacillus sphaericus*, *Enterobacter aerogenes*, *Escherichia coli*, *P. acruginosa*, *S. aureus*, *S. epidermidis*, *S. typhi*, *Shiguella flexneri*, and *Yersinia enterocolitica* [59]. Some of the essential oils commonly used come from *Allium sativum*, *Thymus vulgaris*, *Origanum vulgare*, *Melissa officinalis*, *Cinnamomum zelancium*, and *Lavandula angustifolia* [60].

In a manner similar to their effects on bacteria, essential oils possess the capability to infiltrate and disrupt the balance within fungal cell walls and cytoplasmic membranes, particularly targeting the mitochondria [61]. Proposed mechanisms suggest that essential oils penetrate mitochondrial membranes, altering electron flow within the electron transport system. This disruption, in turn, leads to disturbances in the lipid, protein, and nucleic acid components of fungal cells [62]. Extracts from plants such as *Ocimum basillicum*, *Syzygium aromaticum*, *Citrus aurantium*, *Allium sativum*, *Origanum vulgare*, *Thymus vulgaris*, *Foeniculum vulgare*, *Cymbopogon citratus*, and *Rosmarinus officinalis* have demonstrated their significant antifungal activity against a broad range of fungal human pathogens [63].

Inflammation is the body's reaction to harmful stimuli like infection or tissue damage, and it involves biological, chemical, and physiological mechanisms [64]. Essential oils (EOs) such as chamomile, eucalyptus, rosemary, lavender, and millefolia have been shown to modulate this inflammatory response [65]. They possess the ability to affect antioxidant activity, signaling pathways, cytokines, regulatory transcription factors, and the expression of pro-inflammatory genes [65]. The primary anti-inflammatory properties of essential oils include the inhibition of arachidonic acid metabolism, cytokine production, and the expression of pro-inflammatory genes [65].

5.2 Psychological effects

Generalized anxiety disorder (GAD) is characterized by persistent and excessive worry accompanied by psychic and somatic symptoms [66]. It is a prevalent condition that can significantly impair both personal and social functioning [67]. Current treatments for GAD include cognitive behavioral therapy and medication, primarily benzodiazepines or antidepressants. Essential oils have emerged as a potential new category of treatment for GAD, with animal models showing anxiolytic properties in certain oils such as *Lavandula angustifolia*, *Citrus sinensis*, and *Citrus aurantium* subspecies bergamia [68]. These properties have been replicated in human clinical trials [69]. The method of administration also seems to influence their effectiveness, with inhalation, oral ingestion, and topical application being the most common routes.

Numerous essential oils exert their pharmacological effects on the central nervous system through interactions with serotonin receptors, the GABAergic system, and voltage-gated Na + channels [70]. For instance, inhalation of bergamot (*Citrus bergamia*) oil has been found to regulate the blood pressure and heart rate of healthy volunteers [71]. In palliative care settings, lemon essence has been investigated, showing an increase in heart rate, diastolic blood pressure, and respiratory rate in both conscious and unconscious patients, while lavender oil produced contrasting effects [72]. Interestingly, certain essential oils have been linked to exacerbated anxiety symptoms. Lemon essence, for example, was observed to heighten nociceptive and anxiety responses in rats [73].

Depression, an exceedingly prevalent mental health disorder, manifests through symptoms such as diminished mood, loss of interest, hopelessness, and impaired social functioning [74]. While traditional antidepressant medication primarily operates by modulating neurotransmitters, many patients do not achieve complete symptom remission with monotherapy [75]. Consequently, numerous studies have explored alternative natural products as adjunctive therapies for depression, with St. John's Wort being a prominent example [76]. Research indicates that St. John's Wort is superior to placebo in alleviating depression symptoms and comparably effective to antidepressant medication [77]. Essential oils offer another potential avenue for depression treatment. Lavender oil, in particular, has demonstrated efficacy in mitigating depression-like behavior induced by chronic corticosterone administration [77].

6. Women's use of complementary and alternative therapies in reproductive healthcare

Numerous studies have shown that healthcare consumers worldwide are spending money out of their own pockets on alternative therapies. Women use conventional healthcare services more often than men, so it is not surprising that they make up about two-thirds of healthcare appointments for complementary and alternative therapies. The traditional conceptual frameworks of herbal medicine, homeopathy, and acupuncture are explained, and their common clinical applications in women's reproductive care are discussed.

6.1 Herbal therapies

Women around the world use herbs to address a variety of reproductive health issues, including menstrual problems, infertility, pregnancy discomforts and dysfunctions, labor, and menopause. Every indigenous culture has developed knowledge about local plants and foods that can promote health and cure illnesses. Many popular herbal reference books in the United States reflect European and

Native American traditions, but herbal use in the country also includes influences from Asian traditions. It is important to recognize that various traditions of herbal medicine exist globally.

One reason women's reproductive problems are well-suited to herbal treatment might be that many of these issues are functional, such as the "failure" of cyclic events, physiological adjustments to pregnancy, or changes during perimenopause, rather than infections or surgical emergencies, where Western biomedicine has made significant advances. Most herbal texts classify herbs into standard categories based on their effects [78]. Examples of classifications relevant to midwives include emmenagogues, which induce menstruation, and partus preparators, which reduce false labor pains and promote effective uterine contractions.

Herbal reference books list numerous uses for herbs in women's health care. To discuss the use of herbs in women's health, three clinical issues will be highlighted to illustrate developments in this field: nausea and vomiting during pregnancy, preparation for labor, and menopause.

6.2 Herbal treatments for morning sickness and preparation for labor

The herbs most commonly mentioned for treating nausea during pregnancy are peppermint, spearmint, ginger root, and raspberry leaf. Fennel, chamomile, hops, meadowsweet, and wild yam root are also frequently noted [79]. None of these plants appear on lists of herbs to avoid during pregnancy. Women often try various remedies and may rotate them for increased effectiveness and variety Common sense suggests that the most frequently mentioned herbs are likely the best ones to try first. Herbs are also commonly used in midwifery and maternity care to prepare the uterus for labor and promote effective labor. The most frequently cited herbs for this purpose include raspberry leaves, squaw vine leaves, and blue and black cohosh.

Red raspberry is commonly recommended to prepare for labor and alleviate various pregnancy discomforts. It is noted for its astringent and stimulant properties and is described as a universal remedy for easing childbirth, used by pregnant women across different continents [80]. It is attributed to containing a beneficial substance. Red raspberry is also used to reduce pregnancy nausea, promote easier labor, and treat menstrual pain [80]. Although some reviews find no evidence supporting its effect on smooth muscle function, the plant is considered harmless except for its tannin content. Various over-the-counter herbal products containing red raspberry leaves are available and frequently used for these purposes.

Despite the similarity of their names, black chosh and blue cohosh are two different plants, both native to North America, and have been used for reproductive issues by Native Americans. Recent research has shown that a substance in one of these plants can bind to estrogen receptors and decrease luteinizing hormones in studies with rats, indicating estrogenic effects. This plant has been used to address PMS symptoms, menstrual pain, menopause, and to promote labor.

Blue cohosh is used for various purposes, including as a uterine stimulant and to induce menstruation. Information about its active ingredients highlights caution against self-medication. The plant's effects are due to a compound that constricts coronary blood vessels, posing a risk to heart muscle and causing intestinal spasms in small animals [81]. Given these potent effects, blue cohosh cannot be considered inactive or harmless. Therefore, using it for self-treatment, especially to stimulate uterine contractions or induce menstruation, is not advisable [81].

Pennyroyal, a member of the mint family, is sometimes included in over-the-counter herbal products for inducing labor. However, it has been associated with documented potential for harmful effects [82]. Pennyroyal oil, commonly used to repel fleas, should not be ingested due to its highly toxic nature. The oil can irritate the kidneys and urinary tract, stimulate uterine contractions, act as a central nervous system depressant, and irritate mucous membranes. When used as an emmenagogue or labor preparation, pennyroyal oil has been associated with toxic side effects, including nausea, vomiting, diarrhea, central nervous system depression and stimulation, and convulsions. Individuals considering the use of pennyroyal should strictly use plant material and avoid the essential oil. It is advised that people with kidney disease refrain from using pennyroyal products.

6.3 Black cohosh and menopause

Women have used a certain herb for a variety of gynecologic problems, including hot flashes and depression associated with menopause. It was used by indigenous people for various issues, including gynecologic problems, and was a main ingredient in a well-known nineteenth-century patent medicine. Recent research on the effects of this herb extract on animals has shown vaginal epithelial changes similar to those observed with the administration of estrogen [83]. In a study on the effects of the herb extract on certain hormones in menopausal women, participants who had not received hormonal replacement for at least 6 months experienced hormone-level reductions after 2 months of daily treatment with an oral extract product. Analysis of the product identified three different substances that likely work together to achieve this result. A number of products are available over the counter in health food stores for women who wish to use black cohosh. Other herbs often used during perimenopause include a specific type of ginseng, dong quai, chaste tree berry, licorice root, fennel seed, and red clover [84]. Additionally, some foods have been found to have components that can interact with estrogen receptors, including soybeans, black beans, plums, cherries, dandelion, alfalfa, soybean sprouts, wild yam, and various vegetable oils [83]. Unfortunately, there is insufficient data on the safety of these products when used with and without sources of progesterone.

7. Why people use herbal medicine

The earliest evidence of human use of plants for healing dates back to the Neanderthal period [7]. Currently, an increasing number of patients are turning to herbal medicine, often without informing their clinicians about their concurrent use [85]. There are several reasons why patients choose herbal therapies. Many cite a "sense of control and mental comfort from taking action," which is especially relevant for those with chronic or incurable diseases like diabetes, cancer, arthritis, or AIDS. These patients often feel that conventional medicine has not met their needs. Additionally, patients may resort to home remedies for acute, often self-limiting conditions, such as colds, sore throats, or bee stings, because professional care is not immediately available or is perceived as too inconvenient, costly, or time-consuming [7].

In rural regions, additional cultural factors, such as the environment and local traditions, promote the use of botanical remedies, reflecting a "man–earth relationship." There is a belief that areas where certain diseases are prevalent will also support the growth of plants that can treat these illnesses [7]. In India, a significant portion of the rural population lacks access to modern medical care [86]. Hundreds of primary health centers intended to serve these rural areas suffer from shortages of staff, diagnostic tools, and essential medications. Consequently, the rural population relies heavily on traditional medical systems [86].

Despite the diversification of drug discovery technologies and a decline in funding for natural product-based drug research, compounds sourced from plants and other biological origins continue to be a significant source of new pharmaceuticals. Industrial funding for natural product-based drug discovery decreased between 1984 and 2003, yet the proportion of patents for small molecule drugs derived from natural sources remained stable [87]. A thorough examination of human drugs introduced since 1981 indicates that while a majority were synthetic molecules, a considerable number were either directly derived from natural products or inspired by them. Notably, natural products have made a substantial impact in cancer treatment, with a significant percentage of anticancer drugs tracing their origins back to natural compounds.

Author details

Mehtap Kilic
Turkish Medicines and Medical Devices Agency, Ankara, Turkey

*Address all correspondence to: klcmehtap89@gmail.com

References

[1] Kamboj VP. Herbal medicine. Current Science. 2000;**78**:35-39

[2] Gupta LM, Raina R. Side effects of some medicinal plants. Current Science. 1998;**75**:897-900

[3] Evans M. A Guide to Herbal Remedies. South America: Orient Paperbacks; 1994

[4] Vickers A, Zollman C. ABC of complementary medicine: Herbal medicine. BMJ. 1999;**319**:1050-1053

[5] Tirtha SSS. Overview of ayurveda. In: Khalsa AK, Paon R, editors. The Ayurveda Encyclopedia: Natural Secrets to Healing, Prevention and Longevity. India: Satyaguru Publications; 1998. pp. 3-11

[6] Tyler VE. Phytomedicine: Back to the future. Journal of Natural Products. 1999;**62**:1589-1592

[7] Winslow LC, Kroll DJ. Herbs as medicine. Archives of Internal Medicine. 1998;**158**:2192-2199

[8] Raskin I, Ripoll C. Can an apple a day keep the doctor away? Current Pharmaceutical Design. 2004;**10**:3419-3429

[9] Aanchal B, Chinmayee P. Medicinal properties of phytochemicals and their production. Natural Drugs from Plants. 2021:352-361

[10] Banning M. The carcinogenic and protective effects of food. British Journal of Nursing. 2005;**14**(20):1070-1074

[11] Murakami A, Ohigashi H, Koshimizu K. Anti-tumor promotion with food phytochemicals: A strategy for cancer chemoprevention. Bioscience, Biotechonology and Biochemistry. 1996;**60**(1):1-8

[12] Yasukawa K. Medicinal and edible plants as cancer preventive agents, drug discovery research. In: Vallisuta O, editor. Drug Discovery Research in Pharmacognosy. United Kingdom: Intechopen; 2012

[13] Ngo SN, Williams DB, Head RJ. Rosemary and cancer prevention: Preclinical perspectives. Critical Reviews in Food Science and Nutrition. 2011;**51**(10):946-954

[14] López-Jiménez A, García-Caballero M, Medina MÁ, Quesada AR. Anti-angiogenic properties of carnosol and carnosic acid, two major dietary compounds from rosemary. European Journal of Nutrition. 2013;**52**(1):85-95

[15] Zhou K, Raffoul JJ. Potential anticancer properties of grape antioxidants. Journal of Oncology. 2012;**2012**:803294

[16] Khan SA, Chatterton RT, Michel N, Bryk M, Lee O, Ivancic D, et al. Soy isoflavone supplementation for breast cancer risk reduction: A randomized phase II trial. Cancer Prevention Research. 2012;**5**(2):309-319

[17] Ohta T, Nakatsugi S, Watanabe K, Kawamori T, Ishikawa F, Morotomi M, et al. Inhibitory effects of bifidobacterium-fermented soy milk on 2-amino-1-methyl-6-phenylimidazol[4,5-b]-pyridine-induced rat mammary carcinogenesis, with a partial contribution of its component isoflavones. Carcinogenesis. 2000;**21**(5):937-941

[18] Katz AE. Flavonoid and botanical approaches to prostate health. Journal of Alternative and Complementary Medicine. 2002;**8**(6):813-821

[19] Yogosawa S, Yamada Y, Yasuda S, Sun Q, Takizawa K, Sakai T. Dehydrozingerone, a structural analogue of curcumin, induces cell-cycle arrest at the G2/M phase and accumulates intracellular ROS in HT-29 human colon cancer cells. Journal of Natural Products. 2012;**75**(12):2088-2093

[20] Škrovánková S, Mišurcová L, Machů L. Antioxidant activity and protecting health effects of common medicinal plants. Advances in Food and Nutrition Research. 2012;**67**:75-139

[21] Kurapati KR, Samikkannu T, Kadiyala DB, Zainulabedin SM, Gandhi N, Sathaye SS, et al. Combinatorial cytotoxic effects of *Curcuma longa* and *Zingiber officinale* on the PC-3M prostate cancer cell line. Journal of Basic and Clinical Physiology and Pharmacology. 2012;**23**(4):1-8

[22] Trojan-Rodrigues M. Plants used as antidiabetics in popular medicine in Rio Grande do Sul, southern Brazil. Journal of Ethnopharmacology. 2012;**139**:155-163

[23] Alzugaray D, Alzugaray C. Plantas que curam. São Paulo Três. 1996:260-268

[24] Cordeiro CHG. Interações medicamentosas de fitoterápicos e fármacos: Hypericum perforatum e Piper methysticum. Revista Brasileira de Farmacognosia. 2005;**15**(3):272-278

[25] Hallman-Mikolaczak A, Ebers P. The book of medical knowledge of the 16th century B.C. Egyptians. Archiwum historii i filozofii medycyny/Polskii Towarzystwo Historii Medycyny i Farmacji. 2004;**67**:5-14

[26] Cáceres A. Plantas de Uso Medicinal em Guatemala. 2nd ed. Guatemala: Editorial Universitária; 1999. p. 402

[27] Croteau R. Natural products (secondary metabolites). In: Biochemistry & Molecular Biology of Plants. Rockville: Courier Companies; 2000. pp. 1250-1318

[28] Bruneton J. Pharmacognosie, Phytochimie, Plantes Médicinales. 2nd ed. Paris: Lavoisier; 1993. p. 915

[29] Eisenberg DM. Trends in alternative medicine use in the United States, 1990-1997 results of a follow-up national survey. JAMA. 1998;**280**(18):1569-1575

[30] Santos MS. An aqueous extract of valerian influences the transport of GABA in synaptosomes. Planta Medica. 1994;**60**(3):278-279

[31] Aesculus hippocastanum (Horse chestnut). Alternative Medicine Review. 2009;**14**(3):278-283

[32] Dickson S. An open study to assess the safety and efficacy of Aesculus hippocastanum tablets (Aesculaforce 50 mg) in the treatment of chronic venous insufficiency. Journal of Herbal Pharmacotherapy. 2004;**4**(2):19-32

[33] Lopes CMC. Função hepática em mulheres menopausadas tratadas com extrato seco padronizado do rizoma e raízes de Cimicifuga racemosa L. Revista Brasileira de Medicina. 2009;**66**(8):254-259

[34] Rhyu MR. Black cohosh (Actaea racemosa, Cimicifuga racemosa) behaves as a mixed competitive ligand and partial agonist at the human μ opiate receptor. Journal of Agricultural and Food Chemistry. 2006;**54**(26):9852-9857

[35] Nicoletti MA. Uso popular de medicamentos contendo drogas de origem vegetal e/ou plantas medicinais: principais interações decorrentes. Revista Saúde. 2010;**4**(1):25-39

[36] Racemosa cimicifuga. Alternative Medicine Review. 2003;**8**(2):186-189

[37] Forlenza OV. Ginkgo biloba e memória: Mito ou realidade? Revista de Psiquiatria Clínica. 2003;**30**(6):218-220

[38] Macarenco RSS. Estudo da ação do extrato de Ginkgo biloba e amido hidroxietílico hipertônico na atenuação de alterações decorrentes de isquemia e reperfusão de órgãos esplâncnicos em ratos. Acta Cirurgica Brasileira. 2001;**16**(3):139-145

[39] Czap K. Ginkgo biloba, Alternative Medicine Review Monographs. Thorne Research Inc; 2002. pp. 168-174

[40] Rosenblatt M, Mindel J. Spontaneous hyphema associated with ingestion of Ginkgo biloba extract. The New England Journal of Medicine. 1997;**336**(15):1108

[41] Yunes RA. Fármacos e fitoterápicos: A necessidade do desenvolvimento da indústria de fitoterápicos e fitofármacos no Brasil. Química Nova. 2001;**24**(1):147-152

[42] Hypericum perforatum. Alternative Medicine Review. 2004;**9**(3):318-325

[43] Seely D. Safety and efficacy of Panax ginseng during pregnancy and lactation. Canadian Journal of Clinical Pharmacology. 2008;**15**(1):87-94

[44] Panax ginseng. Alternative Medicine Review. 2009;**14**(2):172-176

[45] Singh YN. Potential for interaction of kava and St. John's Wort with drugs. Journal of Ethnopharmacology. 2005;**100**(2):108-113

[46] Piper methysticum (kava kava). Alternative Medicine Review. 1998;**3**(6):458-460

[47] Segen JC. Dictionary of Alternative Medicine. Stamford, CT: Appleton and Lange; 1998

[48] Gattefossé R-M. Aromatherapy. London: C W Daniel Co Ltd; 1993

[49] Vickers A, Zollman C. ABC of complementary medicine massage therapies. BMJ. 1999;**319**:1254-1257

[50] Essential Oils Market Size, Share & Trends Analysis Report by Application (Cleaning & Home, Medical, Food & Beverages, Spa & Relaxation), by Product, by Sales Channel, and Segment Forecasts, 2019-2025. Grand View Research; 2019

[51] Groot AC, Schmidt E. Essential oils. Dermatitis. 2016;**27**(2):39-42

[52] Ali B, Al-Wabel NA, Shams S, Ahamad A, Khan SA, Anwar F. Essential oils used in aromatherapy. Systematic Reviews. 2015;**5**:601-611

[53] Jimbo D, Kimura Y, Taniguchi M, Inoue M, Urakami K. Effect of aromatherapy on patients with Alzheimer's disease. Psychogeriatrics. 2009;**9**(4):173-179

[54] Lee MY. Essential oils as repellents against arthropods. BioMed Research International. 2018;**2**:6860271-6860279

[55] Marchand L. Integrative and complementary therapies for patients with advanced cancer. Annals of Palliative Medicine. 2014;**3**(3):160-171

[56] Diaz A, Luque L, Badar Z, Kornic S, Danon M. Prepubertal gynecomastia and chronic lavender exposure: Report of three cases. Journal of Pediatric Endocrinology & Metabolism. 2016;**29**(1):103-107

[57] Deyno S, Mtewa AG, Abebe A, Hymete A, Makonnen E, Bazira J, et al. Essential oils as topical anti-infective agents: A systematic review and meta-analysis. Complementary Therapies in Medicine. 2019;**47**:102224

[58] Swamy MK, Akhtar MS, Sinniah UR. Antimicrobial properties of plant essential oils against human pathogens and their mode of action: An updated review. Evidence-based Complementary and Alternative Medicine. 2016;**2016**:3012462

[59] Arora DS, Kaur J. Antimicrobial activity of spices. International Journal of Antimicrobial Agents. 1999;**12**(3):257-262

[60] Burt S. Essential oils: Their antibacterial properties and potential applications in foods a review. International Journal of Food Microbiology. 2004;**94**(3):223-253

[61] Akhtar MS. Antimicrobial activity of essential oils extracted from medicinal plants against the pathogenic microorganisms: A review. Issues in Biological Sciences and Pharmaceutical Research. 2014;**2**:1-7

[62] Arnal-Schnebelen B, Hadji-Minaglou F, Peroteau JF, Ribeyre F, de Billerbeck VG. Essential oils in infectious gynaecological disease: A statistical study of 658 cases. International Journal of Aromatherapy. 2004;**4**:192-197

[63] Kivanç M, Akgül A, Doğan A. Inhibitory and stimulatory effects of cumin, oregano and their essential oils on growth and acid production of *Lactobacillus plantarum* and *Leuconostoc mesenteroides*. International Journal of Food Microbiology. 1991;**13**(1):81-85

[64] de Lavor ÉM, Fernandes AW, de Andrade Teles RB, Leal AE, de Oliveira Júnior RG, Silva GEM, et al. Essential oils and their major compounds in the treatment of chronic inflammation: A review of antioxidant potential in preclinical studies and molecular mechanisms. Oxidative Medicine and Cellular Longevity. 2018;**3**:6468593-6468523

[65] Miguel MG. Antioxidant and anti-inflammatory activities of essential oils: A short review. Molecules. 2010;**15**(12):9252-9287

[66] Haskins JT. Generalized anxiety disorder. Epidemiology, impact of comorbidity, and natural history. Postgraduate Medicine. 1999;**106**(6):3-9

[67] Altunoz U, Kokurcan A, Kirici S, Bastug G, Ozel-Kizil ET. Clinical characteristics of generalized anxiety disorder: Older vs. young adults. Nordic Journal of Psychiatry. 2018;**72**(2):97-102

[68] de Sousa DP, de Almeida Soares Hocayen P, Andrade LN, Andreatini R. A systematic review of the anxiolytic-like effects of essential oils in animal models. Molecules. 2015;**20**(10):18620-18660

[69] Karadag E, Samancioglu S, Ozden D, Bakir E. Effects of aromatherapy on sleep quality and anxiety of patients. Nursing in Critical Care. 2017;**22**(2):105-112

[70] Wang ZJ, Heinbockel T. Essential oils and their constituents targeting the GABAergic system and sodium channels as treatment of neurological diseases. Molecules. 2018;**23**(5):1061-1072

[71] Watanabe E, Kuchta K, Kimura M, Rauwald HW, Kamei T, Imanishi J. Effects of bergamot (Citrus bergamia (Risso) Wright & Arn.) essential oil aromatherapy on mood states, parasympathetic nervous system activity, and salivary cortisol levels in 41 healthy females. Forschende Komplementärmedizin. 2015;**22**(1):43-49

[72] Goepfert M, Liebl P, Herth N, Ciarlo G, Buentzel J, Huebner J. Aroma oil therapy in palliative care: A pilot study with physiological parameters in conscious as well as unconscious patients. Journal of Cancer Research and Clinical Oncology. 2017;**143**(10):2123-2129

[73] Ceccarelli I, Lariviere WR, Fiorenzani P, Sacerdote P, Aloisi AM. Effects of long-term exposure of lemon essential oil odor on behavioral, hormonal and neuronal parameters in male and female rats. Brain Research. 2004;**1001**(1-2):78-86

[74] Cipriani A, Furukawa TA, Salanti G, Chaimani A, Atkinson LZ, Ogawa Y, et al. Comparative efficacy and acceptability of 21 antidepressant drugs for the acute treatment of adults with major depressive disorder: A systematic review and network meta-analysis. Lancet. 2018;**391**(10128):1357-1366

[75] Berton O, Nestler EJ. New approaches to antidepressant drug discovery: Beyond monoamines. Nature Reviews. Neuroscience. 2006;**7**(2):137-151

[76] Maher AR, Hempel S, Apaydin E, Shanman RM, Booth M, Miles JN, et al. St. John's Wort for major depressive disorder: A systematic review. Rand Health Q. 2016;**5**(4):12

[77] Sanchez-Vidana D, Po KK, Fung TK, Chow JK, Lau WK, So PK, et al. Lavender essential oil ameliorates depression-like behavior and increases neurogenesis and dendritic complexity in rats. Neuroscience Letters. 2019;**701**:180-192

[78] French M. The power of plants. Advance for Nurse Practitioners. 1996;**2**:16-21

[79] Stapleton H. Women as midwives and herbalists. In: Tiran D, Mack S, editors. Complementary Therapies for Pregnancy and Childbirth. London: Bailliere Tindall; 1995

[80] Gardner J. Healing yourself During Pregnancy. Freedom (CA): Crossings Press; 1987

[81] Tyler VE. The Honest Herbal. 3rd ed. New York: Pharmaceutical Products Press (an imprint of Haworth Press Inc); 1993

[82] Spoerke DG. Herbal Medications. Santa Barbara (CA): Wood-bridge Press; 1980

[83] Duker EM, Kopanski L, Jarry H, Wuttke W. Effects of extracts from Cimicifuga racemosa on gonadotropin release in menopausal women and ovariectomized rats. Planta Medica. 1991;**57**:420-424

[84] Lien LL, Lien EJ. Hormone therapy and phystoestrogens. Journal of Clinical Pharmacy and Therapeutics. 1996;**21**:101-111

[85] Miller LG. Herbal medicinals: Selected clinical considerations focusing on known or potential drug-herb interactions. Archives of Internal Medicine. 1998;**158**:2200-2211

[86] Mudur G. Mandatory rural practice proposed in India. BMJ. 1995;**311**:1186

[87] Koehn FE, Carter GT. The evolving role of natural products in drug discovery. Nature Reviews. Drug Discovery. 2005;**4**:206-220

Chapter 10

Therapeutic Potential of Medicinal Plants: Current Situation and Outlook

Martins Emeje, Eneojo Ogu, Ifeoma Chidebe, Gautier Roko, Munira Abdullahi and Daniel Sule Bibinu

Abstract

Medicinal plants constitute the major therapeutic sources for the treatment and management of diseases among the large population of the African continent. The application of these plant resources for the management of ailments such as diabetes, cancer, neurodegenerative disorder, malaria, hypertension among others is based on the historical evidence of effectiveness, acceptability, affordability, accessibility and cultural compatibility. Various parts of medicinal plants such as flowers, leaves, stems, bark, roots, seeds, fruits possess therapeutic potentials due to the presence of bioactive substances in them. The therapeutic potentials of these medicinal plants are due to the complex interactions of the bioactive substances with their molecular target structures, such as the transport systems, enzymes and receptors. Currently, many well-known active substances derived from plants are included in medicines through scientific processing procedures that ensure standardization resulting in an improvement over the traditional crude practices among the various African cultures.

Keywords: treatment, historical evidence, ailments, bioactive substances, cultural

1. Introduction

The potency of medicinal plants for healing can be traced back to prehistorical times. Man right in the past relied on nature for food and medicines [1]. Nature served as the repository of diverse biodiversity and a unique laboratory for natural active ingredients of medicinal plants synthesis which man looks to for rescue in times of ailment.

Medicinal plants as major components of the biodiversity have been used in African traditional medicines to provide herbal remedies to different kinds of ailments [2] among the various African cultures.

The application of medicinal plants as the active ingredients of African herbal medicines was rooted in African history, culture belief and religion [2, 3] accepted

IntechOpen

among the various subcultures before the advent of colonization [4] which introduced Western medicines and Western religion that tended to erode the African healing culture [5, 6].

The African healing culture involves the application of the knowledge of medicinal plant healing potentials gained through trial and error experiments, experience and many years of careful observation [1] passed across from one generation to another. This knowledge exists among cultures, tribes and families in the form of local folklore [2]. In preparing the herbal medicines, it was noted that depending upon the individual recipe, all parts of the plant can be utilized, such as the whole plants, seeds, bark, leaves, roots, flowers, stems and fruits [7].

2. Traditional methods of extraction/preparation of medicines from medicinal plants

Historically, the extraction of the therapeutic ingredients of medicinal plant involves variety of methods such as teas, powders, tinctures [2], decoctions, infusions, poultices and digestion. It also included applications like raw plant consumption (without any preparation), juice, salves, vinegars, baths, syrup and inhalation [7].

Teas are prepared by steeping the medicinal plant materials (leaves, roots, flowers or bark). This involved pouring hot water over the plant material in a teapot or infuser and letting it steep for the time recommended usually; 5–7 minutes for flowers and leaves, 10–15 minutes for bark, roots and 3–5 minutes for volatile herbs.

Powders involved drying the medicinal plant parts either the leaves, roots, flower, bark or stem and ground or pulverized then using fine mesh to sieved and removed the chaff [8]. It can be taken as a powder directly, in water, pap, alcohol, etc.

A tincture is prepared by steeping in alcohol from 4 to 6 weeks the medicinal plant materials for use in treatment to extract the medicinal properties.

In decortion, the plant material instead of steeping is boiled in water. A known volume of water is used as a solvent for continuous hot extraction. It involved pouring water onto dried, pulverized and powdered plant materials placed in a clean container and then stirred. The extraction process is hastened by applying heat throughout. Usually, a short duration of about 15 minutes is observed for the process. This process is used for heat stable and water soluble plant material extraction. Usually, the solvent to crude drug ratio is 16:1 or 4:1 [9].

Infusion extraction involves submersing the medicinal plant material in boiling or hot water for some hours to leaches out the therapeutic components from the plant.

Poultices preparations involve grinding into a moist clump, the portion of the medicinal plant materials (roots, leaves or bark) for application on the area affected. Poultices are usually for external applications in treating skin diseases and body swelling while tinctures and infusions are often for internal use except in a few situations where they may be externally applied [7].

Digestion is used for the extraction of readily soluble plant materials. It involves the application of moderate heat during the process of extraction. The mixture of solvent for extraction and powdered plant materials poured into a clean container is placed in an oven at a temperature about 50°C or over water bath with continuous heat application throughout the extraction process to decrease the extraction solvent viscosity and enhanced the bioactive compound removal [9].

2.1 Brief historical evidence of utilization of medicinal plant in Africa

Historical evidence revealed that medicinal plant have been used either as an extract or as a whole plant for the provision of valuable medicines for the treatment of ailments in Africa. Such medicinal plants include the following:

Gum Arabic (*Acacia senegal* L.), which is believed to originate from dried regions and semi-desert of sub-Saharan Africa. Other parts of the world, including North Africa, West Africa and Northern Nigeria, use it as a medicinal plant. For at least four thousand (4000) years ago, and as far back as (3400 B.C.) from the first Egyptian Dynasty, gum Arabic has been used in medicines for both man and animal. Infections such as gonorrhea, upper respiratory tract infections, bleeding, diarrhea, bronchitis, leprosy and typhoid fever have been treated using various parts of the plant [3].

Another important medicinal plant with a documented history of use in Africa which has contributed to poverty alleviation in South Africa is the *Aloe ferox* Mill. known as *Bitter Aloe or Cape Aloe* which originated from Lesotho and South Africa. The plant is used in Africa and Europe as laxative medicine due to the fact that it has anticancer, bitter tonic, antimicrobial, antioxidant and anti-inflammatory attributes [3, 10, 11].

Other African medicinal plants of historical therapeutic values include *Artemisia herba-alba Asso (Med)*—Asteraceae known as Worm-wood. The Worm-wood since ancient times has been used by many cultures in folk medicine. It is used to treat arterial hypertension and diabetes in Moroccan folk medicine [12, 13] and for the treatment of hypertension, neuralgias, diabetes, bronchitis and diarrhea in Tunisia [3]. In folk medicines, *Artemisia herba-alba* tea has been utilized as a hemostatic agents, antispasmodic, analgesic and antibacterial [3].

Worthy of note is *Securidaca longipedunculata* Fresen from the Polygalaceae family an African indigenous medicinal plant exploited for a variety of ailments. Ailments such as malaria, stomach disorder, toothache, headache, sleeping sickness, cough, chest complaints, snakebite and wound are treated using the bark and the root of the plant which are taken orally as a powder or as an infusion. The roots are used as pesticides against storage pests of seeds. Headache, fever and rheumatism are treated with the seeds. Snakebite, venereal diseases and coughs are treated with the leaves while arrow poison and stomach problems are treated with the bark in Nigeria [14]. In Tanzania, the dried bark and root are used for treating nervous system disorders as a purgative. Dried leaves are for the treatment of snakebite, venereal disease, coughs, sores and wounds in East Africa. In Malawi, bilharzia, venereal disease and snakebite, wounds and coughs are treated using the leaves. Ghana uses the root bark for the cure of epilepsy, while impotence and malaria are treated with the plant root in Rhodesia (Zimbabwe) and Bechuanaland now the Republic of Botswana [6].

3. Scientific secret of the therapeutic potentials of medicinal plant

The application of medicinal plants in the cure or treatment of ailments right from the past points to the fact that numerous bioactive substances possessing different therapeutic attributes are present in plants which confer on them the therapeutic potentials.

Most of these bioactive compounds are present in plants not necessarily for the propagation or growth of the plants but as a result of modification requires for the plants adaptation to their habitats, such as protection against diseases, insects, predators or other conditions like stress, drought among others [2].

These bioactive substances are called secondary metabolites and include tannins, lignins, flavonoides, sterols, terpenoids, phenolics, essential oils, alkaloids, glycosides, etc. [15, 16], which are products of primary metabolism (the breakdown and biosynthesis of fats, carbohydrates, nucleic acids and proteins).

To obtain the biosynthetic intermediates which, ultimately, results in the formation of secondary metabolites also known as the bioactive substance, the biosynthesis of the secondary metabolites requires the fundamental processes of glycolysis, Krebs cycle and photosynthesis. The intermediate molecules (acetyl coenzyme A (acetyl-CoA), shikimic acid, mevalonic acid and 1-deoxyxylulose-5-phosphate) are the most important building blocks involved in the biosynthesis of the bioactive compound [2, 17] in medicinal plant.

The therapeutic potentials of these medicinal plants is due to the complex interactions of the bioactive substances with their molecular target structures, such as the transport systems, enzymes and receptors.

With the transport systems, bioactive compounds can interact to influence the absorption, distribution and elimination of nutrients and organic compound and other organic cations [18, 19]. An example is polyphenols from medicinal plants, such as grapes, tea and cocoa, whose presence interferes with the activity and expression of several cell membrane transporters [19].

With the enzymes, bioactive substances can activate or inhibits enzymes [20], modulating metabolic pathways and cellular processes [21]. Plant derivative involved in modulating metabolic pathway and cellular processes is Δ^9-tetrahydrocannabinol (THC), the main psychoactive component of cannabis (*Cannabis sativa* and *Cannabis indica*) which activate G Protein Couple Receptors (GCPRs) cannabinoid 1 (CB1) and cannabinoid 2 (CB2) to which the endocannabinoids (ECBs) bind to and activate [21].

While with the receptors, bioactive compounds can bind to receptors, triggering signaling cascades that regulate various physiological processes [21], such as hormone regulation, neurotransmission and inflammation. Medicinal plant-derived compounds involved in cell signaling as bioactive lipids include carotenoids and phenolics (including flavonoides), terpenoids (including sterols) and cannabinoids (terpenophenol compounds also known as phytocannabinoids) [21].

These bioactive substances interactions can result in several therapeutic effects including the following:

1. Immune system modulation: bioactive compounds such as derivatives of caffeic acid, polysaccharides and alkamides from Echinacea are found to possess immunomodulatory properties. It has been reported that Echinacea interactions with the natural killer (NK) cells, T cells and macrophages increase their immune activity. The two pro-inflammatory cytokines that may be stimulated that are essential for controlling immunological response are interleukin-1 (IL-1) and tumor necrosis factor-alpha (TNF-alpha) [15]. Other bioactive compounds with immunomodulatory activities that regulate immune signaling pathways include triterpenoids, peptidoglycans and polysaccharides from *Ganoderma lucidum* (Reishi mushroom), andrographolides and flavonoids from *Andrographis paniculata*, while ginsenosides from *Panax ginseng* promote immune cell proliferation, and enhance immune responses against infections by modulating cytokine production by regulating function of the immune cell, including T cells, B cells and natural killer (NK) cells [15].

2. Analgesic and Anxiolytic activities: medicinal plants such as *Ganoderma applanatum* (mushroom), *Citrus maxima* (Burm.) and *Echinops kebericho* M. (Asteraceae) contain phytochemicals such as anthraquinone, glycosides, tannins, alkaloids, saponins, flavonoids, phenols and steroid [22], which anxiolytic activities is by mimicking gamma-aminobutyric acid (GABA) activity as a result of the interaction of the phytochemicals with the neurotransmitter receptors [22, 23]. While both the peripheral and central analgesic activities are attributed to the phytochemical inhibition and activation of receptors and transmitters [24].

3. Anti-inflammatory and antioxidant activities: bioactive compounds such as curcumin from turmeric (*Curcuma longa*) possess potent anti-inflammatory potentials by preventing the activation of nuclear factor-kappa B (NF-B) a crucial inflammation regulator. Also, gingerol from the ginger acts by decreasing inflammatory cytokines synthesis, including interleukin-6 (IL-6) and tumor necrosis factor-alpha (TNF-) [15]. Anti-oxidant activities of medicinal plant bioactive compounds such as flavonoid, quercetin from onions and apples are by lipid inhibition and neutralization of reactive oxygen species. Curcumin from turmeric and resveratrol from grapes are other examples [15].

4. Cardiovascular protection: medicinal plants such as turmeric (*Curcuma longa*) has bioactive compounds such as curcumin that have anti-inflammatory, anti-oxidant and lipid lowering effects. It was reported to possess the potentials for stopping atherosclerosis development and lower indicators of inflammation and enhance endothelial functions [25] thereby beneficial to cardiovascular health. Bioactive compounds such as flavonoids, procyanidins and triterpenoids from Hawthorn (*Crataegus* spp.) have been found to demonstrate blood flow improvement, lower blood pressure and heart function improvement, allicin, flavonoids and sulfur compounds from garlic have demonstrated blood pressure lowering activity, and enhance endothelial functions and both LDL and total cholesterol reduction [15]. Others that contribute to cardiovascular health include catechins from green teas.

5. Antimicrobial [21]: bioactive compounds such as berberine from *Berberis* spp., sanguinarine derivatives of alkaloids from the Papaveraceae family. Flavonoids, for example, kaempferol and quercetin, found in plants like *Allium cepa* and *Camellia sinensis* exhibit antibacterial properties by inhibition of essential enzymes and bacterial cell membrane disruption. Growth of fungi like *Candida* spp. and *Aspergillus* spp. have been reported to have been prevented by polyphenols such as the epigallocatechin gallate (EGCG) in green tea (*Camellia sinensis*). Similarly, antiviral activity of some bioactive compounds from flavonoids such as quercetin and hesperidin has been reported. Quercetin and hesperidin are said to inhibit viral pathogen replication. Also, the growth of a number of viruses, including the respiratory syncytial virus (RSV) and the hepatitis C virus (HCV), has been reported to have been prevented by tannins from *Punica granatum* (pomegranate) and *Camellia sinensis* (green tea). The antimicrobial activities of the bioactive compounds from medicinal plants are either by microbial cell membrane disruption leading to lysis and death of cells, inhibition of growth and vital enzymes involved in microbial metabolism and enhancement of the body defense mechanisms against infections by modulating the immune response [15].

6. Anticancer properties: bioactive compounds such as resveratrol a derivative of polyphenols from berries and grapes, epigallocatechin gallate (EGCG) from green teas, alkaloids such as vincristine and vinblastine from *Catharanthus roseus* (Madagascar periwinkle), camptothecin from *Camptotheca acuminata*, paclitaxel a terpenoid from the Pacific yew tree (*Taxus brevifolia*), sulforaphane found in vegetables like cauliflower and broccoli, allyl isothiocyanate from garlic all have been reported to possess anticancer properties which therapeutic activities are through modulation of important signaling pathways for cell apoptosis, growth, inflammation, angiogenesis, metastasis and survival, enzyme systems for tumor growth inhibition, epigenetic modifications and promotion of DNA repair [15].

7. Neuroprotective and neuroregenerative effects: bioactive compounds such as curcumin from turmeric (*Curcuma longa*) have exhibited activity as a neuroprotective compound, its therapeutic activity involved the aggregation of amyloid-beta plaques inhibition and neuroinflammation reduction. Other bioactive compounds for neuroprotective and neuroregenerative disorders such as Parkinson's and Alzheimer's include flavonoids and terpenoids from *Ginkgo biloba*, resveratrol and bacosides from *Bacopa monnieri* [15].

For the development of new drugs and therapies as well as the optimization of traditional herbal remedies, understanding of the complex interactions between bioactive substances and molecular target structures is crucial.

4. Advances in the utilization of bioactive compounds of medicinal plants

The utilization of medicinal plants in the management and treatment of diseases has continue to witness tremendous developments and improvements. Prepared herbal medicines from medicinal plants have been criticized for being crude, lack regulation, lack standardization, have no dose as well as the in ability to describe the mechanisms of action. These mentioned challenges made the use of herbal medicines from plant neglected and it used attributed to the rural populace who were regarded as been poor and could not access Western medications. But today, the emergence of Covid-19 and other terminal diseases, as well as drug resistance ailment, has triggered the quest for herbal medicines from medicinal plant for both developing and developed countries alike. This quest for herbal drugs of natural origin has led to thought-provoking innovations in natural medicine research as well as technological advancement which tend to proffer solutions to those criticisms. Below are some of the advances made in medicinal plant utilization:

a. *Technological advancement in bioactive compound extraction and characterization:* extraction and characterization of medicinal plants bioactive compounds is currently being explored by the researchers using new and advanced technologies which is a great improvement over the crude practices of extraction methods utilized by the ancients. These technologies enable the development of standardized extraction and analysis protocols by the researchers, they allow for new compounds and their structures identification, ensuring bioactive compounds efficient extraction and characterizations, enhancement of medicinal plant-based products quality and efficacy and understanding of biosynthesis of bioactive compound. These technologies include Advanced microscopy and spectroscopy, Supercritical Fluid Extraction (SFE), Microwave-Assisted Extraction (MAE), Phytochemical Analysis Software, Artificial Intelligence (AI) and Machine Learning (ML), High-Performance Liquid Chromatography (HPLC), Mass Spectrometry (MS), Pressurized Liquid Extraction (PLE), Ultra-High-Performance Liquid Chromatography (UHPLC), Nanotechnology approach and Magnetic Resonance (NMR) Spectroscopy [26–29].

b. *Bioinformatic tools*: to accelerate new bioactive compounds discovery and development of drugs from medicinal plant, bioinformatics tools and techniques have been developed to facilitate the analysis and interpretation of large datasets. Over the last two decades, the rapid development of omics-based plant studies has evolved due to the continuous introduction of novel omics concepts and rapid development of sequencing technologies which greatly facilitated the comprehensive dissection of biological processes occurring in plants at the genetic, transcriptional and metabolic levels [30]. At the genetic level, medicinal plants can be explored by the researchers using genome sequencing technology, sequencing and assembling of large medicinal plant genomes have been made easier using next-generation sequencing (NGS) and long-read sequencing technologies, molecular mechanism of medicinal plants and their impact on human health can be understood by genomic insight. These techniques allows for the identification of new bioactive compounds and the understanding of their mechanisms of action [31, 32].

c. *Nanotechnology*: the complaints against herbal medicines have been a lack of dose, standardization, adulteration among others but a novel means of overcoming these challenges is through nanotechnology. It is a "field of applied science and technology which aimed to develop devices and dosage forms in the range of 1 to 100 nm [28]." The field of nanotechnology presents a novel approach for the delivery of herbal drugs thereby overcoming the traditional drug delivery systems drawbacks. Herbal medicines were not given the due attention for development as a novel formulation for a long time as a result of scientific justification and processing difficulties, such as standardization, extraction and identification of individual drug components in complex polyherbal systems that were lacking. However, these scientific needs for herbal medicines in modern medicines have been resolved by modern phytopharmaceutical research which allows for the development of nanoparticles, microemulsions, matrix systems, solid dispersions, liposomes, solid lipid nanoparticles (SLNs), etc., as novel formulations [28].

d. *Artificial intelligence and machine learning:* the application of artificial intelligence and machine learning in medicinal plant research enables the therapeutic properties of medicinal plant extracts and bioactive compounds to be predicted. Identification of new bioactive compounds and extraction methods optimization is facilitated by these techniques [26, 27, 30].

e. *Sustainable domestication and cultivation:* because of the growing need for medicinal plants, their domestication and cultivation become very important because of their economic and ecological significance. More so, deliberate actions needed to be taken to ensure uniformity and consistency of the bioactive compounds supply for drug development. Researchers employed innovative methods of medicinal plant domestication and cultivation such as hydroponics, molecular breeding, agroforestry and vertical farming for the production of a large quantity of medicinal plants using good agricultural cultivation practices thereby, ensuring standard and quality of the bioactive compounds [26, 30].

f. *Pharmacological and toxicological examination*: more comprehensive pharmacological and toxicological studies on medicinal and aromatic plants to assess their efficacy and safety, are being conducted by researchers using *in vitro* and *in vivo* models for the evaluation of medicinal plant extracts and isolated compounds bioactivity and potential toxicity. This help to address the challenges of herbal medicines safety and efficacy issues [26].

4.1 The future outlook of medicinal plants

Large population of people are turning to herbal medicines for its therapeutic value from both developed and developing countries. This development is not necessarily because of poverty or lack of access to Western medicines but due to the realization that several advantages are presented by medicinal plants bioactive compounds such as the ability to cross blood-brain barriers [33], being of natural origin, little or no side effect compared to the Western medications, multiple target effects. Their ability for cellular process modulation, including immune responses, metabolic pathways, oxidative stress and inflammation all enhanced their therapeutic potentials [15].

However, the application of various advancements in medicinal plant research is essential to ensure that the full potential of medicinal plants bioactive compounds is fully realized.

Interdisciplinary collaborations combining traditional knowledge with modern scientific process is required for the future of utilizing medicinal plants bioactive substances. Novel therapies and personalized medicine approaches can be developed from the collaboration which can help in bridging the gap between traditional medicine and evidence-based medicine [15].

Additionally, exciting prospects for enhancing the therapeutic potential of these compounds are provided by advancements in nanotechnology, pharmacogenomics and phytopharmaceutical formulations. The therapeutic outcomes of these compounds can be optimized by improving their bioavailability, targeting specific tissues or cells and tailoring treatments based on individual genetic variations [34].

5. Conclusion

Medicinal plants hold immense therapeutic potentials due to the presence of bioactive compounds. These bioactive compounds conferred on the medicinal plants the healing powers for addressing various health challenges. Evidence of used of medicinal plant by the ancients to cure several ailments abound. With scientific and technological advancements improvements can now be made on the foundation laid by the ancients in the use of herbal medicines. Collaboration and integration of herbal medicine into the healthcare delivery system will further pave the ways for their utilization thus realizing the full therapeutic potentials of medicinal plants.

DOI: http://dx.doi.org/10.5772/intechopen.1005828

Author details

Martins Emeje[1], Eneojo Ogu[1*], Ifeoma Chidebe[1], Gautier Roko[1,2], Munira Abdullahi[1] and Daniel Sule Bibinu[1]

1 Nigeria Natural Medicine Development Agency (NNMDA), Lagos, Nigeria

2 Laboratory of Biology and Molecular Typing in Microbiology, University of Abomey-Calavi, Benin Republic

*Address all correspondence to: eneojo.ogu@nnmda.gov.ng
and ogusamyenes@gmail.com

References

[1] Karunamoorthi K, Jegajeevanram K, Vijayalakshmi J, Mengistie E. Traditional medicinal plants: A source of phytotherapeutic modality in resource-constrained health care settings. Journal of Evidence-Based Complementary & Alternative Medicine. 2013;**18**(1):67-74. DOI: 10.1177/2156587212460241

[2] Krishnaprabu DS. Therapeutic potential of medicinal plants: A review. Journal of Pharmacognosy and Phytochemistry. 2020;**9**(2):2228-2233. DOI: 10.22271/phyto.2020.v9.i2ak.11184

[3] Mahomoodally MF. Evidencebased complementary and alternative medicine traditional medicines in Africa: An appraisal of ten potent African medicinal plants. Evidence-Based Complementary and Alternative Medicine. 2013;**2013**:1-14

[4] Adetunbi RO. African traditions and the modern healthcare delivery system in the contemporary Nigerian Society. African Journal of Culture, History, Religion and Traditions. 2020;**2**(1):1-9

[5] Okigbo RN, Mmeka EC. An appraisal of phytomedicine in Africa. KMITL Science and Technology Journal. 2006;**6**(2):83-94

[6] Schultes RE. Medicinal plants and traditional medicine in Africa. Journal of Ethnopharmacology. 1984;**10**(3):332-333. DOI: 10.1016/0378-8741(84)90026-6

[7] Hamby EB. The roots of healing: Archaeological and historical investigations of African-American Herbal Medicine. PhD dissertation. University of Tennessee; 2004. Available from: https://trace.tennessee.edu/utk_graddiss/4543/

[8] Eneojo O, Martins E. Herbs and spices-based value addition for nutritional and healthy living. In: Herbs Spices—New Perspectives in Human Health and Food Industry [Working Title]. United Kingdom: IntechOpen Limited; 2024. pp. 1-11. DOI: 10.5772/intechopen.1004345

[9] Uttarakhand Open University. Ethnobotany. Haldwani: Uttarakhand Open University; 2017

[10] Jia Y, Zhao G, Jia J. Preliminary evaluation: The effects of Aloe ferox Miller and Aloe arborescens Miller on wound healing. Journal of Ethnopharmacology. 2008;**120**(2):181-189. DOI: 10.1016/j.jep.2008.08.008

[11] Van Staden J. African Herbal Pharmacopoeia, T. Brendler, J.N. Eloff, A. Gurib-Fakim, L.D. Phillips (Eds.), Graphics Press Ltd, Rue des Oursins, Baie du Tombeau, Mauritius (2010). South African Journal of Botany. 2011;77(3):806. DOI: 10.1016/j.sajb.2011.05.005

[12] Tahraoui A, El-Hilaly J, Israili ZH, Lyoussi B. Ethnopharmacological survey of plants used in the traditional treatment of hypertension and diabetes in South-Eastern Morocco (Errachidia province). Journal of Ethnopharmacology. 2007;**110**(1):105-117. DOI: 10.1016/j.jep.2006.09.011

[13] Alami Z, Aynaou H, Alami B, Hdidou Y, Latrech H. Herbal medicines use among diabetic patients in Oriental Morocco. Journal of Pharmacognosy and Phytotherapy. 2015;7(2):9-17. DOI: 10.5897/JPP2014.0338

[14] Lijalem T, Feyissa T. In vitro propagation of *Securidaca longipedunculata* (Fresen) from shoot tip: An endangered medicinal plant. Journal, Genetic Engineering & Biotechnology.

2020;**18**(1):1-10. DOI: 10.1186/s43141-019-0017-0

[15] Dar RA, Shahnawaz M, Ahanger MA, Majid I, ul. Exploring the diverse bioactive compounds from medicinal plants: A review. The Journal of Phytopharmacology. 2023;**12**(3):189-195. DOI: 10.31254/phyto.2023.12307

[16] Oladeji O. The characteristics and roles of medicinal plants: Some important medicinal plants in Nigeria. Natural Products: An Indian Journal. 2016;**12**(3):1-8

[17] Alagoz Y, Gurkok T, Zhang B, Unver T. Manipulating the biosynthesis of bioactive compound alkaloids for next-generation metabolic engineering in opium poppy using CRISPR-Cas 9 genome editing technology. Scientific Reports. 2016;**6**(August):1-9. DOI: 10.1038/srep30910

[18] Vaou N, Stavropoulou E, Voidarou C, et al. Interactions between medical plant-derived bioactive compounds: Focus on antimicrobial combination effects. Antibiotics. 2022;**11**(8):1-23. DOI: 10.3390/antibiotics11081014

[19] Martel F, Monteiro R, Calhau C. Effect of polyphenols on the intestinal and placental transport of some bioactive compounds. Nutrition Research Reviews. 2010;**23**(1):47-64. DOI: 10.1017/S0954422410000053

[20] Cheng YL, Lee CY, Huang YL, et al. We are IntechOpen, the world's leading publisher of open access books built by scientists, for scientists TOP 1%. INTECH. 2016;**11**(tourism):13. Available from: https://www.intechopen.com/books/advanced-biometric-technologies/liveness-detection-in-biometrics

[21] Maccarrone M. Deciphering complex interactions in bioactive lipid signaling. Molecules. 2023;**28**(6):1-13. DOI: 10.3390/molecules28062622

[22] Yimer T, Birru EM, Adugna M, Geta M, Emiru YK. Evaluation of analgesic and anti-inflammatory activities of 80% methanol root extract of *Echinops kebericho* M. (asteraceae). Journal of Inflammation Research. 2020;**13**:647-658. DOI: 10.2147/JIR.S267154

[23] Ahsan MT, Maria NN, Tahmida U, Jasmin AA, Chowdhury DUS. Anxiolytic, analgesic and anti-inflammatory effects of Citrus maxima (Burm.) Merr. Seed extract in Swiss albino mice model. Clinical Phytoscience. 2023;**9**(1):1-10. DOI: 10.1186/s40816-023-00354-7

[24] Hossen SMM, Islam MJ, Hossain MR, Barua A, Uddin MG, Emon NU. CNS anti-depressant, anxiolytic and analgesic effects of Ganoderma applanatum (mushroom) along with ligand-receptor binding screening provide new insights: Multi-disciplinary approaches. Biochemistry and Biophysics Reports. 2021;**27**:101062. DOI: 10.1016/j.bbrep.2021.101062

[25] Jówko E, Sacharuk J, Balasińska B, Ostaszewski P, Charmas M, Charmas R. Green tea extract supplementation gives protection against exercise-induced oxidative damage in healthy men. Nutrition Research. 2011;**31**(11):813-821. DOI: 10.1016/j.nutres.2011.09.020

[26] Ladislau R. What Are the Future Trends in Medicinal Plant Research. LinkedIn; 2023. Available from: https://www.linkedin.com/in/ladislaw-rosenberg-ph-d-7109b14/ [Accessed: April 25, 2024]

[27] Zaky AA, Akram MU, Rybak K, Witrowa-Rajchert D, Nowacka M. Bioactive compounds from plants and by-products: Novel extraction methods,

applications, and limitations. AIMS Molecular Science. 2024;**11**(2):150-188. DOI: 10.3934/molsci.2024010

[28] Lifang Y, Ye Y, Luqi H, Xiuming C, Yuan L. From single- to multi-omics: Future research trends in. Briefings in Bioinformatics. 2022;**24**(1):1-13

[29] Sharma V, Sarkar IN. Bioinformatics opportunities for identification and study of medicinal plants. Briefings in Bioinformatics. 2013;**14**(2):238-250. DOI: 10.1093/bib/bbs021

[30] Cheng QQ, Ouyang Y, Tang ZY, et al. Review on the development and applications of medicinal plant genomes. Frontiers in Plant Science. 2021;**12**(December):1-22. DOI: 10.3389/fpls.2021.791219

[31] Ansari SH, Islam F, Sameem M. Influence of nanotechnology on herbal drugs: A review. Journal of Advanced Pharmaceutical Technology & Research. 2012;**3**(3):142-146. DOI: 10.4103/2231-4040.101006

[32] Ayush G. Medicinal Plants Detection Using ML & DL Project Report Submitted in Partial Fulfillment of the Requirement for the degree of Bachelor of Technology in Computer Science and Engineering/Information Technology. Waknaghat: Jaypee University of Information Technology; 2023

[33] Liu Y, Chen Z, Li A, Liu R, Yang H, Xia X. The phytochemical potential for brain disease therapy and the possible nanodelivery solutions for brain access. Frontiers in Oncology. 2022;**12**(June):1-11. DOI: 10.3389/fonc.2022.936054

[34] Kapoor N, Bhatti E, Kaur N. Therapeutic potential of medicinal plants derived nanoparticles: A review. International Journal of Multidisciplinary Research. 2019;**5**(5):199-201

Chapter 11

Traditional Uses, Essential Oil Chemical Composition, and Biological Activities of Moroccan Lavenders

Soulaimani Bouchra, Ayoub Amssayef, Abbad Imane, Abbad Abdelaziz and Hassani Lahcen

Abstract

Lavandula is a genus of small herbs and sub-shrubs belongs to the Lamiaceae family, one of the most economically important plant families, which includes approximately 236 genera and nearly 7200 species. The *Lavandula* genus contains about 34 species widely distributed globally, mainly in the Mediterranean region, and used from ancient time to cure diverse diseases. The essential oils (EOs) obtained from species of this genus are widely used in perfumery, cosmetics, food processing, as well as in aromatherapy products due to their multiple biological properties. This chapter reports the traditional uses, chemical composition, and biological activities of EOs extracted from *Lavandula* species growing wild and/or cultivated in Morocco. The chemical composition of Moroccan *Lavandula* EOs is mainly composed of monoterpenes. The majority of EOs extracted from lavender are characterized by a high antimicrobial power, especially those with a richness in phenolic compounds, particularly carvacrol. Some species have been reported to have a very powerful anti-oxidant effect, while others have an important acaricidal or/and insecticidal activities.

Keywords: Moroccan lavender, traditional use, essential oil, chemical composition, biological activities

1. Introduction

The Lamiaceae (Labiatae) is a large family of dicotyledonous flowering plants, comprising about 236 genera and over 7200 species and subspecies. Among, the genus *Lavandula* is one of the most economically important plants of the family, with approximately 39 species, many hybrids, and nearly 400 registered cultivars [1]. The species of the genus *Lavandula*, commonly called "Khzama" in Arabic "Lavender" in English, or "Lavande" in French, generally include both spontaneous and cultivated forms, widely distributed in the Mediterranean basin, the Canary Islands, Cape Verde Islands, Madeira Islands, North Africa, Southwest Asia, the Arabian Peninsula, and tropical Northeast Africa [2, 3]. In Morocco, this genus is represented by nine species of which five are endemics (*Lavandula maroccana* Murb, L. *rejdalii* Upson et Jury, L. *mairei* Humbert Var, *L. pedunculata* subsp. *atlantica* (Braun-Blanquet), and *L. tenuisecta* Coss. Ex Ball) [1, 3, 4] and two cultivated species (*L. angustifolia* and *L. latifolia*).

Moroccan lavenders have been used in traditional pharmacopeia in different forms to treat several illnesses, including digestive, respiratory, gastro-intestinal, genital, nervous, urinary, inflammatory, and pulmonary diseases [5–7]. Different plant parts of these lavenders are also used for the preparation of herbal tea and some traditional meals, and for cosmetic purposes [8]. The essential oils (EOs) from different Moroccan lavender species have been reported to possess many biological properties such as antibacterial, antifungal, insecticidal, acaricidal, and antioxidant activities [9–13]. Oxygenated and hydrocarbons monoterpenes such as linalool, carvacrol, 1,8-cineole, β-ocimene, terpinen-4-ol, and camphor constitute the principal chemical constituents of the EOs extracted from Moroccan lavenders [10–13]. The aim of the present chapter is to provide a comprehensive summary on the traditional uses, EO chemical compositions, and the main biological activities of the *Lavandula* species growing wild or cultivated in Morocco.

2. Taxonomic presentation of the genus *Lavandula*

The taxonomy of the genus *Lavandula* has been particularly well described by Upson and Andrews [1]. It includes more than 39 species and 79 intraspecific and hybrid taxa, allowing for classification into three subgenera (i.e., Lavandula, Fabricia, and Sabaudia), comprising eight sections, respectively: Lavandula, Dentatae, Stoechas/Pterostoechas, Subnudae, Chaetostachys, Hasikenses, and Sabaudia [1]. In Morocco, the genus *Lavandula* is represented by nine native species, five of which are endemics, represented by *L. maroccana* Murb, *L. rejdalii* Upson et Jury, *L. mairei* Humbert Var, *L. pedunculata* subsp. *atlantica* (Braun-Blanquet), and *L. tenuisecta* Coss. Ex Ball [3, 4]. Pterostoechas is the most diverse and represented section in Morocco with six native species, including four endemics. Stoechas section is represented by two native species, while the section Dentatae is represented by only one species which is *L. dentata* [1, 14]. The main cultivated *Lavandula* species in Morocco are fine or true lavender (*L. angustifolia*) and spike lavender (*L. latifolia*), which belong to the *Lavandula* section and *Lavandula* subgenera [1, 4].

3. Methodology

The electronic databases Web of Science, Scopus, SciFinder, Pubmed, and Google Scholar were used to search the traditional uses, EO chemical composition, and biological activities of Moroccan *Lavandula*. The search keywords used were: *Lavandula*, Morocco, ethnobotany, essential oils, chemical composition, biological activities, antimicrobial, antibacterial, antifungal, antioxidant, insecticidal, and anti-inflammatory activities. All works published on Moroccan *Lavandula* species in different languages (French or English) were taken into consideration, and then the articles was rigorously selected according to the focus of the study.

4. Traditional use

In the traditional Moroccan pharmacopeia, lavenders are used as medicinal, aromatic, culinary, and/or cosmetic herbs. Generally, in traditional Moroccan medicine, lavenders are the most recommended herbs for the treatment of colds, flu, coughs, diarrhea, gastrointestinal disorders, and urinary infections [15]. Dried flowers have also been used since time immemorial under pillows or in sachets to promote sleep and relaxation. However, there is a clear difference in their therapeutic uses depending on the region and species involved. At the level of the locality of Oulmes (Mid-Atlas), a relatively humid and cold region in winter, rheumatism is the pathology most treated by lavender species as anti-inflammatory remedies, while in the Western High Atlas, lavender leaves and flowers are used in the form of decoction for the treatment of broncho-pulmonary, gastrointestinal, and urogenital diseases [6]. In El Maghzen (High Atlas), the flowers of *L. dentata* or "Timzuria" in Tamazirt are extensively used in infusion to treat headaches, stomach, menstrual pain, and some gynecological problems. *L. dentata* is also used by local women with henna for tattooing or to color hair [8]. Leaves and flowers of *L. angustifolia* and *L. stoechas* are used in infusion or decoction against hypertension and diabetes in southeast Morocco, mainly the province of Errachidia [16]. According to a survey conducted in the city of Meknes, *L. multifida* was listed among the plants used in the treatment of different oral diseases [5]. Moreover, an ethnobotanical study in five area of the province of Guelmim showed that *L. maroccana* is widely used against many health problems, particularly rheumatism, hair care, and gastrointestinal diseases [7].

5. Essential oils of lavenders

5.1 Generalities on the EOs of lavender

The EOs extracted from lavender have a great demand and interest in perfumery, aromatherapy, and cosmetics. These EOs, as of many aromatic and medicinal plants, are essentially composed of terpene compounds, particularly mono- and sesquiterpenes [1, 17], and are essentially stored in specialized structures (glandular trichomes) [18]. These trichomes consist of a few basal epidermal cells topped by secretory cells generally numbering 2 for caped glandular trichomes and 8 for peltate glandular trichomes (**Figure 1a**) [19]. The terpene compounds produced by these cells are stored under their cuticle, this is why the calyxes and leaves of the plant usually need to be rubbed to burst the glands and subsequently release their fragrance. Glandular trichomes are much more abundant and denser on the flower calyx than on the leaves. There are other types of trichomes (tector trichomes) largely abundant in lavenders in the form of branched hairs. However, these types of trichomes do not produce terpenes. Therefore, EOs and terpene compounds can be extracted from lavender leaves and inflorescences by different distillation methods (hydro-distillation and steam distillation). In general, the steam generated during distillation degrades the cuticle of the glandular trichomes and subsequently carries away the volatile compounds [19]. The color of EOs from lavenders varies from yellow to red-orange, with yields ranging from 0.01% to 7.2% [20]. This variability may be related to many intrinsic and/or extrinsic factors, including geographic origin, harvesting period (seasonal variation), plant age, EO extraction method, and plant genetic characteristics [21–24].

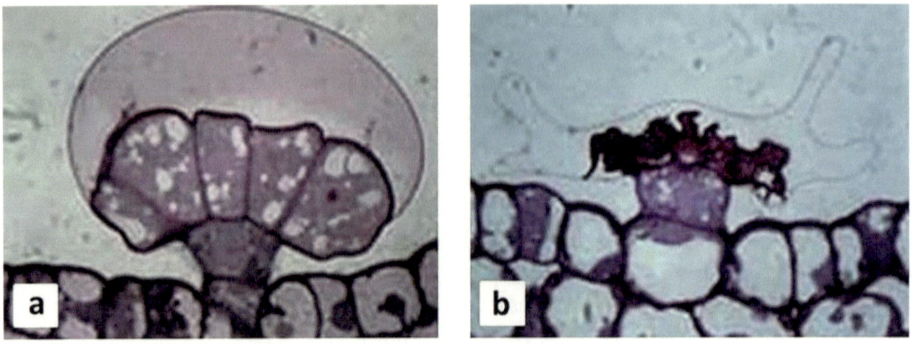

Figure 1.
Light microscope image of lavender glandular trichome before (a) and after (b) EO extraction.

5.2 Chemical composition of lavender EOs

The chemical investigations carried out on the EOs of different Moroccan lavenders showed different volatile profiles, dominated essentially by oxygenated and hydrocarbon monoterpene classes, while sesquiterpenes (oxygenated or/and hydrocarbon) are generally present in low proportions (**Table 1** and **Figure 2**). Carvacrol

Species	Used part	Main compounds	Reference
L. maroccana	AP	Carvacrol (78%), 2-Methoxy-4-vinylphenol (2.5%), Spathulenol (2.2%)	[25]
	AP	Carvacrol (76.98%), Methoxy-4-vinylphenol (3.04%,) Spathulenol (2.2)	[26]
	L, F, St	Carvacrol (26.5–35.2%), β-Bisabolene (18.9–25%), Camphor (2.4–53%)	[27]
	AP	Carvacrol (37.1%), β-Bisabolene (27.2%), Camphor (4.7%), Spathulenol (4,3%), Linalool (4.1%)	[28]
	AP	Carvacrol (42.08%), Camphor (17.95%), Fenchone (12.05%)	[29]
	AP	carvacrol (44.58–55.12%), p-cymen-8-ol (4.84–6.41%), α-farnesene (4.11–4.74%) and 2-methoxy-4-vinylphenol (3.71–5.35%)	[30]
L. rejdalii	AP	Linalool (32.03%), Carvacrol (19.61%), Camphor (11.03%)	[31]
L. mairei	AP	Carvacrol (78%), Terpinolene (3.2%), Octen-3-ol (2.3%)	[23]
	AP	Carvacrol (77.32%)	[9]
L. tenuisecta	AP	Camphor (26.9%), Fenchone (22.7%), 1,8-Cineole (18.1%)	[32]
	F, L, St	Camphor (20.9–26.4%), 1,8-Cineole (19.4–38.1%), Fenchol (16–22%)	[33]
L. pedunculata subsp. atlantica	AP	Camphor (50.4%), Fenchone (14.1%), Camphene (5.6%)	[34]
	WP	Camphor (53.1%), 1,8-Cineole (6.5%), Camphene (6.1%)	[35]
	B	camphor (44.16%), 1 –epi-cubenol (8.61%), fenchone (7.48%), camphene (6.45%) and α-pinene (4.86%)	[13]
	AP	Camphor (74.51%), Fenchone (27.06%)	[29]

Species	Used part	Main compounds	Reference
	AP	Camphor (46.36%), α-Pinene (10.74%), Camphene (5.74%)	[36]
	AP	Camphor (30.8%), α-Pinene (14.8%), Camphene (14.6%), Fenchone (7.5%)	[37]
L. coronopifolia	—	Carvacrol (48.9%), E-Caryophyllene (10.8%), Caryophyllene oxide (7.7%)	[38]
	AP	Carvacrol (48.9%), E-caryophyllene (10.8%), caryophyllene oxide (7.7%)	[39]
L. dentata	AP	1, 8-Cineole (41.28%), Sabinene (13.69%), Bicycle [3.1.0] hexan-3-Ol, 4-methylene-1-(1-methylethyl) (6.76%), Myrtenal (5.11%), α-Pinene (4.05%)	[40]
	—	1,8-Cineole (49.82%), Camphor (6.31%), α-Pinene (4.12%)	[12]
	WP	Camphor (50.3%), trans-Pinocarveol (6.2%), β-Eudesmol (4.1%), Borneol (3.0%), Linalool (2.2%)	[35]
	AP	Camphor (49.75%), 1,8-Cineole (39.84%), cis-Linalool oxide (1.17%)	[36]
	AP	Linalool (45.06%), Camphor (15.62%), Borneol (8.28%), 1,8-Cineole (7.24%), γ-Terpineol (7.01%), Linalool acetate (6.01)	[10]
L. multifida	L, St	Carvacrol (44.3%), ß-bisabolene (31.9%), caryophyllene oxide (5.8%)	[41]
	AP	1,8-Cineole (28.11%), camphor (11.57%), endo-borneol (7.82%), linalyl acetate (5.22%)	[42]
	AP	Carvacrol (57.9–59.0%), Carvacrol methyl ether (7–7.6%), p-Cymen-8-ol (3.9–4.7%), Caryophyllene oxide (2.1–2.7%)	[43]
	AP	Carvacrol (47.62%), β-Bisabolene (9.01%), Dodecyl acrylate (8.37%), Linalool (7.42%), Menthone (4.98%), β-Caryophyllene (3.34%), β-Pinene (3.21%)	[44]
L. stoechas	AP	10s,11s-Himachala-3(12),4-diene (23.62%), Cubenol (16.19%), Methyl eugenol (6.19%) δ-Cadinene (5.31%), Myrtenyl acetate (4.96%)	[45]
	AP	Fenchone (31.81%), Camphor (29.60%), Terpineol (13.14%), Menthone (8.96%), 1,8-Cineole (5.88%)	[11]
	AP	Camphor (18–39%), Fenchone (9–30%)	[46]
	AP	Camphor (43.97%), Fenchone (30.39%), camphene (4.09%), Borneol (2.92%), α-Pinene (2.84%)	[47]
	AP	Fenchone (31.8%), Camphor (29.6%), Terpineol (13.1%), Menthone (8.9%)	[48]
	AP	Fenchone (29.77%), Camphor (24.9%)	[49]
	L	L-Fenchone (14.39%), G-1-Cadinene aldehyde (10.61%), Viridiflorol (8.54%), Bornyl acetate (8.39%), and Myrtenyl acetate (3.77%)	[50]
	L	Cubebol (22.68%), Camphor (22.29%), Borneol (5.15%), Muurol-5-en-4-one <cis-14-nor- > (4.21%), L-Fenchone (4.03%), Silphiperfol-5-ene (3.27%)	
	L	t-Muurolol (18.44%), Cubebol (16.07%), Camphor (13.39), Muurol-5-en-4-one (cis-14-nor-) (6.84), Selina-3,7(11)-diene (4.5%), 3-Adamantan-1-yl-butan-2-one (4.39%)	

Species	Used part	Main compounds	Reference
L. angustifolia	AP	Linalool (21.81%), 1,8-Cineole (18.07%) Camphor (11.89%), Linalyl acetate (10.21%), Borneol (8.47%), α-Terpineol (5.00%)	[51]
	—	Linalool (32.23%), Linalyl acetate (14.23%), Geraniol (5.8%), Lavandulyl acetate (4.8%), Camphor (4.21%), β-Caryophyllene (4.2%), Terpinen-4-ol (3.4%)	[12]
	F	Linalool (44.67%), Linalyl acetate (42.00%), Camphor (6.02%), 1,8-Cineole (5.30%)	[52]
	WP	Linalyl acetate (44.96%), Linalool (44.64%), Caryophyllene oxide (3.15%)	[53]
	AP	1,8-Cineole (39.05%), Camphor (24.21%), Borneol (8.29%)	[29]

Table 1.
Chemical composition of Moroccan lavender EOs.

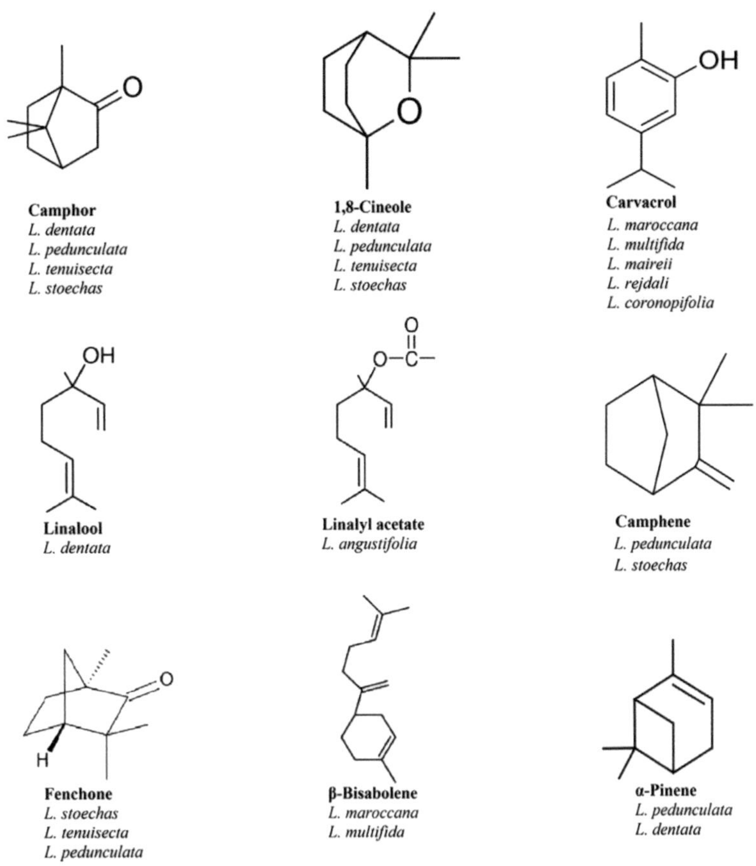

Figure 2.
Main compounds identified in Moroccan lavender EOs.

constituted the major compound in the EOs of lavender species of the section Pterostoechas in particular, *L. maroccana, L. mairei, L. coronopifolia,* and *L. multifida* with percentages ranging from 26.5 to 78.0% [23, 25, 27–29, 38, 43, 44]. The EO of

L. rejdali is composed mainly by linalool (32.03%), carvacrol (19.61%), and camphor (11.03%) [31]. The EO of *L. tenuisecta* is dominated by camphor (20.9–26.9%), 1,8-cineole (18.1–38.1%), fenchone (22.7%), and/or fenchol (16–22%) [32, 33]. These compounds in addition to terpineol and menthone have been detected also in the chemical profiles of *L. stoechas* EOs as major constituents [11, 46–48]. However, a different chemical profile characterized by the dominance of 10s,11s-himachala-3(12),4-diene (23.62%), cubenol (16.19%), methyl eugenol (6.19%), δ-cadinene (5.31%), and myrtenyl acetate (4.96%) has been reported for the EO of *L. stoechas* collected in northern Morocco [45]. Camphor (30.8–74-51%) was found as the predominant compound in most EOs of *L. pedunculata* subsp. *atlantica* in addition to fenchone, camphene, 1,8-cineole and α-pinene in highly variable content [13, 34, 35, 37]. In contrast, the EO of cultivated *L. angustifolia* was found to be dominated mainly by linalool and linalyl acetate in addition to the main detected constituents in the EOs of *L. tenuisecta* and *L. pedunculata* subsp. *atlantica* [12, 51–53].

5.3 Biological activities of lavender EOs

5.3.1 Antimicrobial activity

The current issues with conventional antimicrobials, along with the emergence of drug-resistance observed in recent years among many pathogenic strains to these synthetic products, have prompted the search for alternatives primarily based on natural constituents. Numerous studies have shown that EOs extracted from lavender species have proven to be an effective and efficient antimicrobial agent that could serve as an excellent substitute to overcome the use of synthetic antimicrobials. According to our analysis of studies conducted on Moroccan lavender EOs, we found that these volatile fractions are much more studied for their antimicrobial properties and most of them showed strong activities against many pathogenic strains (bacteria, yeasts, and fungi) (**Table 2**). The EOs of *L. maroccana* and *L. maireii* characterized by high levels of carvacrol have proven broad-spectrum antimicrobial activities and were effective at low concentrations especially against Gram-positive bacterial strains [23, 25, 26, 54]. For instance, the investigations carried out on the EOs extracted from *L. maroccana* showed interesting antimicrobial potency against many pathogenic bacteria and yeast strains (MICs = 0.60–18.416 mg/mL) [25, 26, 54]. In another study, El Hamdaoui et al. [23] evaluated the antibacterial activity of EOs from wild and cultivated *L. maireii* against six bacterial strains and reported that both EOs possess high inhibitory effect (MIC ranged from 0.80 to 1.00 mg/mL). Similarly, Ghanimi et al. [55] reported a potent antibacterial effect for the EO extracted from wild *L. maireii.* According to the study carried out by Ait Said et al. [38], the EO obtained from *L. coronopifolia* exhibited interesting antibacterial effect regarding multi-drug resistant clinical isolates of 11 pathogenic bacteria (IZ = 13.0 ± 0.57–22.0 ± 1.52 mm and MICs = 1.00–4.00%). Moreover, Sayout et al. [32] reported the antibacterial activity of *L. tenuisecta* EO against eight resistant bacteria. However, this Moroccan endemic lavender EO showed moderate to week effects against tested strains (MICs = 6.25–25.00 mg/L), except for *Salmonella spp.* against which it did not show any activity. Similarly, Sayout et al. [34] reported in another study a relatively moderate antibacterial effect of EO obtained from *L. pedunculata* on nine bacterial strains (MICs = 3.13–25.00 mg/L). Radi et al. [56] evaluated the antimicrobial effect of *L. pedunculata* against six bacteria, three yeasts, and two fungi, and the results showed that the EO possess remarkable antimicrobial effectiveness, with MIC values ranged between 2 and 30 μL/mL. In other

Species	Strains	IZ (mm)	MIC	MBC	Reference
L. maroccana	*Staphylococcus aureus (CCMMB3)*	13.00 ± 0.10	4.604 mg/mL	4.604 mg/mL	[25]
	Micrococcus luteus (ATCC 10,240)	15.00 ± 0.20	2.302 mg/mL	2.302 mg/mL	
	Bacillus subtilis (ATCC 9524)	23.00 ± 0.05	2.302 mg/mL	2.302 mg/mL	
	Escherichia coli (ATCC 8739)	9.00 ± 0.25	9.208 mg/mL	9.208 mg/mL	
	Pseudomonas aeruginosa (DSM, 50090)	13.00 ± 0.40	18.416 mg/mL	18.416 mg/mL	
	Klebsiella pneumoniae	7.00 ± 0.12	4.604 mg/mL	9.208 mg/mL	
	Candida albicans CCMML4	18.00 ± 0.70	4.604 mg/mL	4.604 mg/mL	
	Candida glabrata CCMM-L7	22.00 ± 0.90	4.604 mg/mL	4.604 mg/mL	
	Candida krusei CCMM-L10	19.00 ± 0.31	4.604 mg/mL	4.604 mg/mL	
	Candida parapsilosis CCMM-L18	19.00 ± 0.81	4.604 mg/mL	9.208 mg/mL	
	Escherichia coli (ATCC 8739)	9.00 ± 0.25	9.208 mg/mL	9.208 mg/mL	[26]
	Pseudomonas aeruginosa (DSM, 50090)	13.00 ± 0.40	4.604 mg/mL	9.208 mg/mL	
	Klebsiella pneumoniae	7.00 ± 0.12	18.416 mg/mL	18.416 mg/mL	
	Staphylococcus aureus (CCMMB3)	10.55 ± 0.96	0.125%	0.125%	[54]
	Escherichia coli (ATCC 8739)	9.59 ± 0.27	0.25%	0.25%	
	Pseudomonas aeruginosa (DSM, 50090)	9.00 ± 0.67	2.50%	2.50%	

Species	Strains	IZ (mm)	MIC	MBC	Reference
	Staphylococcus aureus (CCMMB3)	14.16 ± 0.22–24.12 ± 0.26	0.60–1.25 mg/mL	0.60–1.25 mg/mL	[30]
	Micrococcus luteus (ATCC 10,240)	20.83 ± 0.49–22.17 ± 0.78	0.60 mg/mL	0.60 mg/mL	
	Bacillus subtilis (ATCC 9524)	20.00 ± 0.33–24.90 ± 0.67	0.30 mg/mL	0.30 mg/mL	
	Escherichia coli (ATCC 8739)	11.00 ± 0.67–14.17 ± 1.22	0.60–1.25 mg/mL	0.60–1.25 mg/mL	
	Pseudomonas aeruginosa (DSM, 50090)	08.70 ± 0.47–10.27 ± 0.49	0.60 mg/mL	0.60 mg/mL	
	Klebsiella pneumoniae	14.50 ± 0.20–16.37 ± 0.42	2.50–5.00 mg/mL	2.50–10.0 mg/mL	
	Candida albicans CCMML4	21.07 ± 0.64–23.00 ± 0.33	0.60–1.25 mg/mL	1.25 mg/mL	
	Candida glabrata CCMM-L7	22.17 ± 0.56–23.07 ± 0.36	0.60–1.25 mg/mL	1.25 mg/mL	
	Candida krusei CCMM-L10	20.17 ± 0.36–23.50 ± 0.33	0.60 mg/mL	0.60–1.25 mg/mL	
	Candida parapsilosis CCMM-L18	18.13 ± 0.24–20.33 ± 0.44	1.25 mg/mL	1.25 mg/mL	
	Escherichia coli ATCC 8739	—	14.12 mg/mL	—	[29]
	Salmonella spp	—	14.12 mg/mL	—	
	Staphylococcus aureus CCMM-B3	—	3.53 mg/mL	—	
L. mairei	*Listeria innocua (CECT 4030)*	34.6 ± 4.7–35.3 ± 4.1	0.90 mg/mL	0.90 mg/mL	[23]
	Listeria monocytogenes (CECT 4032)	34.6 ± 2–35.6 ± 2	0.80 mg/mL	0.85 mg/mL	
	Staphylococcus aureus (CECT 976)	23.5 ± 0.7–24.5 ± 0.7	1.20 mg/mL	1.20 mg/mL	
	Bacillus subtilis (DSM 6633)	25.5 ± 0.7	0.60 mg/mL	0.60 mg/mL	
	Proteus vulgaris (CECT 484) Pseudomonas aeruginosa (CECT 118)	23.5 ± 0.7–24.0 ± 0.0	0.60 mg/mL	0.60 mg/mL	
		27.0 ± 0	1.00 mg/mL	1.00 mg/mL	

Species	Strains	IZ (mm)	MIC	MBC	Reference
	Escherichia coli	13 ± 0.2	0.156 mg/mL		[55]
	Klebsiella pneumonia	16 ± 0.5	0.039 mg/ml		
	Staphylococcus aureus	15 ± 0.5	0.078 mg/mL		
	Pseudomonas aeruginosa	10 ± 0.1	0.624 mg/mL		
	Acinetobacter baumannii	10 ± 0.2	0.624 mg/mL		
	Citrobacter koseri	13 ± 0.86	0.078 mg/mL		
	Acinetobacter baumannii	28.67 ± 1.15–40 ± 2.00	0.39–3.125 μL/mL	0.39–3.125 μL/mL	[9]
L. tenuisecta	*Staphylococcus aureus P637*	10.00–25.00	6.25 mg/L	12.50 mg/L	[32]
	Escherichia coli P1420	10.00–25.00	6.25 mg/L	25.000 mg/L	
	Enterobacter aerogenes P1260	10.00–25.00	16.66 mg/L	33.33 mg/L	
	Pseudomonas aeruginosa P1418	10.00–25.00	12.50 mg/L	25.000 mg/L	
	Klebsiella pneumoniae LA726	10.00–25.00	12.50 mg/L	12.50 mg/L	
	Klebsiella oxytoca BU9399	10.00–25.00	12.50 mg/L	25.00 mg/L	
	Salmonella spp. S	0.00	—	—	
	Acinetobacter baumannii PDP533	10.00–25.00	12.50 mg/L	50.00 mg/L	
	Enterobacter cloacae P1374	10.00–25.00	25.00 mg/L	50.00 mg/L	
L. pedunculata	*Staphylococcus aureus P637*	15	12.50 mg/L	25.00 mg/L	[34]
	Escherichia coli P1420	19	12.50 mg/L	50.00 mg/L	
	Enterobacter aerogenes P1260	36	16.67 mg/L	50.00 mg/L	
	Pseudomonas aeruginosa P1418	12	20.00 mg/L	33.33 mg/L	
	Klebsiella pneumoniae LA726	21	3.13 mg/L	25.00 mg/L	
	Klebsiella oxytoca BU9399	26	25.00 mg/L	50.00 mg/L	
	Salmonella spp.	29	12.50 mg/L	16.67 mg/L	
	Acinetobacter baumannii PDP533	23	12.50 mg/L	25.00 mg/L	
	Enterobacter cloacae P1374	27	25.00 mg/L	50.00 mg/L	

Species	Strains	IZ (mm)	MIC	MBC	Reference
	Escherichia coli (ATCC 4157)	14.5–26.7	5.00 μg/mL	—	[35]
	Pseudomonas aeruginosa (ATCC 27853)	14.5	5.00 μg/mL	—	
	Staphylococcus aureus (ATCC 25923)	26.7	5.00 μg/mL	—	
	Streptococcus fasciens (ATCC 29212)	14.5–26.7	20.00 μg/mL	—	
	Escherichia coli ATCC 8739	—	4.84 mg/mL	—	[29]
	Salmonella spp	—	4.84 mg/mL	—	
	Staphylococcus aureus CCMM-B3	—	9.68 mg/mL	—	
	Escherichia coli (Ec01)	12.3 ± 2.3	—	—	[36]
	Escherichia coli (Ec02)	9.0 ± 1.2	—	—	
	Klebsiella pneumoniae (Kp01)	6.0 ± 0.0	—	—	
	Klebsiella pneumoniae Kp02)	9.3 ± 0.9	—	—	
	Pseudomonas aeruginosa (Ps01)	0.0 ± 0.0	—	—	
	Pseudomonas aeruginosa (Ps02)	0.0 ± 0.0	—	—	
	Pseudomonas aeruginosa	6	—	—	[13]
	Escherichia Coli (EC1)	0	—	—	
	Escherichia Coli (EC2)	0	—	—	
	Escherichia Coli (EC3)	6	—	—	
	Staphylococcus aureus (Staph A1)	12	—	—	
	Staphylococcus aureus (Staph A2)	0	—	—	
	Staphylococcus blanc (Staph B)	14	—	—	
	Proteus	10	—	—	
	Klebsiella pneumonia	8	—	—	

Species	Strains	IZ (mm)	MIC	MBC	Reference
	Escherichia coli	08 ± 0.5–14 ± 0.1	6.00 µL/mL	8.00 µL/mL	[56]
	Staphylococcus aureus	20 ± 0.18–35 ± 0.3	2.00 µL/mL	4.00 µL/mL	
	Salmonella thyphi	09 ± 08–15 ± 05	6.00 µL/mL	6.00 µL/mL	
	Acinetobacter baumanii	11 ± 00–20 ± 0.1	10.00 µL/mL	10.00 µL/mL	
	Enterobacter cloacae	07 ± 0.9–14 ± 0.5	6.00 µL/mL	6.00 µL/mL	
	Shigella dysenteria	10 ± 0–15 ± 0.8	6.00 µL/mL	6.00 µL/mL	
	Candida albican	23 ± 0.5	20 µL/mL	20 µL/mL	
	Candida glabrata	25 ± 2.1	20 µL/mL	20 µL/mL	
	Candida ssp	18 ± 0.1	30 µL/mL	30 µL/mL	
	Aspergillus fisheri	23 ± 0.2	20 µL/mL	20 µL/mL	
	Fusarum solani	06 ± 00	—	—	
L. coronopifolia	*Acinetobacter baumannii*	22.0 ± 1.52	1%	2%	[38]
	Klebsiella pneumoniae subsp. pneumoniae	15.0 ± 1.00	2%	4%	
	Klebsiella ornithinolytica	16.0 ± 0.50	4%	4%	
	Escherichia coli	13.0 ± 0.57	4%	4%	
	Hafnia alvei	16.0 ± 0.57	4%	4%	
	Salmonella spp.	13.0 ± 0.57	4%	4%	
	Enterobacter aerogenes	13.0 ± 0.57	4%	4%	
	Enterobacter cloacae	19.0 ± 1.15	2%	4%	
	Providencia rettgeri	14.5 ± 0.70	2%	2%	
	Citrobacter freundii	19.0 ± 1.15	2%	2%	
	Staphylococcus aureus (MRSA)	16.0 ± 1.00	1%	2%	

DOI: http://dx.doi.org/10.5772/intechopen.1005486

Species	Strains	IZ (mm)	MIC	MBC	Reference
L. dentata	*Salmonella sp (1)*	20	—		[40]
	Salmonella sp (2)	15	—		
	Neisseria meningitidis (1)	50	0.041 mg/mL		
	Neisseria meningitidis (2)	21	0.04187 mg/mL		
	Enterobacter cloacae	15	0.04187 mg/mL		
	Klebsiella pneumoniae (1)	20	0.167 mg/mL		
	Klebsiella pneumoniae (2)	38	0.04187 mg/mL		
	Heamophilus influezae(1)	28	—		
	Heamophilus influezae (2)	50	—		
	Pseudomonas aeruginosa ATCC12228	0	10.00 mg/mL		
	Pantoea sp	15	0.083 mg/mL		
	Escherichia coli	20	0.167 mg/mL		
	Escherichia coli	12	0.041 mg/mL		
	Escherichia coli ATCC125922	15	0.167 mg/mL		
	Escherichia coli	11	0.167 mg/mL		
	Escherichia coli	11	0.167 mg/mL		
	Proteus mirabilis	18	0.041 mg/mL		
	Staphylococcus aureus ATCC 25923	22	0.167 mg/mL		
	Staphylococcus aureus	16	0.041 mg/mL		
	Streptococcus sp	50	0.338 mg/mL		
	Streptococcus pneumoniae	43	0.041 mg/mL		
	Listeria monocytogenes	70	—		

Species	Strains	IZ (mm)	MIC	MBC	Reference
	Escherichia coli (ATCC 4157)	13.5–25.25	5.00 µg/mL	—	[35]
	Pseudomonas aeruginosa (ATCC 27853)	13.5	5.00 µg/mL	—	
	Staphylococcus aureus (ATCC 25923)	25.25	10.00 µg/mL	—	
	Streptococcus fasciens (ATCC 29212)	13.5–25.25	20.00 µg/mL	—	
	Escherichia coli (Ec01)	12 ± 2.1	—	—	[36]
	Escherichia coli (Ec02)	9.6 ± 0.1	—	—	
	Klebsiella pneumoniae (Kp01)	6.0 ± 0.0	—	—	
	Klebsiella pneumoniae Kp02)	8.3 ± 0.9	—	—	
	Pseudomonas aeruginosa (Ps01)	0.0 ± 0.0	—	—	
	Pseudomonas aeruginosa (Ps02)	0.0 ± 0.0	—	—	
	Alternaria alternata	—	˃ 40 µg/mL	—	[10]
	Botrytis cinerea	—	5 µg/mL	—	
	Fusarium oxysporum	—	˃ 40 µg/mL	—	
	Escherichia coli	14 ± 0.5	0.156 mg/mL	—	[55]
	Klebsiella pneumonia	14 ± 0.5	0.156 mg/mL	—	
	Staphylococcus aureus	18 ± 0.5	0.039 mg/mL	—	
	Pseudomonas aeruginosa	12 ± 0.4	0.156 mg/mL	—	
	Acinetobacter baumannii	13.3 ± 0.1	0.312 mg/mL	—	
	Citrobacter koseri	15.5 ± 0.9	0.039 mg/mL	—	

Species	Strains	IZ (mm)	MIC	MBC	Reference
L. multifida	*Bacillus subtilis DCM 6633*	12.500 ± 0,707	2%	>4%	[44]
	Staphylococcus Aureus MBLA	14.500 ± 0,707	1%	2%	
	Staphylococcus Aureus ATCC 25923	16.000 ± 2828	1%	>4%	
	Listeria innocua CECT 4030	11.000 ± 1414	>4%	>4%	
	Listeria monocytogenes CECT 4032	8.500 ± 0,707	>4%	>4%	
	Escherichia coli K12 MBLA	9.500 ± 0,707	>4%	>4%	
	Escherichia coli CECT 4076	9.500 ± 0,707	4%	>4%	
	Proteus mirabilis IH	12.500 ± 0,707	4%	>4%	
	Proteus vulgaris CECT 484	11.500 ± 0,707	4%	>4%	
	Pseudomonas aeruginosa IH	0	—	—	
	Staphylococcus aureus	20 ± 0.01	2 mg/mL	0.5 mg/mL	[41]
	Staphylococcus epidermidis	14.66 ± 0.44	2 mg/mL	2 mg/mL	
	Klebsiella pneumoniae	11 ± 0.01	4 mg/mL	4 mg/mL	
	Acinetobacter baumannii	10.16 ± 0.22	4 mg/mL	4 mg/mL	
	Escherichia coli	9 ± 0.01	2 mg/mL	2 mg/mL	
	Staphylococcus aureus ATCC 29213	—	0.78 mg/mL	0.78 mg/mL	[42]
	Listeria monocytogenes ATCC 13932	—	0.78 mg/mL	0.78 mg/mL	
	Bacillus subtilis ATCC 6633	—	0.78 mg/mL	0.78 mg/mL	
	Escherichia coli ATCC 25922	—	1.56 mg/mL	3.12 mg/mL	
	Salmonella typhimurium ATCC 700408	—	6.25 mg/mL	12.5 mg/mL	
	Pseudomonas aeruginosa ATCC 27853	—	25 mg/mL	25 mg/mL	

Species	Strains	IZ (mm)	MIC	MBC	Reference
L. stoechas	*Salmonella enterica subsp. enterica serovar Senftenberg (STCC 4563),*	14.8 ± 0.17	14.0 µL/mL	>56.0 µL/mL	[45]
	Escherichia coli O157:H7,	20.7 ± 0.45	14.0 µL/mL	14.0 µL/mL	
	Escherichia coli (STCC 471)	16.2 ± 0.60	21.0 µL/mL	>56.0 µL/mL	
	Yersinia enterocolitica (STCC 4315)	12.5 ± 1.70	14.0 µL/mL	>56.0 µL/mL	
	Staphylococcus aureus (STCC 976)	28.0 ± 0.70	2 µL/mL	14.0 µL/mL	
	Enterococcus faecium (STCC 4932)	29.5 ± 0.50	2.0	14.0	
	Listeria monocytogenes (STCC 4031)	29.5 ± 0.50	8.0	14.0	
	Listeria. monocytogenes EGD-e	37.5 ± 2.50	0.5	8.0	
	Bacillus subtilis (STCC 4071)	34.0 ± 1.40	4.0	8.0	
	Staphylococcus aureus MBLA	21 ± 0.25	0.5%	0.5%	[11]
	Staphylococcus aureus CECT 976	<21	2%	2%	
	Staphylococcus aureus CECT 994	<21	1%	1%	
	Listeria monocytogenes serovar 4b CECT 4032	23 ± 0.85	0.25%	0.25%	
	Proteus mirabilis CECT	<21	1%	1%	
	Pseudomonas aeruginosa IH	<21	>2%	>2%	
	Bacillus subtilis DSM 6633	<21	2%	2%	
	Escherichia coli K12	<21	0.5%	0.5%	
	Escherichia coli	12 ± 0.2	0.156 mg/mL	—	[55]
	Klebsiella pneumonia	16.3 ± 0.6	0.039 mg/mL	—	
	Staphylococcus aureus	18 ± 0.1	0.039 mg/mL	—	
	Pseudomonas aeruginosa	14 ± 0.3	0.156 mg/mL	—	
	Acinetobacter baumannii	15.6 ± 0.3	0.156 mg/mL	—	
	Citrobacter koseri	14 ± 0.5	0.039 mg/mL	—	

DOI: http://dx.doi.org/10.5772/intechopen.1005486

Species	Strains	IZ (mm)	MIC	MBC	Reference
	Bacillus subtilis DSM 6633	20.66 ± 1.15–25 ± 4.35	6.25–25 mg/mL	˃ 50 mg/mL	[50]
	Staphylococcus aureus CECT 976	6 ± 0.00–7.36 ± 0.57	—	—	
	Proteus mirabilis INH	18.66 ± 1.15–22.66 ± 0.57	12.25–˃ 50 mg/mL	25–˃ 50 mg/mL	
	Escherichia coli K12	6 ± 0.00–10.66 ± 0.57	3.12–12.5 mg/mL	˃ 50 mg/mL	
	Pseudomonas aeruginosa CECT 118	13.33 ± 1.15–19 ± 1.00	—	—	
	Candida albicans	19.00 ± 1.0–25.33 ± 0.5	—	—	
	Micrococcus luteus (clinical isolate)	27.0 ± 0.5	0.25%	0.031%	[49]
	Bacillus subtilis (ATCC 6633)	24.0 ± 0.3	0.015%	0.015%	
	Pseudomonas aeruginosa (ATTC 27853)	14.0 ± 1.9	0.5%	0.5%	
	Escherichia coli (ATCC 25922)	28.5 ± 1.4	0.125%	0.125%	
	Salmonella enterica (clinical isolate)	25.0 ± 3.3	0.125%	0.125%	
	Candida albicans (clinical isolate)	25.3 ± 0.1	0.125%	0.125%	
L. angustifolia	*Escherichia coli ATCC 25922*	26.67–43	3.33 µL/mL	10.67 µL/mL	[51]
	Staphylococcus aureus ATCC 25923	30.67–41	1.33 µL/mL	6.67 µL/mL	
	Pseudomonas aeruginosa ATCC 27853	8.67–16	42.67 µL/mL	85.33 µL/mL	
	Enterococcus faecalis	17	10 µL/mL	10 µL/mL	[53]
	Escherichia coli	15	10 µL/mL	10 µL/mL	
	Klebsiella pneumoniae	13	10 µL/mL	10 µL/mL	
	Streptococcus D	12	5 µL/mL	5 µL/mL	
	Escherichia coli ATCC 8739	—	7.93 mg/mL	—	[29]
	Salmonella spp	—	7.93 mg/mL	—	
	Staphylococcus aureus CCMM-B3	—	15.96 mg/mL	—	

Species	Strains	IZ (mm)	MIC	MBC	Reference
	Escherichia coli	10 ± 0.1–40 ± 0.14	4.00 μL/mL	6.00 μL/mL	[56]
	Staphylococcus aureus	15 ± 0.8–30 ± 0	2.00 μL/mL	4.00 μL/mL	
	Salmonella thyphi	11 ± 0.1–20 ± 0.1	4.00 μL/mL	6.00 μL/mL	
	Acinetobacter baumanii	11 ± 0.12–40 ± 00	6.00 μL/mL	6.00 μL/mL	
	Enterobacter cloacae	10 ± 0.1–24 ± 0.6	4.00 μL/mL	4.00 μL/mL	
	Shigella dysenteria	08 ± 0–14 ± 0.17	6.00 μL/mL	6.00 μL/mL	
	Candida albican	52 ± 0.1	20 μL/mL	20 μL/mL	
	Candida glabrata	22 ± 0.2	30 μL/mL	30 μL/mL	
	Candida ssp	33 ± 1.2	20 μL/mL	20 μL/mL	
	Aspergillus fisheri	20 ± 1.3	20 μL/mL	20 μL/mL	
	Fusarum solani	40 ± 2.1	20 μL/mL	20 μL/mL	

Table 2.
Antimicrobial activity of Moroccan lavender EOs.

investigation, N'dédianhoua et al. [36] reported that *L. pedunculata subsp. atlantica* and *L. dentata* EOs showed inhibitory action against *E. coli* and *K. pneumoniae* strains (ZI between 6 and 12 mm) using the agar diffusion method. Ghanimi et al. [55] compared the antibacterial activity of EOs extracted from three Moroccan lavenders, namely *L. dentata, L. stoechas,* and *L. maireii* against five Gram-negative strains (*E. coli, P. aeruginosa, K. pneumoniae, C. koseri, and A. baumanni*) and the Gram-positive *S. aureus*, and showed that the three studied EOs possess strong antibacterial activity (MICs = 0.039–0.156 mg/mL). *L. dentata* EO was reported to have also total inhibitory effect on mycelial growth of the fungus *Botrytis cinerea* [10]. Studies on *L. stoechas* have shown that its EO exhibited potent antimicrobial activity against strains of *S. enterica, E. coli, Y. enterocolitica, S. aureus, E. faecium, L. monocytogenes, P. mirabilis,* and *B. subtilis* [11, 45]. In addition, Hachlafi et al. [49] demonstrated the antibacterial effect of *L. stoechas* EO regarding six bacteria, with MICs ranging from 0.015 to 0.125%. In contrast, *L. multifida* EO showed moderate inhibitory activity against *S. aureus, B. subtilis, P. mirabilis, P. vulgaris,* and *E. coli* ($1\% \leq MIC \leq 4\%$) [44]. Concerning cultivated *L. angustifolia,* the investigations carried out on its EO showed interesting antibacterial and anticandidal activities with comparable MIC values (MICs = 1.33–30 μL/mL) [29, 53, 56].

The antimicrobial activity of Moroccan lavender EOs is strongly related to the presence of oxygenated monoterpenes, including carvacrol, camphor, 1,8-cineole, linalool, fenchone, and terpineol. It has been reported that these monoterpenes are capable of disrupting the outer membrane of bacteria, releasing lipopolysaccharides and increasing cytoplasmic membrane permeability, resulting in ATP leakage [57–59]. These terpene compounds also act on yeast and fungi by blocking, hyphal transition, expression of genes encoding efflux pumps, and ergosterol biosynthesis [60–63]. Hydrocarbon monoterpenes (camphene, α-pinene, caryophyllene, and β-bisabolene) present in the EOs of some lavender species in varying proportions have also been reported to have a part in this antimicrobial activity.

5.3.2 Antioxidant activity

Antioxidants derived from natural products have attracted special interest in recent years, as they are recognized as safe and are subject to less stringent regulatory requirements than the synthetic ones widely available in the market (e.g., Butylated Hydroxyanisole (BHA), Butylated Hydroxytoluene (BHT), and Propyl Gallate (PG). These compounds are unfortunately known to have long-term toxicological effects and uncertain health safety [64]. Terpene compounds, which are dominants in the EOs of many medicinal and aromatic plants, have strong antioxidant activities due to their high redox potential. The antioxidant properties of EOs from the *Lavandula* species have been mainly attributed to the content of some well-known compounds, mainly carvacrol, camphor, 1,8-cineole, linalool, fenchone, camphene, and α-pinene. According to our literature search (**Table 3**), the EOs of five Moroccan lavender species have been described as exhibiting antioxidant effects. In particular, the EO of *L. stoechas* showed a much stronger reducing capacity on the DPPH free radical (IC50 = 785.38 ± 9.04 μg/mL) and FRAP (EC_{50} = 107.53 ± 1.74 μg/mL) [11]. However, the other studies performed on EOs of the same species showed moderate to strong activity using DPPH, FRAP, TAC, and β-carotene/linoleic acid bleaching reduction assays [45, 55]. *L. mairei* and *L. pedunculata* EOs also showed high antioxidant activity against DPPH and FRAP [13, 23, 55]. Sayout et al. [33] showed that the antioxidant property of lavender EOs varies depending on the plant part. For example, the EO

Species	Aassays	Results	References
L. mairei	DPPH FRAP	IC_{50} = 107.54 µg/mL IC_{50} = 5.22 µg/ml	[23]
	DPPH FRAP TAC	IC_{50} = 6.62 mg/ml EC_{50} = 13.4 mg/ml 125.9 mg AAE/g EO	[55]
L. tenuisecta	DPPH FRAP	IC_{50} = 2.15–11.5 mg/mL EC_{50} = 2.27–9.15 mg/mL	[33]
L.dentata	DPPH FRAP TAC	IC_{50} = 12.95 mg/mL EC_{50} = 11.88 mg/mL 81.28 ± 2.28 mg AAE/g EO	[10]
	DPPH FRAP TAC	IC_{50} = 4.75 mg/mL EC_{50} = 9.23 mg/mL 262.1 mg AAE/g EO	[55]
L. stoechas	DPPH FRAP β-Carotene bleaching	$IC_{50} = {}^{>}$ 5.00 µL/ml $IC_{50} = {}^{>}$ 10.00 µL/ml IC_{50} = 5.00 µL/ml	[45]
	DPPH FRAP	IC_{50} = 785.38 ± 9.04 µg/mL EC_{50} = 107.53 ± 1.74 µg/mL	[11]
	DPPH FRAP TAC	IC_{50} = 3.11 mg/ml EC_{50} = 6.88 mg/ml 443.2 mg AAE/g EO	[55]
	FRAP ABTS	4.82 ± 1.52–15.73 ± 3.26 mg AAE/g EO $IC_{50} = {}^{<}$ 10.00 µg/ml	[50]
L. multifida	DPPH H_2O_2 Xanthine oxidase	15.23 ± 0.05 µg/mL 34.81 ± 0.01 µg/mL 19.74 ± 0.08 µg/mL	[42]
L. pedunculata	DPPH FRAP	IC_{50} = 21.14 mg/ml EC_{50} = 8.65 mg/ml	[13]

Table 3.
Antioxidant activity of Moroccan lavender EOs.

obtained from the flowers of *L. tenuisecta* showed significantly higher antioxidant capacity than those extracted from the leaves and stems. On the other hand, the antioxidant effect of *L. dentata* EOs showed moderate activity in the DPPH, FRAP, and TAC tests [10, 55]. In general, the antioxidant activity of lavender EOs seems to be mainly related to their chemical composition, in particular to the nature of their major compounds. On the other hand, the antioxidant effects of some minority compounds and their synergy with the majority ones remain as well not negligible.

5.3.3 Biopesticide activity

The increasing spread of pests that attack agricultural crops continues to negatively impact the economies of many countries. The continued and increasing use of synthetic crop protection products is also a concern due to the increasing resistance of these pests to the used chemical pesticides, as well as to human health and environmental safety issues. Research dedicated to the discovery of natural products to be used to protect agricultural crops and their products in storage, is constantly growing

Species	Biological activity	Pests	Results	Reference
L. maroccana	Acaricidal	*Varroa destructor*	LC_{50} = 2,49 41 μL/L air LC_{90} = 8,41 μL/L air	[28]
L. pedunculata	Acaricidal	*Hyalomma aegyptium*	LD_{50} = 0,505 μL/mL for larvae LD_{50} = 0,0036 μL/mL for nymphs	[37]
L. coronopifolia	Insecticidal	*Ceratitis capitata*	LC_{50} = 86.339 μL/g LC_{90} = 236.0747 μL/g	[39]
L. dentata	Larvicidal	*Culex pipiens*	LC_{50} = 2670 μg/ml LC_{90} = 7400 μg/ml	[12]
	Insecticidal	*Callosobruchus maculatus*	LC_{50} = 4.01 μL/L d'air	[10]
L. stoechas	Antileishmanial	*Leishmania major* *L. infantum* *L. tropica*	CI_{50} = 0,9 ± 0,45% (v/v) CI_{50} = 7 ± 0.54% (v/v) CI_{50} = > 10% (v/v)	[11]
	Insecticidal	*Anopheles labranchiae*	LC_{50} = 112,51 mg/L	[65]
L. angustifolia	Larvicidal	*Culex pipiens*	LC_{50} = 140 μg/mL LC_{90} = 450 μg/mL	[12]

Table 4.
Biocidal activity of Moroccan lavender EOs.

as agricultural losses worsen year after year. The EOs of Lavender species have shown promising insecticidal effects on many arthropods (**Table 4**). As an example, the EOs of *L. pedunculata* and *L. stoechas* have shown insecticidal and repellent effects against the red flour beetle (*Tribolium castaneum*), a secondary pest of great economic and agricultural importance [66]. *L. dentata* EO also showed significant insecticidal and repellent potential on pea weevil (*Callosobruchus maculatus*) adults in both fumigation and contact tests [10]. The biopesticidal activity of lavender EOs has also been demonstrated against some species of mosquitoes and parasites responsible for the transmission of many diseases and pathogens (e.g., *Culex pipiens* L. 1758). EOs of *L. dentata* and *L. angustifolia* showed insecticidal effects at low concentrations on *C. pipiens* larvae [12]. In addition, *L. stoechas* EO exhibited significant larvicidal properties on the malaria vector (*Anopheles labranchiae*) [65] and antiparasitic effects against *Leishmania major*, responsible for the zoonotic cutaneous leishmaniasis disease [11]. Acaricidal effects against adults of *Varroa destructor* and different life stages of *Hyalomma aegyptium* were shown by the EOs of *L. maroccana* and *L. pedunculata* subsp. *atlantica*, respectively [28, 37]. Generally, the biopesticidal properties of lavender EOs have been attributed to the presence of some terpenic constituents, mainly 1,8-cineole, camphor, α-pinene, camphene, linalool, and fenchone.

6. Conclusions

This chapter represents an overview on traditional use of Moroccan lavenders, chemical profiles, and the main biological activities of their Eos. The Moroccan *Lavandula* species have been used in folk medicine for a long time. It is used in different forms to treat several diseases such as diabetes, digestive, genital, urinary, skin, and broncho-pulmonary diseases. The chemical compositions of the EOs from Moroccan *Lavandula* species are rich sources of oxygenated monoterpenes including carvacrol, camphor, 1,8-cineole, fenchone, fenchol, terpineol, and linalool. Furthermore, some hydrocarbon monoterpenes such as camphene, β-bisabolene, terpinolene, and caryophyllene, also characterized the chemical profiles of *Lavandula* EOs. As regards the pharmacological properties, many investigations reported several activities for Moroccan *Lavandula* species, essentially antimicrobial (antibacterial and antifungal), antioxidant, insecticidal, and larvicidal activities. Interestingly, the EOs rich phenolic compounds, particularly carvacrol showed a high antibacterial, antifungal, and antioxidant activities, while others species have generally an important acaricidal or/and insecticidal activities.

Conflict of interest

The authors declare no conflict of interest.

Author details

Soulaimani Bouchra[1*], Ayoub Amssayef[2], Abbad Imane[3], Abbad Abdelaziz[1] and Hassani Lahcen[1]

1 Laboratory of Microbial Biotechnologies, Agrosciences and Environment, Faculty of Sciences Semlalia, Cadi Ayyad University, Marrakech, Morocco

2 Euromed University of Fez (UEMF), Fez, Morocco

3 Faculty of Sciences Semlalia, Cadi Ayyad University, Marrakech, Morocco

*Address all correspondence to: bouchrasoulaimanigebc@gmail.com

References

[1] Upson T, Andrews S. The Genus Lavandula. Portland: Timber Press; 2004. 456 p

[2] Upson TM. Systematics of the Genus Lavandula L. (Lamiaceae) [Ph.D. Thesis]. Reading, UK: University of Reading; 1997

[3] Upson T. The taxonomy of the genus Lavandula L. In: Lis-Balchim M, editor. Lavender, the Genus Lavandula. New York: Taylor & Francis; 2002. pp. 2-34

[4] Fennane M, Ibn Tattou M, Ouyahya A, El Oulaidi J. Flore pratique du Maroc, Manuel de détermination des plantes vasculaires. Vol. 2. Rabat: Institut Scientifique; 2007. 636 p

[5] Harouak H, Ibijbijen J, Nassiri L. Comparison between medicinal plants used against oral diseases and pharmaceutical dental products in Morocco. Annals of Dental Specialty. 2019;7(2):1-4

[6] Bachiri L, Labazi N, Daoudi A, Ibijbijien J, Nassiri L, Echchegadda G, et al. Etude ethnobotanique de quelques lavandes marocaines spontanées. International Journal of Biological and Chemical Sciences. 2015;**9**(3):1308-1318. DOI: 10.4314/ijbcs.v9i3.16

[7] Afrokh M, Tahrouch S, ELMehrach K, Fahmi F, Bihi MA, Weber-Ravn H, et al. Ethnobotanical, phytochemical and antioxidant study of fifty aromatic and medicinal plants. Chemical Data Collections. 2023;**43**:100984. DOI: 10.1016/J.CDC.2022.100984

[8] Montanari B. Aromatic, medicinal plants and vulnerability of traditional herbal knowledge in a Berber community of the high atlas mountains of Morocco. Plant Diversity and Resources. 2014;**36**(3):388-402

[9] Laktib A, Nayme K, El Hamdaoui A, Timinouni M, Hassi M, Alla AA, et al. Antibacterial activity of *Lavandula mairei* Humbert essential oil against Carbapenem-resistant *Acinetobacter baumannii*. Mediterranean Journal of Infection, Microbes and Antimicrobials. 2022;**11**(1):12. DOI: 10.4274/mjima.galenos.2021.2021.3

[10] El Abdali Y, Agour A, Allali A, Bourhia M, El Moussaoui A, Eloutassi N, et al. *Lavandula dentata* L.: Phytochemical analysis, antioxidant, antifungal and insecticidal activities of its essential oil. Plants. 2022;**11**(3):311. DOI: 10.3390/plants11030311

[11] Bouyahya A, Et-Touys A, Abrini J, Talbaoui A, Fellah H, Bakri Y, et al. *Lavandula stoechas* essential oil from Morocco as novel source of antileishmanial, antibacterial and antioxidant activities. Biocatalysis and Agricultural Biotechnology. 2017;**12**:179-184. DOI: 10.1016/j.bcab.2017.10.003

[12] El-Akhal F, Ramzi A, Farah A, Ez Zoubi Y, Benboubker M, Taghzouti K, et al. Chemical composition and larvicidal activity of *Lavandula angustifolia* subsp. *angustifolia* and *Lavandula dentata* spp. *dentata* essential oils against *Culex pipiens* Larvae, vector of west nile virus. Psyche: A Journal of Entomology. 2021;**2021**:1-7. DOI: 10.1155/2021/8872139

[13] Chroho M, El Karkouri J, Hadi N, Elmoumen B, Zair T, Bouissane L. Chemical composition, antibacterial and antioxidant activities of the essential oil of *Lavandula pedunculata* from

Khenifra Morocco. IOP Conference Series: Earth and Environmental Science. 2022;**1090**(1):012022. DOI: 10.1088/1755-1315/1090/1/012022

[14] Upson TM, Jury SL. A revision of native Moroccan species of *Lavandula L.* section Pterostoechas Ging.(Lamiaceae). Taxon. 2002;**51**(2):309-327

[15] Haddad PS, Depot M, Settaf A, Chabli A, Cherrah Y. Comparative study on the medicinal plants most recommended by traditional practitioners in Morocco and Canada. Journal of Herbs Spices & Medicinal Plants. 2003;**10**(3):25-45. DOI: 10.1300/J044v10n03_04

[16] Tahraoui A, El-Hilaly J, Israili ZH, Lyoussi B. Ethnopharmacological survey of plants used in the traditional treatment of hypertension and diabetes in south-eastern Morocco (Errachidia province). Journal of Ethnopharmacology. 2007;**110**(1):105-117. DOI: 10.1016/j.jep.2006.09.011

[17] Wells R, Truong F, Adal AM, Sarker LS, Mahmoud SS. Lavandula essential oils: A current review of applications in medicinal, food, and cosmetic industries of lavender. Natural Product Communications. 2018;**13**(10):1403-1417

[18] Perrin A, Colson M. L'appareil sécréteur des lavandes et des lavandins. Parfum cosmétiques, arômes. 1986;**69**:61-63

[19] Iriti M, Colnaghi G, Chemat F, Smadja J, Faoro F, Visinoni FA. Histo-cytochemistry and scanning electron microscopy of lavender glandular trichomes following conventional and microwave-assisted hydrodistillation of essential oils: A comparative study. Flavour and Fragrance Journal. 2006;**21**(4):704-712. DOI: 10.1002/FFJ.1692

[20] Aprotosoaie AC, Gille E, Trifan A, Luca VS, Miron A. Essential oils of Lavandula genus: A systematic review of their chemistry. Phytochemistry Reviews. 2017;**16**(4):761-799. DOI: 10.1007/s11101-017-9517-1

[21] Jamali CA, Kasrati A, Bekkouche K, Hassani L, Wohlmuth H, Leach D, et al. Phenological changes to the chemical composition and biological activity of the essential oil from Moroccan endemic thyme (*Thymus maroccanus* Ball). Industrial Crops and Products. 2013;**49**:366-372. DOI: 10.1016/j.indcrop.2013.05.016

[22] Sefidkon F, Abbasi K, Khaniki GB. Influence of drying and extraction methods on yield and chemical composition of the essential oil of *Satureja hortensis*. Food Chemistry. 2006;**99**(1):19-23. DOI: 10.1016/j.foodchem.2005.07.026

[23] El Hamdaoui A, Msanda F, Boubaker H, Leach D, Bombarda I, Vanloot P, et al. Essential oil composition, antioxidant and antibacterial activities of wild and cultivated *Lavandula mairei* Humbert. Biochemical Systematics and Ecology. 2018;**76**:1-7. DOI: 10.1016/j.bse.2017.11.004

[24] Sellami IH, Wannes WA, Bettaieb I, Berrima S, Chahed T, Marzouk B, et al. Qualitative and quantitative changes in the essential oil of *Laurus nobilis* L. leaves as affected by different drying methods. Food Chemistry. 2011;**126**(2):691-697. DOI: 10.1016/j.foodchem.2010.11.022

[25] Soulaimani B, Nafis A, Kasrati A, Rochdi A, Mezrioui N, Abbad A, et al. Chemical composition, antimicrobial activity and synergistic potential of essential oil from endemic *Lavandula*

maroccana (Mill.). South African Journal of Botany. 2019;**125**(2019):202-206. DOI: 10.1016/j.sajb.2019.07.030

[26] Soulaimani B, El Hidar N, El Fakir SB, Mezrioui N, Hassani L, Abbad A. Combined antibacterial activity of essential oils extracted from *Lavandula maroccana* (Murb.), *Thymus pallidus* Batt. and *Rosmarinus officinalis* L. against antibiotic-resistant Gram-negative bacteria. European Journal of Integrative Medicine. 2021;**43**:101312. DOI: 10.1016/j.eujim.2021.101312

[27] Ouarhach A, Costa J, Romane A. Chemical profiling of *Lavandula maroccana* of Morocco. Chemistry of Natural Compounds. 2020;**56**(2):348-350. DOI: 10.1007/s10600-020-03028-9

[28] Alahyane H, Ouknin M, Aboussaid H, El Messoussi S, Costa J, Majidi L. Biological activities of essential oils from Moroccan plants against the honey bee ectoparasitic mite, *Varroa destructor*. International Journal of Acarology. 2022;**48**(1):50-56. DOI: 10.1080/01647954.2021.2015436

[29] Nafis A, Ouedrhiri W, Iriti M, Mezrioui N, Marraiki N, Elgorban AM, et al. Chemical composition and synergistic effect of three Moroccan lavender EOs with ciprofloxacin against foodborne bacteria: A promising approach to modulate antimicrobial resistance. Letters in Applied Microbiology. 2021;**72**(6):698-705. DOI: 10.1111/lam.13460

[30] Soulaimani B, Meddich A, Lahbouki S, Abbad I, Ouarghidi A, Mezrioui NE, et al. Arbuscular mycorrhizal fungi associated with endemic Moroccan lavender (*Lavandula maroccana* Murb.): Effects on plant growth, volatile oil composition and antimicrobial activity. Journal of Essential Oil-Bearing Plants. 2023;**2023**(26):534-546. DOI: 10.1080/0972060X.2023.2220367

[31] Gharby S, Asdadi A, Ibourki M, Hamdouch A, Ainane T, Hassani LAI. Chemical characterization of the essential oil from aerial parts of *Lavandula rejdalii* Upson & Jury, a medicinal plant endemic to Morocco. Journal of Essential Oil-Bearing Plants. 2020;**23**(6):1422-1427. DOI: 10.1080/0972060X.2020.1870575

[32] Sayout A, Ouarhach A, Dilagui I, Soraa N, Romane A. Antibacterial activity and chemical composition of essential oil from *Lavandula tenuisecta* Coss.ex Ball. An endemic species from Morocco. European Journal of Integrative Medicine. 2020;**33**:101017. DOI: 10.1016/j.eujim.2019.101017

[33] Sayout A, Ouarhach A, Romane A. Antioxidant properties and chemical composition of *Lavandula tenuisecta*, an endemic species of Morocco. Chemistry of Natural Compounds. 2020;**56**(6):1148-1150. DOI: 10.1007/s10600-020-03251-4

[34] Sayout A, Ouarhach A, Rabie R, Dilagui I, Soraa N, Romane A. Evaluation of antibacterial activity of *Lavandula pedunculata* subsp. *atlantica* (braun-blanq.) romo essential oil and selected terpenoids against resistant bacteria strains–structure–activity relationships. Chemistry & Biodiversity. 2020;**17**(1):e1900496. DOI: 10.1002/cbdv.201900496

[35] Bouazama S, Harhar H, Costa J, Desjobert JM, Talbaoui A, Tabyaoui M. Chemical composition and antibacterial activity of the essential oils of *Lavandula pedunculata* and *Lavandula dentata*. Journal of Materials and Environmental Science. 2017;**8**(6):2154-2160

[36] N'dédianhoua KS, Majdouli K, Khabbal Y, Zaïr T. Chemical composition

and antibacterial activity of Lavandula species *L. dentata* L., *L. pedunculata* Mill and *Lavandula abrialis* essential oils from Morocco against food-borne and nosocomial pathogens. International Journal of Innovation and Applied Studies. 2014;**7**(2):774

[37] Laghzaoui EM, Kasrati A, Abbad A, Leach D, Spooner-Hart R, El Mouden EH. Acaricidal properties of essential oils from Moroccan plants against immature ticks of *Hyalomma aegyptium* (Linnaeus, 1758); an external parasite of the spur-thighed tortoise (Testudo graeca). International Journal of Acarology. 2018;**44**(7):315-321. DOI: 10.1080/01647954.2018.1520918

[38] Ait Said L, Zahlane K, Ghalbane I, El Messoussi S, Romane A, Cavaleiro C, et al. Chemical composition and antibacterial activity of *Lavandula coronopifolia* essential oil against antibiotic-resistant bacteria. Natural Product Research. 2015;**29**(6):582-585. DOI: 10.1080/14786419.2014.954246

[39] Ouarhach A, Ait Said L, Aboussaid H, Ghalbane I, El Messoussi S, Romane A. Evaluation of insecticidal activity of *Lavandula coronopifolia* essential oil against the Mediterranean fruit fly *Ceratitis capitata* Wiedemann (Diptera: Tephritidae). South African Journal of Botany. 2022;**149**:748-753. DOI: 10.1016/J.SAJB.2022.05.026

[40] Imelouane B, Elbachiri A, Ankit M, Benzeid H, Khedid K. Physico-chemical compositions and antimicrobial activity of essential oil of eastern Moroccan *Lavandula dentata*. International Journal of Agriculture and Biology. 2009;**11**(2):113-118

[41] Elmakaoui A, Bourais I, Oubihi A, Nassif A, Bezhinar T, Shariati MA, et al. Chemical composition and antibacterial activity of essential oil of *Lavandula multifida*. Journal of Microbiology, Biotechnology and Food Sciences. 2022;**11**(6):e7559-e7559. DOI: 10.55251/jmbfs.7559

[42] Al-mijalli SH, Elsharkawy ER, Abdallah EM, Hamed M, El Omari N, Mahmud S, et al. Determination of volatile compounds of *Mentha piperita* and *Lavandula multifida* and investigation of their antibacterial, antioxidant, and antidiabetic properties. Evidence-Based Complementary and Alternative Medicine. 2022;**2022**:9. DOI: 10.1155/2022/9306251

[43] Znini M, Paolini J, Majidi L, Desjobert J-M, Costa J, Lahhit N, et al. Evaluation of the inhibitive effect of essential oil of *Lavandula multifida* L., on the corrosion behavior of C38 steel in 0.5 M H2SO4 medium. Research on Chemical Intermediates. 2012;**38**(2):669-683. DOI: 10.1007/s11164-011-0407-7

[44] Douhri B, Douhri H, Farah A, Idaomar M, Senhaji NS, Abrini J. Phytochemical analysis and antibacterial activity of essential oil of *Lavandula multifidi* L. International Journal of Science and Innovative Research. 2014;**1**:116-126

[45] Cherrat L, Espina L, Bakkali M, Pagán R, Laglaoui A. Chemical composition, antioxidant and antimicrobial properties of *Mentha pulegium, Lavandula stoechas* and *Satureja calamintha* Scheele essential oils and an evaluation of their bactericidal effect in combined processes. Innovative Food Science and Emerging Technologies. 2014;**22**:221-229. DOI: 10.1016/J.IFSET.2013.12.016

[46] Zrira S, Benjilali B. The constituents of the oils of *Lavandula stoechas* L. ssp. atlantica Br.-Bl. and L. stoechas ssp. stoechas from Morocco. Journal of

Essential Oil Research. 2003;**15**(2):68-69. DOI: 10.1080/10412905.2003.9712066

[47] Ez-zoubi A, Ez zoubi Y, Ramzi A, Fadil M, El Ouali Lalami A, Farah A. Ethanol and glycerol green emulsifying solvent for the formation of a *Lavandula stoechas* essential oil/β-cyclodextrin inclusion complex: Mixture design and adulticidal activity against *Culex pipiens*. Heliyon. 2022;**8**(8):e10204. DOI: 10.1016/j.heliyon.2022.e10204

[48] Bouyahya A, Dakka N, Lagrouh F, Abrini J, Bakri Y. In vitro antiproliferative and antidermatophyte activities of essential oils from three Moroccan medicinal plants. Journal of Biologically Active Products from Nature. 2018;**8**(3):144-153. DOI: 10.1080/22311866.2018.1496032

[49] El Hachlafi N, Benkhaira N, Hamad Al-Mijalli S, Naceiri Mrabti H, Abdnim R, Abdallah EM, et al. Phytochemical analysis and evaluation of antimicrobial, antioxidant, and antidiabetic activities of essential oils from Moroccan medicinal plants: *Mentha suaveolens, Lavandula stoechas,* and *Ammi visnaga*. Biomedicine & Pharmacotherapy. 2023;**164**:114937. DOI: 10.1016/j.biopha.2023.114937

[50] Benali T, Lemhadri A, Harboul K, Chtibi H, Khabbach A, Jadouali SM, et al. Chemical profiling and biological properties of essential oils of *Lavandula stoechas* L. collected from three Moroccan sites: In vitro and in silico investigations. Plants. 2023;**12**(6):1413. DOI: 10.3390/plants12061413

[51] Moussi Messaoudi I, Houda F, Said Amal AH, Kaotar N, Mohammed T, Imane R, et al. Phytochemical composition and antibacterial activity of Moroccan *Lavandula angustifolia* Mill. Journal of Essential Oil-Bearing Plants. 2017;**20**(4):1074-1082. DOI: 10.1080/0972060X.2017.1363000

[52] Alnamer R, Alaoui K, Houcine Bouidida E, Benjouad A, Cherrah Y. Toxicity and psychotropic activity of essential oils *of Rosmarinus officinalis* and *Lavandula officinalis* from Morocco. Journal of Biologically Active Products from Nature. 2011;**1**(4):262-272. DOI: 10.1080/22311866.2011.10719093

[53] Talbaoui A, Jamaly N, Il Idrissi A, Bouksaim M, Gmouh S, El Moussaouiti M, et al. Chemical composition and antibacterial activity of essential oils from six Moroccan plants. Journal of Medicinal Plants Research. 2012;**6**(31):4593-4600. DOI: 10.5897/jmpr10.078

[54] Soulaimani B, Abbad I, Varoni E, Iriti M, Mezrioui N-E, Hassani L, et al. Optimization of antibacterial activity of essential oil mixture obtained from three medicinal plants: Evaluation of synergism with conventional antibiotics and nanoemulsion effectiveness. South African Journal of Botany. 2022;**151**:900-908. DOI: 10.1016/j.sajb.2022.11.010

[55] Ghanimi R, Ouhammou A, El Atki Y, Cherkaoui M. Antioxidant and antibacterial activities of essential oils from three Moroccan species (*Lavandula mairei* Humbert, *Lavandula dentata* L. and, *Lavandula stoechas* L.). Journal of Pharmaceutical Research International. 2021;**33**:64-71. DOI: 10.9734/JPRI/2021/v33i45B32779

[56] Radi FZ, Zekri N, Drioiche A, Zerkani H, Boutakiout A, Bouzoubaa A, et al. Volatile and non-volatile chemical compounds and biological power of the genus Lavandula: Case of two Moroccan lavenders *Lavandula angustifolia* Mill. (cultivated lavender) and *Lavandula pedunculata* (Mill.) Cav. (spontaneous lavender). Egyptian Journal of

Chemistry. 2022;**65**(3):273-294. DOI: 10.21608/ejchem.2021.82036.4053

[57] Ultee A, Bennik MHJ, Moezelaar R. The phenolic hydroxyl group of carvacrol is essential for action against the food-borne pathogen *Bacillus cereus*. Applied and Environmental Microbiology. 2002;**68**(4):1561-1568. DOI: 10.1128/AEM.68.4.1561-1568.2002

[58] Mulyaningsih S, Sporer F, Zimmermann S, Reichling J, Wink M. Synergistic properties of the terpenoids aromadendrene and 1,8-cineole from the essential oil of *Eucalyptus globulus* against antibiotic-susceptible and antibiotic-resistant pathogens. Phytomedicine. 2010;**17**(13):1061-1066. DOI: 10.1016/j.phymed.2010.06.018

[59] Abd El-Baky RM, Hashem ZS. Eugenol and linalool: Comparison of their antibacterial and antifungal activities. African Journal of Microbiology Research. 2016;**10**(44):1860-1872. DOI: 10.5897/AJMR2016.8283

[60] Ivanov M, Kannan A, Stojković DS, Glamočlija J, Calhelha RC, Ferreira ICFR, et al. Camphor and eucalyptol—Anticandidal spectrum, antivirulence effect, efflux pumps interference and cytotoxicity. International Journal of Molecular Sciences. 2021;**22**(2):483. DOI: 10.3390/ijms22020483

[61] Ahmad A, Khan A, Bharathi NP, Hashmi AA, Khan LA, Manzoor N. Impaired ergosterol biosynthesis mediated fungicidal activity of oil based tin polymer. Medicinal Chemistry Research. 2011;**20**(8):1141-1146. DOI: 10.1007/s00044-010-9449-4

[62] Lima IO, de Oliveira Pereira F, de Oliveira WA, de Oliveira Lima E, Menezes EA, Cunha FA, et al. Antifungal activity and mode of action of carvacrol against *Candida albicans* strains. Journal of Essential Oil Research. 2013;**25**(2):138-142. DOI: 10.1080/10412905.2012.754728

[63] Manoharan RK, Lee J-H, Kim Y-G, Kim S-I, Lee J. Inhibitory effects of the essential oils α-longipinene and linalool on biofilm formation and hyphal growth of *Candida albicans*. Biofouling. 2017;**33**(2):143-155. DOI: 10.1080/08927014.2017.1280731

[64] Liu R, Mabury SA. Synthetic phenolic antioxidants: A review of environmental occurrence, fate, human exposure, and toxicity. Environmental Science & Technology. 2020;**54**:11706-11719, 11719. DOI: 10.1021/acs.est.0c05077

[65] El Ouali Lalami A, El-Akhal F, Maniar S, Ez Zoubi Y, Taghzouti K. Chemical constituents and larvicidal activity of essential oil of *Lavandula Stoechas* (Lamiaceae) from Morocco against the malaria vector *Anophelesl Labranchiae* (Diptera: Culicidae). International Journal of Pharmacognosy and Phytochemical Research. 2016;**8**(3):505-511

[66] Bachiri L, Bouchelta Y, Bouiamrine EH, Echchegadda G, Ibijbijen J, Nassiri L. Valorization as bioinsecticide of the essential oils of two indigenous lavender species in Morocco: *Lavandula stoechas* and *Lavandula pedunculata*. International Journal of Herbal Medicine. 2018;**6**(1):86-90